Pathogenesis and Management of Alzheimer's Disease

Pathogenesis and Management of Alzheimer's Disease

Edited by Elliot Cooper

STATES
ACADEMIC PRESS
www.statesacademicpress.com

States Academic Press,
109 South 5th Street,
Brooklyn, NY 11249, USA

Visit us on the World Wide Web at:
www.statesacademicpress.com

ISBN: 978-1-63989-405-5

Cataloging-in-Publication Data

Pathogenesis and management of alzheimer's disease / edited by Elliot Cooper.
p. cm.
Includes bibliographical references and index.
ISBN 978-1-63989-405-5
1. Alzheimer's disease. 2. Alzheimer's disease--Pathogenesis.
3. Alzheimer's disease--Treatment. I. Cooper, Elliot.

RC523 .P38 2022
616.831--dc23

Table of Contents

Preface

This book aims to highlight the current researches and provides a platform to further the scope of innovations in this area. This book is a product of the combined efforts of many researchers and scientists, after going through thorough studies and analysis from different parts of the world. The objective of this book is to provide the readers with the latest information of the field.

Alzheimer's disease is a medical condition in which the normal functioning of the brain is hampered. Some of the common symptoms of this disease are loss of memory, unstable behavior and language problems. The patients also have difficulty in executing complex tasks and recognizing people. The major characteristics of Alzheimer's disease are tangles and plaques in the brain. The disease is broadly categorized into three stages, mild, moderate and severe. The dependency on others for everyday tasks increases as the disease gets more severe. It is diagnosed with the help of procedures such as neurologic function tests, genetic testing, cognitive and memory tests, and CT scan and MRI scan. This book unfolds the innovative aspects of research on Alzheimer's disease which will be crucial for the progress of this field in the future. Also included herein is a detailed explanation of the various ways of managing this disease. Those in search of information to further their knowledge will be greatly assisted by this book.

I would like to express my sincere thanks to the authors for their dedicated efforts in the completion of this book. I acknowledge the efforts of the publisher for providing constant support. Lastly, I would like to thank my family for their support in all academic endeavors.

Editor

1

Tau Oligomers as Potential Drug Target for Alzheimer Disease (AD) Treatment

Rakez Kayed
University of Texas Medical Branch
USA

1. Introduction

The microtubule-associated protein tau is required for microtubule assembly, axonal transport, neurite outgrowth, and stability of microtubules (Binder *et al.* 1985). Tau self-assembly, aggregation, and accumulation in neurofibrillary tangles (NFTs) are major pathological hallmarks of Alzheimer disease (AD) and other neurodegenerative diseases (Lee *et al.* 2001, Alonso *et al.* 2008). Although the importance of tau in AD and other tauopathies is well established (Iqbal *et al.* 2009, Ballatore *et al.* 2007, Haroutunian *et al.* 2007) still unanswered is whether NFTs are the primary neurotoxic factor (Brunden *et al.* 2008, Marx 2007, Kayed & Jackson 2009).

Despite the poor correlation between NFTs and disease progression, and evidence showing, that neuronal loss in AD actually precedes NFTs formation research until recently focused on them and other large meta-stable inclusions composed of aggregated hyperphosphorylated tau protein. Lately, the significance and toxicity of NFTs have been challenged and new aggregated tau entity has emerged as the true pathogenic species in tauopathies and a possible mediator of Aβ toxicity in AD. Tau intermediate aggregate (tau oligomers; aggregates of an intermediate that is between monomers and NFTs in size) can cause neurodegeneration and memory impairment in the absence of Aβ. This exciting body of evidence includes results from human brain samples, transgenic mouse and cell-based studies, thus tau oligomers present a new and novel drug target for AD treatment.

In this chapter, we summarize the characterization and toxicity of tau oligomers; discuss the evidence supporting their critical role in AD pathogenesis, and the potential and challenges for targeting them by immunotherapy and drug discovery as a novel approach for AD treatment

2. Tau oligomer formation

A key early finding about tau in NFTs accumulated in AD and non-AD tauopathies was the fact that it is abnormally phosphorylated (Spires-Jones *et al.* 2009, Grundke-Iqbal *et al.* 1986). The sequence of early tau phosphorylation suggests that there are events prior to NFT formation that are specific to particular phosphorylated tau epitopes, leading to conformational changes and cytopathological alterations. Using phosphorylation dependent tau antibodies, three stages of NFT development were introduced: *(1)* pre-NFT, *(2)* intra-, and *(3)* extra-neuronal NFT. The pre-NFT state, in which neurons display nonfibrillar, punctate regions in the cytoplasm, dendrites, somata, and nuclei, was observed especially with phospho-tau antibodies TG3 (pT231), pS262, and pT153. Intraneuronal NFTs were homogeneously stained with fibrillar tau structures, which were most prominently stained with pT175/181, 12E8 (pS262/pS356), pS422, pS46, pS214 antibodies. Extracellular NFTs, which contain substantial filamentous tau, are most prominently stained with AT8 (pS199/pS202/pT205), AT100 (pT212/pS214), and PHF-1 (pS396/pS404) antibodies, which also stain intracellular NFT. Moreover, the severity of AD and neuronal loss correlates with the patterns of tau phosphorylation in NFT(Augustinack *et al.* 2002, Trinczek *et al.* 1995).

Tau hyperphosphorylation is thought to be an early event in the cascade leading from soluble to insoluble tau protein, but evidence demonstrating that hyperphosphorylation is sufficient for filament formation is lacking. Why does hyperphosphorylation promote aggregation of tau proteins into abnormal filaments? One possibility is that the negative charge imparted by phosphorylation neutralizes the basic charges of tau, thus facilitating intermolecular interaction and aggregation (Alonso *et al.* 2001a, Alonso *et al.* 2001b). An alternative explanation is that hyperphosphorylation detaches tau from microtubules, thus increasing the pool of unbound tau. Unbound, hyperphosphorylated tau may compete with microtubules for binding to normal tau and other microtubule associated proteins, thereby sequestering them and enhancing disassembly of microtubules (Alonso et al. 2001a). As compared to microtubule-bound tau, this unbound tau may be more degradation-resistant and more likely to aggregate. Reduced proteolysis of hyperphosphorylated tau may also increase the pool of soluble tau available for formation of paired helical filaments (PHF). Thus, abnormal phosphorylation of tau may result in an increase in the total cellular pool of tau, and may change its solubility, thus negatively regulating stability of microtubules (Litersky & Johnson 1992, Litersky & Johnson 1995, Litersky *et al.* 1993).

One important contributor to tau phosphorylation and NFT formation may be amyloid. The "amyloid cascade" hypothesis holds that the accumulation of Aβ peptides in senile plaques results in the formation of NFTs and neuronal cell death (Busciglio *et al.* 1995). In primary neuronal cultures, Aβ is capable of inducing tau phosphorylation (Busciglio et al. 1995). Aβ42 fibrils induced formation of neurofibrillary tangles in P301L tau transgenic mice (Gotz *et al.* 2001), and pre-aggregated Aβ42 induced PHF formation mediated by distinct phospho-epitopes of tau in cells overexpressing wild-type and mutant forms of human tau (Ferrari *et al.* 2003, Pennanen & Gotz 2005). Aβ oligomers, but not the soluble or fibrillar forms of Aβ, induced tau hyperphosphorylation in cells overexpressing human tau(De Felice *et al.* 2008); this phenomenon is not Aβ-specific, but rather conformation specific, as demonstrated by the ability of soluble oligomers from a non-disease related protein, hen egg white lysozyme, to mimic tau hyperphosphorylation induced by Aβ aggregates(Vieira *et al.* 2007).

Amyloid formation is a complex process that involves many morphologically and conformationally distinct species. The critical role of soluble amyloid oligomers in neurodegeneration has become generally accepted for multiple neurodegenerative diseases (Haass & Selkoe 2007, Brunden et al. 2008, Glabe 2006, Glabe 2008). Very little is known about tau oligomers, because reliable methods for preparing homogeneous populations of tau oligomers are lacking, which prevents researchers from studying them and testing chemical and other approaches to combating their formation and toxicity.

Unlike Aβ peptide,which is highly prone to aggregation and spontaneously forms amyloid in vitro, tau is an unfolded, soluble protein. In vitro aggregation of tau into filaments can be achieved using high concentrations and via the addition of promoters (Avila *et al.* 2004,

Barghorn *et al.* 2005, Barghorn & Mandelkow 2002). Mechanistic studies of full-length tau protein aggregation and filament formation in vitro have revealed striking similarities to Aβ aggregation; tau aggregates via either a nucleation-dependent mechanism (Congdon & Duff 2008) or the formation of intermediates (Xu *et al.*). In vitro, amyloid fibrils can accelerate the aggregation of the same protein via a nucleation-dependent mechanism, i.e., "seeding" (Jarrett *et al.* 1993, Kelly 2000). Seeding refers to the addition of a substoichiometric amount of fibrils, intact or sonicated, to a monomeric solution of the same protein, thus increasing the rate of conversion to amyloid fibrils. Lately, we and others have reported methods for preparing homogeneous Aβ and α-synuclein amyloid species (e.g., oligomers and fibrils) (Kayed *et al.* 2003, Kayed *et al.* 2007). These techniques provide an opportunity to test the effectiveness of different amyloid species as seeds. We have observed that amyloid oligomers similar to fibrils, can seed and induce monomer aggregation and oligomer formation (Kayed et al. 2007, Kayed & Glabe 2006). As we mentioned above it is well established that aggregated Aβ makes an important contribution to tau phosphorylation and aggregation in animal models and cell cultures. These experiments have used aggregated Aβ, which is likely to contain different prefibrillar and fibrillar Aβ aggregates. We recently demonstrated that Aβ42 and α-synuclein oligomer seeds induce the conversion of unstructured,monomeric human recombinant tau into β-sheet rich toxic tau oligomers(Lasagna-Reeves *et al.* 2010). This study show the ability of oligomer to cross-seed in vitro and induce tau aggregation

Tau oligomers prepared by this novel method were largely SDS-stable apparent trimers and display a spherical morphology similar to oligomers formed by other amyloidogenic proteins (Kayed & Glabe 2006, Kayed *et al.* 2004). When shaken in PBS buffer for longer periods of time, tau oligomers prepared by this method continue to aggregate and eventually form tau filaments. Biophysical characterization of tau oligomers demonstrates that tau oligomers are β-sheet rich with minimal ellipticity as compared with the natively unfolded monomeric tau, which shows a random coil with minimal ellipticity(Lasagna-Reeves et al. 2010).

Dynamic oligomers represent a toxic amyloid species that is conformationally distinct from fibrils and monomers. Targeting oligomers is a challenge that requires reliable protocols and reagents. Further investigations and analysis are needed to elucidate the synergy between different oligomer species and the contribution of amyloid oligomers to the induction of tau aggregation and to understand fully the role of tau oligomers in tauopathies.

2.1 Tau oligomers toxicity in vivo

The correlation between NFT in the brains of AD patients the disease progression remains contentious. Many studies have shown corelation between NFT and disease progresstion (Braak & Braak 1991, Delacourte & Buee 2000, Morsch *et al.* 1999, Bretteville & Planel 2008, Congdon & Duff 2008, Arriagada *et al.* 1992, Bird *et al.* 1999, Hernandez & Avila 2008, Rankin & Gamblin 2008, Cash *et al.* 2003, Tabaton *et al.* 1989). Other stereological studies show that neuronal loss actually exceeds NFT formation (Gomez-Isla et al. 1997, Terry 2000, van de Nes *et al.* 2008, Vogt *et al.* 1998). This and the exciting data published in the last half decade, emerging from biochemical, cell-based and transgenic mouse studies suggest that pre-filament forms of tau may be the most toxic and pathologically significant form of tau aggregates (Brunden et al. 2008, Marx 2007, Kayed *et al.* 2009, Meraz-Rios *et al.* 2009). This evolutionary transition was overdue in the tau field and similar to the transition witnessed for Aβ in the last 15 years driven by the characterization of Aβ intermediate species and their crucial role in Aβ-mediated toxicity (Harper *et al.* 1997, Roher *et al.* 1993, Walsh & Selkoe 2004, Walsh & Selkoe 2007).

Analogous to Aβ oligomers, tau oligomers have been shown to be neurotoxic when applied extracellularlly to cultured neuronal cells (Lasagna-Reeves et al. 2010) and to provoke an increase in intracellular calcium levels (Gomez-Ramos *et al.* 2006, Gomez-Ramos *et al.* 2008). Detailed characterization of newly developed tau animal models suggests that tau oligomers play a key role in eliciting neurodegeneration and behavioral impairments. These phenotypes are concurrent with accumulation of soluble aggregated tau species and dissociated from the accumulation of NFT (Brunden et al. 2008). Cell death and synaptic lesions occurred independently of NFT formation (h-tau mice) expressing non-mutant human tau (Andorfer et al. 2005, Polydoro et al. 2009); hippocampal synapse loss, impaired synaptic function and microgliosis precede the formation of NFT in the P301S mutant human tau transgenic mouse model (P301S Tg) (Yoshiyama et al. 2007), similar resuls were found in (Tau(RD)/deltaK280) mouse model, (Mocanu *et al.* 2008), fly model (Wittmann *et al.* 2001) and zebra fish model (Paquet *et al.* 2009). Tau oligomers were biochemically characterized in JNPL3 mice expressing human tau with the P301L mutation, and the conditional model (rTg4510) expressing the same P301L human tau mutant; surprisingly, the accumulation of oligomeric tau correlated best with neuronal loss and behavioral deficits in these models, whereas NFT did not. These findings suggest that the accumulation of tau oligomers, behavioral deficits and neuronal loss precede the formation NFT (Berger et al. 2007, Spires et al. 2006). Tau oligomers were biochemically characterized in post mortem human brain, and a correlation between disease progression and the accumulation of granular tau oligomers in the brains of AD patients was reported. Moreover, increased levels of tau oligomers detected in the frontal cortex at very early stage of the disease (Braak stage I), when clinical symptoms of AD and NFT are believed to be absent. This finding suggests that an increase in tau oligomer levels occurs before NFT formation and before individuals manifest clinical symptoms of AD (Maeda et al. 2007, Maeda et al. 2006). Tau-positive fine granules (TFGs) resembling tau oligomers were found in the cerebral white matter of post mortem tissue from the parkinsonism-dementia complex of guam (PDC) tauopathy (Yamazaki et al. 2005). The data discussed here support the notion that soluble oligomers of amyloid proteins including tau are the acutely toxic structures of these proteins, rather than insoluble aggregates such as plaques and tangles. This concept has become more generally accepted for multiple neurodegenerative diseases including AD and tauopathies (Haass & Selkoe 2007, Brunden et al. 2008).

Recently, we investigated the neurotoxiciy of different forms of tau in vivo by injecting well characterized oligomers , fibrils, or monomers of full length recombinant h-tau-441 (2N4R) into the hippocampus of C57BL/6 wild-mice. We found that the mice injected with tau oligomers presented with memory deficits in their performance of the novel-object recognition task, (Lasagna-Reeves 2010) which is widely used for evaluating memory in AD mouse models (Huang et al., 2006; Mouri et al., 2007; Scholtzova et al., 2008; Zhang et al., 2006). These observations correlate with previous studies in humans and primates that have shown hippocampal lesions to result in impaired object recognition (Reed and Squire, 1997; Zola et al., 2000).We also showed the loss of synaptic-related proteins and mitochondrial respiratory chain components in conjunction with the activation of the mitochondrial dysfunction markers and the pro-apoptotic protein caspase-9. Our results strongly suggest that tau oligomers result in learning impairment through the disruption of synaptic and mitochondrial functions. If we take into consideration these studies and the novel data presented above, we can postulate that tau oligomers generated intracellularly could be released either by binding and local rupture of the membrane, or after cell death. The oligomers in the extracellular space could be taken up by healthy neurons in the vicinity disrupt normal activity like lysosomal function and stimulate further aggregation of functional monomeric tau. Thus, understanding the negative impact of tau oligomers in neuronal damage, specifically in reference to important cellular mechanisms, such as mitochondrial and synaptic function, will likely be of great importance to understanding the relevant disease processes and progression in AD and other tauopathies.

2.1.1 Tau based therapies

The important role of tau in neurodegenerative diseases, supports tau as a potential target for the development of disease modifying therapeutics. Therapeutic approaches targeting tau include, (1) interference with the splicing machinery to decrease the four-repeat tau isoforms, (2) activation of proteolytic or proteasomal degradation pathways, (3) prevention/reduction of tau hyperphosphorylation using inhibitors of tau kinases, (4) pharmacological stabilization of microtubule networks, (5) inhibition of tau aggregation by small molecules, and (6) tau-directed immunotherapy (Schneider & Mandelkow 2008).

Inhibition of tau hyperphosphorylation: This approach to treat AD was first introduced in 1998 (Gong & Iqbal 2008). Although a kinase inhibitor was shown to reduce tau hyperphosphorylation and the formation of soluble aggregated tau and to prevent motor deficits in mice expressing mutant human tau (Iqbal & Grundke-Iqbal 1998), a major drawback to targeting kinases is that these enzymes are commonly found throughout the body playing normal physiological roles and their inhibition may have unwanted side effects.

Activation of proteolytic or degradation pathway: Tau was found to be sensitive to calpain protolysis (Johnson *et al.* 1989). Recently, puromycin-sensitive aminopeptidase (PSA), which was identified by a genetic screen as a modifier of tau pathology (Abazov *et al.* 2006), was shown to be effective in degrading both recombinant and PHF tau purified from AD brain(82)

Stabilization of microtubules: Microtubule-binding drugs could be beneficial in treating tauopathies by functionally substituting for the MT-binding protein tau (Trojanowski *et al.* 2005). Paclitaxel, a drug know to bind and stabilize microtubule, was tested in transgenic mice and showed to be effective in restoring axonal transport and ameliorating motor impairments (Zhang *et al.* 2005)

Inhibition of tau aggregation by small molecules: The last decade has witnessed a renaissance of interest in inhibitors of tau aggregation as potential disease-modifying drugs. A search for non-toxic, cell penetrant inhibitors of tau aggregation capable of crossing the blood-brain barrier (BBB) was performed using a high throughput screen, which resulted in the identification of more than 139 hits (Pickhardt *et al.* 2005, Larbig *et al.* 2007). This and the recent report of a phase-II clinical trial with the tau aggregation inhibitor MTC (ma ethylene blue derivative) could hold promise for the validation of the concept. The research on tau aggregation inhibitors was recently reviewed (Bulic et al. 2009).

Tau clearance by immunotherapy: Tau immunotherapy is a new concept (Sigurdsson 2009). A few reports of tau immunotherapy in animal models have been published, all using active vaccination (Boimel *et al.* , Asuni *et al.* 2007, Boutajangout *et al.* 2010). In these reports, the authors used tau fragments phosphorylated at positions commonly associated with NFT, such as Ser396 and Ser404. Behavioral analysis showed improved performance after immunization as compared to controls, biochemical and immunohistochemical i analyses showed reduction of both soluble and insoluble tau species, moreover the studies showed reduction of phosphorylated NFTs in the brains of these animals. One study clearly demonstrated that antibodies were able to cross the blood-brain barrier and bind to phosphorylated tau (Asuni et al. 2007). Although the use of phosphorylated tau antigens seems promising for vaccination studies, such an approach mainly targets NFTs, rather than pre-filament tau species (tau oligomers) which form at early stages of NFT development (Kayed & Jackson 2009, Kayed 2010).

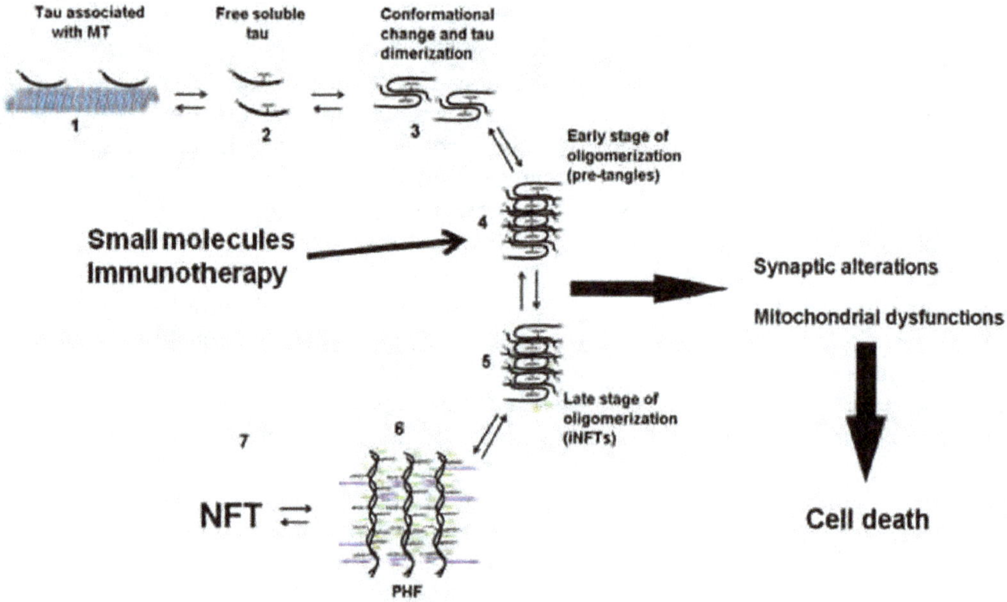

Fig. 1. Schematic presentation of tau aggregation, and the potential therapeutic approaches targeting tau oligomers.

3. Conclusion

Despite extensive efforts to develop anti amyloid treatments the results have, been disappointing. This led to the resurgence of tau as a potential therapeutic target for the treatment of AD. The question remains, which form of tau is the best target? The elegant studies over the past decade argue that soluble tau oligomers represent the primary pathological species of tau, therefore elucidating the pathways and mechanisms triggering their formation and understanding their mechanisms of toxicity are of immense importance. Studies focused on developing anti tau therapies must dissect the targets and better illuminate mechanisms of action for such approaches on each tau entity. As a starting point, it is important to evaluate the effects of immunotherapy and other therapeutic approaches on tau oligomers, this will be helpful for optimization of these approaches and may lead to the development of disease modifying therapies for AD and other neurodegenerative diseases.

4. Acknowledgment

Supported by the Cullen Trust, the Alzheimer`s Drug Discovery foundation (ADDF), and the Mitchell Center to Neurodegenerative Diseases. I am grateful for Dr. Cristian Lasagna-Reeves, and Prof. George Jackson for their helpful suggestions.

5. References

Abazov, V. M., Abbott, B., Abolins, M. et al. (2006) Search for neutral Higgs bosons decaying to tau pairs in pp[over] collisions at sqrt[s]=1.96 TeV. *Phys Rev Lett,* 97, 121802.

Alonso, A., Zaidi, T., Novak, M., Grundke-Iqbal, I. and Iqbal, K. (2001a) Hyperphosphorylation induces self-assembly of tau into tangles of paired helical filaments/straight filaments. *Proc Natl Acad Sci U S A,* 98, 6923-6928.

Alonso, A. C., Li, B., Grundke-Iqbal, I. and Iqbal, K. (2008) Mechanism of tau-induced neurodegeneration in Alzheimer disease and related tauopathies. *Curr Alzheimer Res,* 5, 375-384.

Alonso, A. D., Zaidi, T., Novak, M., Barra, H. S., Grundke-Iqbal, I. and Iqbal, K. (2001b) Interaction of tau isoforms with Alzheimer's disease abnormally hyperphosphorylated tau and in vitro phosphorylation into the disease-like protein. *J Biol Chem,* 276, 37967-37973.

Andorfer, C., Acker, C. M., Kress, Y., Hof, P. R., Duff, K. and Davies, P. (2005) Cell-cycle reentry and cell death in transgenic mice expressing nonmutant human tau isoforms. *J Neurosci,* 25, 5446-5454.

Arriagada, P. V., Growdon, J. H., Hedley-Whyte, E. T. and Hyman, B. T. (1992) Neurofibrillary tangles but not senile plaques parallel duration and severity of Alzheimer's disease. *Neurology,* 42, 631-639.

Asuni, A. A., Boutajangout, A., Quartermain, D. and Sigurdsson, E. M. (2007) Immunotherapy targeting pathological tau conformers in a tangle mouse model reduces brain pathology with associated functional improvements. *J Neurosci,* 27, 9115-9129.

Augustinack, J. C., Schneider, A., Mandelkow, E. M. and Hyman, B. T. (2002) Specific tau phosphorylation sites correlate with severity of neuronal cytopathology in Alzheimer's disease. *Acta Neuropathol,* 103, 26-35.

Avila, J., Perez, M., Lucas, J. J., Gomez-Ramos, A., Santa Maria, I., Moreno, F., Smith, M., Perry, G. and Hernandez, F. (2004) Assembly in vitro of tau protein and its implications in Alzheimer's disease. *Curr Alzheimer Res,* 1, 97-101.

Ballatore, C., Lee, V. M. and Trojanowski, J. Q. (2007) Tau-mediated neurodegeneration in Alzheimer's disease and related disorders. *Nat Rev Neurosci,* 8, 663-672.

Barghorn, S., Biernat, J. and Mandelkow, E. (2005) Purification of recombinant tau protein and preparation of Alzheimer-paired helical filaments in vitro. *Methods Mol Biol,* 299, 35-51.

Barghorn, S. and Mandelkow, E. (2002) Toward a unified scheme for the aggregation of tau into Alzheimer paired helical filaments. *Biochemistry,* 41, 14885-14896.

Berger, Z., Roder, H., Hanna, A. et al. (2007) Accumulation of pathological tau species and memory loss in a conditional model of tauopathy. *J Neurosci,* 27, 3650-3662.

Binder, L. I., Frankfurter, A. and Rebhun, L. I. (1985) The distribution of tau in the mammalian central nervous system. *J Cell Biol,* 101, 1371-1378.

Bird, T. D., Nochlin, D., Poorkaj, P. et al. (1999) A clinical pathological comparison of three families with frontotemporal dementia and identical mutations in the tau gene (P301L). *Brain,* 122 (Pt 4), 741-756.

Boimel, M., Grigoriadis, N., Lourbopoulos, A., Haber, E., Abramsky, O. and Rosenmann, H. Efficacy and safety of immunization with phosphorylated tau against neurofibrillary tangles in mice. *Exp Neurol,* 224, 472-485.

Boutajangout, A., Quartermain, D. and Sigurdsson, E. M. (2010) Immunotherapy targeting pathological tau prevents cognitive decline in a new tangle mouse model. *J Neurosci,* 30, 16559-16566.

Braak, H. and Braak, E. (1991) Neuropathological stageing of Alzheimer-related changes. *Acta Neuropathol,* 82, 239-259.

Bretteville, A. and Planel, E. (2008) Tau aggregates: toxic, inert, or protective species? *J Alzheimers Dis,* 14, 431-436.

Brunden, K. R., Trojanowski, J. Q. and Lee, V. M. (2008) Evidence that non-fibrillar tau causes pathology linked to neurodegeneration and behavioral impairments. *J Alzheimers Dis,* 14, 393-399.

Bulic, B., Pickhardt, M., Schmidt, B., Mandelkow, E. M., Waldmann, H. and Mandelkow, E. (2009) Development of tau aggregation inhibitors for Alzheimer's disease. *Angew Chem Int Ed Engl,* 48, 1740-1752.

Busciglio, J., Lorenzo, A., Yeh, J. and Yankner, B. A. (1995) beta-amyloid fibrils induce tau phosphorylation and loss of microtubule binding. *Neuron,* 14, 879-888.

Cash, A. D., Aliev, G., Siedlak, S. L. et al. (2003) Microtubule reduction in Alzheimer's disease and aging is independent of tau filament formation. *Am J Pathol,* 162, 1623-1627.

Congdon, E. E. and Duff, K. E. (2008) Is tau aggregation toxic or protective? *J Alzheimers Dis,* 14, 453-457.

De Felice, F. G., Wu, D., Lambert, M. P. et al. (2008) Alzheimer's disease-type neuronal tau hyperphosphorylation induced by A beta oligomers. *Neurobiol Aging,* 29, 1334-1347.

Delacourte, A. and Buee, L. (2000) Tau pathology: a marker of neurodegenerative disorders. *Curr Opin Neurol,* 13, 371-376.

Ferrari, A., Hoerndli, F., Baechi, T., Nitsch, R. M. and Gotz, J. (2003) beta-Amyloid induces paired helical filament-like tau filaments in tissue culture. *J Biol Chem,* 278, 40162-40168.

Glabe, C. G. (2006) Common mechanisms of amyloid oligomer pathogenesis in degenerative disease. *Neurobiol Aging,* 27, 570-575.

Glabe, C. G. (2008) Structural classification of toxic amyloid oligomers. *J Biol Chem,* 283, 29639-29643.

Gomez-Isla, T., Hollister, R., West, H., Mui, S., Growdon, J. H., Petersen, R. C., Parisi, J. E. and Hyman, B. T. (1997) Neuronal loss correlates with but exceeds neurofibrillary tangles in Alzheimer's disease. *Ann Neurol,* 41, 17-24.

Gomez-Ramos, A., Diaz-Hernandez, M., Cuadros, R., Hernandez, F. and Avila, J. (2006) Extracellular tau is toxic to neuronal cells. *FEBS Lett,* 580, 4842-4850.

Gomez-Ramos, A., Diaz-Hernandez, M., Rubio, A., Miras-Portugal, M. T. and Avila, J. (2008) Extracellular tau promotes intracellular calcium increase through M1 and M3 muscarinic receptors in neuronal cells. *Mol Cell Neurosci,* 37, 673-681.

Gong, C. X. and Iqbal, K. (2008) Hyperphosphorylation of microtubule-associated protein tau: a promising therapeutic target for Alzheimer disease. *Curr Med Chem,* 15, 2321-2328.

Gotz, J., Chen, F., van Dorpe, J. and Nitsch, R. M. (2001) Formation of neurofibrillary tangles in P301l tau transgenic mice induced by Abeta 42 fibrils. *Science,* 293, 1491-1495.

Grundke-Iqbal, I., Iqbal, K., Tung, Y. C., Quinlan, M., Wisniewski, H. M. and Binder, L. I. (1986) Abnormal phosphorylation of the microtubule-associated protein tau (tau) in Alzheimer cytoskeletal pathology. *Proc Natl Acad Sci U S A,* 83, 4913-4917.

Haass, C. and Selkoe, D. J. (2007) Soluble protein oligomers in neurodegeneration: lessons from the Alzheimer's amyloid beta-peptide. *Nat Rev Mol Cell Biol,* 8, 101-112.

Haroutunian, V., Davies, P., Vianna, C., Buxbaum, J. D. and Purohit, D. P. (2007) Tau protein abnormalities associated with the progression of alzheimer disease type dementia. *Neurobiol Aging,* 28, 1-7.

Harper, J. D., Wong, S. S., Lieber, C. M. and Lansbury, P. T. (1997) Observation of metastable Abeta amyloid protofibrils by atomic force microscopy. *Chem Biol,* 4, 119-125.

Hernandez, F. and Avila, J. (2008) Tau aggregates and tau pathology. *J Alzheimers Dis,* 14, 449-452.

Iqbal, K. and Grundke-Iqbal, I. (1998) Tau phosphatase activity as a therapeutic target for AD. *Drug News Perspect,* 11, 10-14.

Iqbal, K., Liu, F., Gong, C. X., Alonso, A. D. and Grundke-Iqbal, I. (2009) Mechanisms of tau-induced neurodegeneration. *Acta Neuropathol,* 118, 53-69.

Jarrett, J. T., Berger, E. P. and Lansbury, P. T., Jr. (1993) The carboxy terminus of the beta amyloid protein is critical for the seeding of amyloid formation: implications for the pathogenesis of Alzheimer's disease. *Biochemistry,* 32, 4693-4697.

Johnson, G. V., Jope, R. S. and Binder, L. I. (1989) Proteolysis of tau by calpain. *Biochem Biophys Res Commun,* 163, 1505-1511.

Kayed, R. (2010) Anti-tau oligomers passive vaccination for the treatment of Alzheimer's disease. *Hum Vaccin,* 6, 47-51.

Kayed, R. and Glabe, C. G. (2006) Conformation-dependent anti-amyloid oligomer antibodies. *Methods Enzymol,* 413, 326-344.

Kayed, R., Head, E., Sarsoza, F. et al. (2007) Fibril specific, conformation dependent antibodies recognize a generic epitope common to amyloid fibrils and fibrillar oligomers that is absent in prefibrillar oligomers. *Mol Neurodegener,* 2, 18.

Kayed, R., Head, E., Thompson, J. L., McIntire, T. M., Milton, S. C., Cotman, C. W. and Glabe, C. G. (2003) Common structure of soluble amyloid oligomers implies common mechanism of pathogenesis. *Science,* 300, 486-489.

Kayed, R. and Jackson, G. R. (2009) Prefilament tau species as potential targets for immunotherapy for Alzheimer disease and related disorders. *Curr Opin Immunol,* 21, 359-363.

Kayed, R., Pensalfini, A., Margol, L., Sokolov, Y., Sarsoza, F., Head, E., Hall, J. and Glabe, C. (2009) Annular protofibrils are a structurally and functionally distinct type of amyloid oligomer. *J Biol Chem,* 284, 4230-4237.

Kayed, R., Sokolov, Y., Edmonds, B., McIntire, T. M., Milton, S. C., Hall, J. E. and Glabe, C. G. (2004) Permeabilization of lipid bilayers is a common conformation-dependent activity of soluble amyloid oligomers in protein misfolding diseases. *J Biol Chem,* 279, 46363-46366.

Kelly, J. W. (2000) Mechanisms of amyloidogenesis. *Nat Struct Biol*, 7, 824-826.

Larbig, G., Pickhardt, M., Lloyd, D. G., Schmidt, B. and Mandelkow, E. (2007) Screening for inhibitors of tau protein aggregation into Alzheimer paired helical filaments: a ligand based approach results in successful scaffold hopping. *Curr Alzheimer Res*, 4, 315-323.

Lasagna-Reeves, C. A., Castillo-Carranza, D. L., Guerrero-Muoz, M. J., Jackson, G. R. and Kayed, R. (2010) Preparation and characterization of neurotoxic tau oligomers. *Biochemistry*, 49, 10039-10041.

Lasagna-Reeves, C. A. C.-C., D.L. Clos, A.L. Sengupta, U. Jackson, G.R. Kayed. R. (2010) Tau oligomers impair memory and induce synaptic and mitochondrial dysfunction in wild type mice. *Society for Neuroscience, San Diego, USA. November 2010.*

Lee, V. M., Goedert, M. and Trojanowski, J. Q. (2001) Neurodegenerative tauopathies. *Annu Rev Neurosci*, 24, 1121-1159.

Litersky, J. M. and Johnson, G. V. (1992) Phosphorylation by cAMP-dependent protein kinase inhibits the degradation of tau by calpain. *J Biol Chem*, 267, 1563-1568.

Litersky, J. M. and Johnson, G. V. (1995) Phosphorylation of tau in situ: inhibition of calcium-dependent proteolysis. *J Neurochem*, 65, 903-911.

Litersky, J. M., Scott, C. W. and Johnson, G. V. (1993) Phosphorylation, calpain proteolysis and tubulin binding of recombinant human tau isoforms. *Brain Res*, 604, 32-40.

Maeda, S., Sahara, N., Saito, Y. et al. (2007) Granular tau oligomers as intermediates of tau filaments. *Biochemistry*, 46, 3856-3861.

Maeda, S., Sahara, N., Saito, Y., Murayama, S., Ikai, A. and Takashima, A. (2006) Increased levels of granular tau oligomers: an early sign of brain aging and Alzheimer's disease. *Neurosci Res*, 54, 197-201.

Marx, J. (2007) Alzheimer's disease. A new take on tau. *Science*, 316, 1416-1417.

Meraz-Rios, M. A., Lira-De Leon, K. I., Campos-Pena, V., De Anda-Hernandez, M. A. and Mena-Lopez, R. (2009) Tau oligomers and aggregation in Alzheimer's disease. *J Neurochem*.

Mocanu, M. M., Nissen, A., Eckermann, K. et al. (2008) The potential for beta-structure in the repeat domain of tau protein determines aggregation, synaptic decay, neuronal loss, and coassembly with endogenous Tau in inducible mouse models of tauopathy. *J Neurosci*, 28, 737-748.

Morsch, R., Simon, W. and Coleman, P. D. (1999) Neurons may live for decades with neurofibrillary tangles. *J Neuropathol Exp Neurol*, 58, 188-197.

Paquet, D., Bhat, R., Sydow, A. et al. (2009) A zebrafish model of tauopathy allows in vivo imaging of neuronal cell death and drug evaluation. *J Clin Invest*, 119, 1382-1395.

Pennanen, L. and Gotz, J. (2005) Different tau epitopes define Abeta42-mediated tau insolubility. *Biochem Biophys Res Commun*, 337, 1097-1101.

Pickhardt, M., von Bergen, M., Gazova, Z., Hascher, A., Biernat, J., Mandelkow, E. M. and Mandelkow, E. (2005) Screening for inhibitors of tau polymerization. *Curr Alzheimer Res*, 2, 219-226.

Polydoro, M., Acker, C. M., Duff, K., Castillo, P. E. and Davies, P. (2009) Age-dependent impairment of cognitive and synaptic function in the htau mouse model of tau pathology. *J Neurosci*, 29, 10741-10749.

Rankin, C. A. and Gamblin, T. C. (2008) Assessing the toxicity of tau aggregation. *J Alzheimers Dis*, 14, 411-416.

Roher, A. E., Palmer, K. C., Yurewicz, E. C., Ball, M. J. and Greenberg, B. D. (1993) Morphological and Biochemical Analyses of Amyloid Plaque Core Proteins Purified from Alzheimer Disease Brain Tissue. *Journal of Neurochemistry,* 61, 1916-1926.

Schneider, A. and Mandelkow, E. (2008) Tau-based treatment strategies in neurodegenerative diseases. *Neurotherapeutics,* 5, 443-457.

Sigurdsson, E. M. (2009) Tau-focused immunotherapy for Alzheimer's disease and related tauopathies. *Curr Alzheimer Res,* 6, 446-450.

Spires-Jones, T. L., Stoothoff, W. H., de Calignon, A., Jones, P. B. and Hyman, B. T. (2009) Tau pathophysiology in neurodegeneration: a tangled issue. *Trends Neurosci,* 32, 150-159.

Spires, T. L., Orne, J. D., SantaCruz, K., Pitstick, R., Carlson, G. A., Ashe, K. H. and Hyman, B. T. (2006) Region-specific dissociation of neuronal loss and neurofibrillary pathology in a mouse model of tauopathy. *Am J Pathol,* 168, 1598-1607.

Tabaton, M., Cammarata, S., Manetto, V., Perry, G. and Mancardi, G. (1989) Tau-reactive neurofibrillary tangles in cerebellar cortex from patients with Alzheimer's disease. *Neurosci Lett,* 103, 259-262.

Terry, R. D. (2000) Do neuronal inclusions kill the cell? *J Neural Transm Suppl,* 59, 91-93.

Trinczek, B., Biernat, J., Baumann, K., Mandelkow, E. M. and Mandelkow, E. (1995) Domains of tau protein, differential phosphorylation, and dynamic instability of microtubules. *Mol Biol Cell,* 6, 1887-1902.

Trojanowski, J. Q., Smith, A. B., Huryn, D. and Lee, V. M. (2005) Microtubule-stabilising drugs for therapy of Alzheimer's disease and other neurodegenerative disorders with axonal transport impairments. *Expert Opin Pharmacother,* 6, 683-686.

van de Nes, J. A., Nafe, R. and Schlote, W. (2008) Non-tau based neuronal degeneration in Alzheimer's disease -- an immunocytochemical and quantitative study in the supragranular layers of the middle temporal neocortex. *Brain Res,* 1213, 152-165.

Vieira, M. N., Forny-Germano, L., Saraiva, L. M., Sebollela, A., Martinez, A. M., Houzel, J. C., De Felice, F. G. and Ferreira, S. T. (2007) Soluble oligomers from a non-disease related protein mimic Abeta-induced tau hyperphosphorylation and neurodegeneration. *J Neurochem,* 103, 736-748.

Vogt, B. A., Vogt, L. J., Vrana, K. E., Gioia, L., Meadows, R. S., Challa, V. R., Hof, P. R. and Van Hoesen, G. W. (1998) Multivariate analysis of laminar patterns of neurodegeneration in posterior cingulate cortex in Alzheimer's disease. *Exp Neurol,* 153, 8-22.

Walsh, D. M. and Selkoe, D. J. (2004) Oligomers on the brain: the emerging role of soluble protein aggregates in neurodegeneration. *Protein Pept Lett,* 11, 213-228.

Walsh, D. M. and Selkoe, D. J. (2007) A beta oligomers - a decade of discovery. *J Neurochem,* 101, 1172-1184.

Wittmann, C. W., Wszolek, M. F., Shulman, J. M., Salvaterra, P. M., Lewis, J., Hutton, M. and Feany, M. B. (2001) Tauopathy in Drosophila: neurodegeneration without neurofibrillary tangles. *Science,* 293, 711-714.

Xu, S., Brunden, K. R., Trojanowski, J. Q. and Lee, V. M. Characterization of tau fibrillization in vitro. *Alzheimers Dement,* 6, 110-117.

Yamazaki, M., Hasegawa, M., Mori, O., Murayama, S., Tsuchiya, K., Ikeda, K., Chen, K. M., Katayama, Y. and Oyanagi, K. (2005) Tau-positive fine granules in the cerebral white matter: a novel finding among the tauopathies exclusive to parkinsonism-dementia complex of Guam. J Neuropathol Exp Neurol, 64, 839-846.

Yoshiyama, Y., Higuchi, M., Zhang, B. et al. (2007) Synapse loss and microglial activation precede tangles in a P301S tauopathy mouse model. Neuron, 53, 337-351.

Zhang, B., Maiti, A., Shively, S. et al. (2005) Microtubule-binding drugs offset tau sequestration by stabilizing microtubules and reversing fast axonal transport deficits in a tauopathy model. Proc Natl Acad Sci U S A, 102, 227-231.

2

Hypotension in Subcortical Vascular Dementia, a New Risk Factor – Wasn't It Hypertension?

Rita Moretti, Francesca Esposito, Paola Torre,
Rodolfo M. Antonello and Giuseppe Bellini
Medicina Clinica, Ambulatorio Complicanze Internistiche Cerebrali, Dipartimento Universitario Clinico di Scienze Mediche Tecnologiche e Traslazionali, Università degli Studi di Trieste,
Italy

1. Introduction

The identification of additional genetic susceptibility genes in the etiology of AD and the metabolic mechanisms leading to differences in age of onset and disease pathogenesis are active areas of current susceptibility. Although all the contributing factors may never be known, scientists have identified several common threads. They include: age (more than 65 years old), sex (women are more likely than men are to develop the disease, in part because they live longer), toxicity (such as overexposure to certain trace metals, such as aluminum), head injury (serious traumatic injury to the head, for example, a concussion with a prolonged loss of consciousness) may be a risk factor for Alzheimer's), hormone replacement therapy (the exact role hormone replacement therapy may play in the development of dementia isn't yet clear; throughout the 1980s and '90s, evidence seemed to show that estrogen supplements given after menopause could reduce the risk of dementia; results from the large-scale Women's Health Initiative Memory Study indicated an increased risk of dementia for women taking estrogen after age 65: the verdict is not yet in on whether estrogen affects the risk of dementia if given at an earlier age), lifestyle (the same factors that put you at risk of heart disease, such as high blood pressure and high cholesterol, may also increase the likelihood that you'll develop Alzheimer's disease, poorly controlled diabetes is another risk factor). Atrial fibrillation, systolic hypertension, and angina have been associated with more rapid decline in cognition, while history of coronary artery bypass graft surgery, diabetes, and antihypertensive medications were associated with a slower rate of decline, and may represent modifiable risk factors for secondary prevention in Alzheimer disease. There was an age interaction such that systolic hypertension, angina, and myocardial infarction were associated with greater decline with increasing baseline age. The attenuated decline for diabetes and coronary artery bypass graft surgery may be due to selective survival. Some of these effects appear to vary with age (Mielke et al., 2007). There is an overlap of risk factors between VaD and AD, so much so that it raises some serious questions about vascular contributions to AD. Recognition that cerebrovascular disease causing dementia may be modified by treatment of cerebrovascular risk factors serves as an important tool for investigating various treatments aimed at secondary prevention of vascular cognitive impairment (Moretti et al., 2008). Some individuals presenting cerebrovascular pathology probably have some component of Alzheimer's Disease (AD) pathology as part of their dementia; this relationship supports the possible interaction between cerebrovascular disease, aging and the degenerative process (see data and Literature in: Brookmeyer et al., 1998). Various factors may influence the nature and severity of brain degeneration. The degree of cerebral grey matter damage, neuronal death, and survival will be dictated by the multiplicity, size, and laterality of the tissue injury or the extent of vascular disease (Kalaria, 1996; Kalaria, 2010). Anatomical features of the circulation, including the size of vessels and vascular wall cellular elements, e.g., arterioles versus capillaries, are important factors in defining the pathology. The distribution territories of the anterior, posterior, and middle cerebral and the lenticulo-striate arteries affect different structures, including the angular gyrus, the caudate nucleus and medial thalamus in the dominant hemisphere, the amygdala, and the hippocampus, all structures implicated in forms of cognitive impairment (Kalaria, 2010; Ferrer et al, 2008). The origin and degree of vascular occlusion or injury and whether this results in ischemic or hemorrhagic lesions are further factors that define the extent and severity of damage. Alterations in specific genes associated with systemic disease or brain-specific proteins and environmental or lifestyle factors may further modify the course of degeneration. On the other hand, vascular dementia is defined simply as the syndrome of dementia due to brain vascular disease (Hebert et al., 2003). Numerous epidemiological studies show a high prevalence of vascular brain injury amongst the elderly (Wolf et al., 1991; Wu et al., 2002) and recent evidence supports a strong association between vascular risk factors and dementia (Vermeer et al, 2003; Chui, 1989). Overall in the Western world, vascular disease is the second most common cause of dementia (Skoog et al., 1993). However in the very elderly, aged 85 years and older, there is a high risk of both stroke and Alzheimer's disease, and the prevalence of VaD is reported to be slightly higher than that of Alzheimer's disease (46.9% and 43.5%, respectively, with some patients possibly having mixed forms of dementia) (Skoog et al., 1993). Vascular dementia is a heterogeneous syndrome, grouping together a broad category of patients in whom various manifestations of cognitive decline are attributed to cerebral- or cardio-vascular disease. The National Institute of Neurological Disorders and Stroke and the Association Internationale pour la Recherche et l'Enseignement en Neurosciences (NINDS-AIREN) (Roman et al, 1993) elaborated a clinical and diagnostic tool, the so- called NINDS-AIREN criterium. It lists different pathologies, in order to identify patients with different subtypes of VaD: multi-infarct dementia (multiple large and complete infarcts); post-hemorrhage dementia, and subcortical VaD (small-vessel disease). According to NINDS-AIREN, the subcortical VaD (sVaD) is mainly due to lacunar infarct, occurring in distribution of small arteriole, usually in the white matter, basal ganglia, thalamus and pons, or to microinfarct - not seen on macroscopic examination, small area of cystic or non-cystic necrosis surrounded by astrocytes. Incomplete infarct may also be present, due to a selective loss of neurons, myelin, and oligodendrocytes, without cystic necrosis, occurring in the periphery of major artery distribution infarcts (e.g., penumbra) or in deep white matter. Incomplete white matter infarcts are associated with myelin pallor, astrocytosis, and a variable degree of axonal loss. Subcortical VaD now incorporates the old entities 'lacunar state' and 'Binswanger disease' and relates to small vessel disease and hypoperfusion resulting in focal and diffuse ischaemic white matter lesions and incomplete ischaemic injury (Erkinjuntti et al 1997; Pantoni et al., 2000). Assaying cerebrovascular risk factors probably can't be used for diagnosis of microvascular VaD, but the more risk factors there are might have some predictive value. There is an uncanny overlap of risk factors between VaD and AD, so much so that it raises some serious questions about vascular contributions to AD. Hypertension has often been observed to be a risk factor for VaD (Brookmeyer et al., 1998; Hebert et al., 2000) and sometimes for AD (Posner et al., 2002; LAuner et al., 1995; Morris et al. 2001) although not always (van Dijck et al., 2004). Hypertension leads to changes in arterioles and eventually to arteriolar occlusive disease and then on to infarction. Hypertension's effects on the brain in VaD or AD could also be related to changes in blood flow or blood-brain-barrier integrity. In fact, a number of epidemiological studies show strong associations between elevations in middle-life blood pressure and the prevalence of later life cognitive impairment and dementia. Increase in systolic blood pressure levels has been associated with more severe periventricular and subcortical white matter lesions (van Dijck et al., 2004). People with poorly controlled hypertension had a higher risk of severe white matter lesions than those without hypertension. But, it clearly merged that a potential negative effect of decreasing diastolic blood pressure level on the occurrence of severe periventricular white matter lesions should be taken into account. Recent large observational studies have suggested that high blood pressure may also play a role in Alzheimer's disease and in the so-called mixed forms of dementia, also defined as overlapping syndromes (vascular/degenerative dementia). The mechanisms linking hypertension to Alzheimer's disease remain to be elucidated, but white matter lesions seen on cerebral magnetic resonance imaging appear to be a good marker of this association (Brookmeyer et al., 1998; Ferrer et al., 2008; Tzourio, 2007). Hypertension leads to changes in arterioles and eventually to arteriolar occlusive disease and then on to infarction, and consequent brain parenchima degeneration (Skoog et al., 1993; 1Hebert et al., 2000; Posner et al., 2002). A large number of epidemiological studies show strong associations between elevations in middle-life blood pressure and the prevalence of later life cognitive impairment and dementia. Early evidence suggest that treatment hypertension in the elderly may be quite successful in reducing incident dementia. In the Syst-Eur trial (Forette et al., 1998), given the high percentage of elderly suffering with untreated hypertension, are that secondary prevention treatment trials such as Syst-Eur might have a substantial impact on cognitive impairment. Indeed, high blood pressure may accelerate cerebral white matter lesions (Yamamoto et al., 1998; Schmidt et al., 1999), but white matter lesions have been found to be facilitated also by excessive fall in blood pressure, (Kario et al., 1996; Nakamura et al., 1995; Watanabe et al., 1996; Chamorro et al., 1997), including orthostatic dysregulation (Matsubayashi et al., 1997) and postprandial hypotension (Kohara et al., 1999). The traditional general practice teaches that "the lower the blood pressure is, the better is the prognosis"; nevertheless, low blood pressure as a predictor of increased mortality has been described in a 5-year prospective study in Finland (Mattila et al. 1988) as well as paradoxical survival of elderly men with high blood pressure (Brookmeyer et al., 1988; 33Langer et al., 1989). Notwithstanding all of this, interpretations of these so-called J-shaped curves between blood pressure, and mortality have always been viewed with caution and skepticism by epidemiologists and statisticians (Fletcher & Bulpitt, 1992; Glynn et al., 1995). Chronic low blood pressure has been positively associated with a number of clinical symptoms and psychosomatic distress—including unexplained fatigue, depression, and anxiety—and with minor psychiatric morbidity (de Buyzere et al., 1998). A causal relationship between low blood pressure and low mood remains uncertain, but a vicious circle should not be excluded (de Buyzere et al., 1998). Zhu et al. (1998) observed that there was a correlation between systolic pressure reduction and cognitive decline in women, which was not accounted for by other factors. Baseline blood pressure level was not significantly related to cognitive decline in that sample with initial good cognition. The Authors speculated that blood pressure reduction might be an early change of the dementing process (see also literature in Gorelick, 1997), even if no clear statement merges on this point (Ferrer et al., 2008). Ruitenberg et al. (2001) found out that lower systolic and diastolic blood pressures at baseline were associated with a higher risk of dementia at follow-up. This association was observed across all age strata, in men as well in woman and both in Alzheimer's disease and vascular dementia. Subjects with incident dementia also decreased more in blood pressure level than in persons without dementia, even if not significantly (Ruitenberg et al., 2001). This may reflect that low blood pressure causes or contributes to dementia or that incipient dementia leads a drop in blood pressure (Ruitenberg et al., 2001). The authors suggested that for the first part of the proposition, they observed an inverse association between blood pressure and dementia mainly in subjects, who used antihypertensive medication (Ruitenberg et al., 2001). This may indicate that their hypertension was longer lasting, and perhaps that these patients were more susceptible to pressure drops, causing inadequate cerebral blood flow. That would be particularly important in vulnerable areas, such as watershed zones and white matter. A second explanation given by the authors (Ruitenberg et al., 2001) was that low pressure might be a consequence of an incipient dementia. The Authors found that blood pressure was lower in subjects with manifest dementia, and those with dementia, who presented lower pressure, declined more rapidly. The possible explanation given by these Authors (Ruitenberg et al., 2001) is that several areas are involved in pressure regulation; Burke et al. (1994) reported a strong correlation between the decrease of the number of C1 neurones in the medulla oblongata and blood pressure dysregulation in Alzheimer patients. Guo et al. (1999) examined whether initially low blood pressure is related to the incidence of dementia and showed that individuals with baseline systolic pressure of 140 mmHg or less had a significantly higher risk of dementia and Alzheimer's disease. That was the first study that has reported clearly an association between relatively low systolic pressure and increased incidence of dementia with a particular presumable sufferance of brain parenchima, generally hypoperfused in dementia patients (Brown & Frackowiak, 1991), related to an impairment of the cerebral autoregulation, secondary to the degenerative disorder. The direct consequence would be a sequential ulterior reduction of blood pressure, due to dysregulation, which might accelerate the lowering of blood perfusion, altered regulation flow capacity, and therefore the underlying degenerative process (Forette et al., 1998 Bolster et al., 2001; Nilsson et al., 2007). Starting from these studies, we would like to prove if hypotension is a key point in vascular dementia patients, and if this aspect reflects its importance in the daily living assistance.

2. Subjects and methods

2.1 Patients

Study subjects were men and women aged 68–94 years, entering in Cognitive Disorder Unit Evaluation of the University of Trieste, with Mini-Mental State Examination (MMSE) scores of at least 14 (Folstein et al., 1975) and satisfying the fourth edition of the Diagnostic and Statistical Manual of Mental Disorders (APA, 2000) for dementia, recruited from June 1st

2007 to December 31st 2010. We have examined 2657 patients, who have been diagnosed as suffering from Mild Cognitive Impairment, Alzheimer's Disease, Frontal Lobe Dementia, Lewy Body Dementia and Parkinson - dementia complex. 1047 patients suffered from vascular dementia: 183 have been diagnosed as Multi-Infarct Dementia. 864 patients suffered from subcortical vascular dementia: these study subjects satisfied the criteria for probable VaD in accordance with the NINDS-AIREN criteria (Roman et al., 1993). A patient was diagnosed as having subcortical VaD (sVaD) when the CT/MRI scan showed moderate to severe ischemic white matter changes (Erkinjunnti et al., 2000) and at least one lacunar infarct. Brain CT-scans or MRI images were randomized and assessed independently, after the radiologist's opinion, by neurologists (RM, PT). Patients were not included in the study if they showed signs of normal pressure hydrocephalus, previous brain tumors, previous diagnosis of major stroke or brain hemorrhage. We did not include patients with white matter lesions, caused by specific etiologies, such as multiple sclerosis, brain irradiation, collagen vascular disease, and genetic forms of vascular dementia (such as CADASIL or CARASIL). Patients with previous major psychiatric illness (i.e. schizophrenia, bipolar disorders, psychosis, compulsive-obsessive disorders, etc) or central nervous system disorders and alcoholism were excluded too.

2.2 Study design

This was a prospective cohort study, designed to investigate gait (balance and equilibrium) disorders, behavioral alterations, drug intake of a subcortical dementia population. Study subjects were 646 men and women, diagnosed as previously stated as subcortical vascular dementia (sVaD), not bedridden, aged 68-94 years outpatients, recruited from June, 1st 2007 to December, 31st 2010, who underwent a standardized baseline assessment that included a detailed history, a physical examination, laboratory tests and psychiatric evaluations. The physical examination included evaluations of pulse rate and rhythm, blood pressure, heart size and sounds, peripheral pulses, retinal vessel and carotid artery evaluation, electrocardiographic evaluation, and chest X-ray. The physical examination was repeated at every visit; electrocardiographic evaluation and laboratory tests were repeated every 3 months. Caregivers have been instructed to measure blood pressure 3 times/week, baseline and after two minutes in hortostatism and write the evaluation in a diary, which we checked at each visit. Patients in both groups were allowed to continue any previous therapy (e.g. cholinesterase inhibitors, antihypertensive, antidyslipidemic, antidiabetic drugs). (Table 1). Patients were divided in two groups: those with hypertension history and at baseline, who progressively registered low blood pressure (415 patients) and those with hypertension history, who maintained elevated values of systolic/diastolic pressure (398 patients). From this point, the former will be defined as group A, the latter as group B. All patients were followed with periodical neurological and neuropsychological examinations. Visits were scheduled to take place every four months. A complete neuropsychological examination was conducted at baseline, and every 6 months; every 12 months' results were compared. The trial was conducted in accordance with the Declaration of Helsinki and with the Ethics Guidelines of the Institute.

2.3 Outcome measures

Global performance was assessed using the Ten Point Clock test (Manos, 1997) at every visit. Behavioral symptoms were assessed using the Neuropsychiatric Inventory (NPI)

(Cummings et al., 1994) at every visit. In particular, we have examined sub-item "apathy", from the complex of NPI evaluation system. The Complex activities of daily living were evaluated by the Instrumental activity of Daily living (IADL) (Lawton & Brody, 1969). Frontal Battery has been evaluated every three months (Dubois et al., 1997). Mobility problems were assessed by the Tinetti scale for equilibrium/balance and gait (Tinetti, 1986) at every visit. Hachinski Ischemic score (HIS) was done (Hachinski et al., 1973). Patients were registered for their medical intake and for their blood pressure diaries.

2.4 Statistical analyses

Statistical analyses were performed using the Statistical Package for the Social Sciences (SPSS, version 16.0). Within- and between -group changes from baseline to 12, 24 and 36 months were tested using the Wilcoxon Signed Ranks test. This was done for the overall scores for each efficacy variable. Spearman's rank correlation analyses were performed between behavioral outcome measures (NPI), Tinetti scale, Ten Point Clock Test (TPCT), FAB assessment score, Apathy, and BI. Results are presented as mean changes from baseline with standard deviations, and P-values are presented where appropriate.

3. Results

We have examined 2657 patients, who have been diagnosed as suffering from Mild Cognitive Impairment, Alzheimer's Disease, Frontal Lobe Dementia, Lewy Body Dementia and Parkinson - dementia complex. 1047 patients suffered from vascular dementia: 183 have been diagnosed as Multi-Infarct Dementia. 864 patients suffered from subcortical vascular dementia. These patients, 415 men and 449 women, were included in the study (Table 1).

Age in years (mean ± SD)	72.4 ± 5.8
Gender (male/female)	401/412
Education level in years (mean ± SD)	10.4 ± 2.3
Concomitant illnesses (N.+ % patients)	
Essential hypertension	794 (97.6%)
Diabetes mellitus, type 2	236 (29.1%)
Ischaemic cardiopathy/valvular failure/arrythmias	413 (50.8%)
Chronic obstructive bronchopathy	205 (25.2%)
Neoplasia	36 (4.4%)

Table 1. Baseline characteristics of patients.

Their mean age was 72.4 + 5.8 years, and they had a mean education level of 10.4 + 2.3 years. The diagnosis was based on historical information and neuropsychological assessment and supported by findings on structural (CT or magnetic resonance) imaging. Subsequent follow-up of subjects has reinforced the clinical diagnoses in all cases. Brain CT-scans or MRI images were available for all the 864 selected patients; all the patients attended CT scans, 246 patients did, moreover, MRI studies. These 246 patients were requested by us to complete their diagnostic route with MRI sequences, in case of not adequate imaging acquisition, or not convincing data. Thirty one patients died during follow-up; twenty patients did not have a caregiver, who could guarantee adequate compliance, and therefore have been excluded, after the first year from the study. All the other 813 patients (401 men and 412 women) completed the full 36-month study. Patients were allowed to continue any previous therapy (e.g. antihypertensive, antidyslipidemic, antidiabetic drugs) (Table 2).

Drug utilization mg/day	baseline	12 months	24 months	36 months
ACE inhibitor	**412 patients**	**292 patients**	**203 patients**	173 patients
Sartan	**283 patients**	**169 patients**	**179 patients**	143 patients
Calcium antagonists	**345 patients**	**172 patients**	**167 patients**	158 patients
Two or more (Antihypertensive) drugs together	**246 patients**	0	0	0
Antidiabetic medication	**186 patients**	**251 patients**	**198 patients**	105 patients
Antiplatetelet drugs	**321 patients**	**349 patients**	**430 patients**	349 patients
ASA	**247 patients**	**344 patients**	**376 patients**	389 patients
Digoxin	**223 patients**	**215 patients**	**175 patients**	125 patients
Diuretics	**153 patients**	**187 patients**	**178 patients**	196 patients
Thiazide diuretics	**165 patients**	**143 patients**	**189 patients**	110 patients
Lipid lowering drugs	**156 patients**	**189 patients**	**265 patients**	311 patients
Nitroglycerine or analogue	**234 patients**	**254 patients**	**209 patients**	148 patients
Bronchodilators	**121 patients**	**87 patients**	**97 patients**	104 patients
A combination of the above therapies	**512 patients**	**683 patients**	**545 patients**	**631patients**

Table 2. A synopsis of the drugs employed by the two groups of patients at baseline

During the follow-up, the patients were prescribed neuroleptics and/or benzodiazepines (Table 3).

Drug utilization	baseline	12 months	24 months	36 months
Benzodiazepines	**144 patients**	**289 patients**	**276 patients**	314 patients
Typical neurolpetics	**78 patients**	**356 patients**	**498 patients**	577 patients
Atypical neurolpetics	**24 patients**	**115 patients**	**167 patients**	345 patients
Two or more drugs	203 patients	345 patients	406 patients	567 patients

Table 3. A synopsis of the SNC drugs employed by the patients

The patients were homogeneously recruited and no demographical/social/ cultural/clinical difference distinguish from each other. Patients were divided in two groups: those with hypertension history and at baseline, who progressively registered low blood pressure (415 patients), and those with hypertension history, who maintained elevated values of systolic/diastolic pressure (398 patients). From this point, the former will be defined as group A, the latter as group B. Two neurologists of the group revised all the imaging, employing the Blennow et al. (1991) scale for CT scans and the Scheltens et al. (1993) scale for MRI imaging. There was 94.2% inter-rater agreement for the independent assessment of the scans (kappa=0.76). Considering the global health conditions, there was an obvious deterioration in the patients as evidenced by the increase of the daily drug uptake (Table 3). Main scores obtained by the patients, during the follow-up have been reported in table 4 as mean and SD . Particularly, the results obtained in the FAB scale, Tinetti Scale, apathy (as sub-score of NPI) have been reported in table 4a which reports the differences within Group A, in the follow-up; in table b, it has been reported the differences within Group B during follow-up; in table 4c it has been reported the differences between the two groups in the follow-up. According to a Wilcoxon Signed Ranks test, there was a general worsening of the cognitive, behavioral and instrumental capacities of the patients observed in the 36 months of follow-up within the two groups (table 4a and 4b). It has been showed that there was an evident difference between groups, as evidenced in table 4c: no significant difference has been registered between the two groups at baseline, a part from the performance obtained at the FAB test ($p<0.05$). At twelve, twenty four and thirty six months, the differences between the two groups were significant ($p<0.01$) as demonstrated by table 4c.

Tests	Baseline		12 months		24 months		36 months	
	Group A	Group B	Group A	Group B	Group A	Group B	Group A	Group B
TPCT	7.7 ± 0.2	7.4 ± 0.5	6.1 ± 0.1	6.8 ± 0.3	5.4 ± 0.2	6.1 ± 0.5	4.1 ± 0.1	5.9 ± 0.6
NPI	24.5 ± 3.2	23.5 ± 2.4	41.4 ± 2.1	34.5 ± 3.2	66.4 ± 1.1	64.5 ± 2.7	86.3 ± 9.1	74.5 ± 3.2
Apathy (NPI)	6.6± 0.2	6.2 ± 0.4	8.3 ± 0.1	6.8 ± 0.6	9.2 ± 0.5	7.9 ± 0.7	11.1± 0.2	9.6± 0.1
FAB	13.3 ± 1.2	14.1 ± 1.1	10.3 ± 0.5	11.1 ± 1.1	9.3 ± 0.9	10.8 ± 1.3	8.4 ± 0.2	10.1 ± 0.9
Barthel Index	89.1 ± 5.3	87.1 ± 6.2	81.1 ± 1.2	83.1 ± 2.4	76.8 ± 6.1	81.1 ± 4.1	61.1 ± 7.3	69.1 ± 4.3
Tinetti score	21.8 ± 1.8	22.1 ± 1.1	18.3 ± 1.4	21.4 ± 1.4	17.7 ± 1.5	21.1 ± 0.5	15.7 ± 1.6	19.1± 1.1
Hachinski Ischemic Score	7.6 ± 0.1	8.1 ± 0.3	6.4 ± 0.11	7.9 ± 0.1	6.2 ± 0.3	7.3 ± 0.1	6.2 ± 0.1	6.9 ± 0.3

Table 4. Tests results in the patients observed during follow-up

Tests	12 months vs baseline	24 months vs baseline	36 months vs baseline
TPCT	0.9 ± 0.3 p<0.01	5.4 ± 0.1 p<0.01	3.6 ± 0.2 p<0.01
NPI	-16.9 ± 1.3 p<0.01	-41.9 ± 4.3 p<0.01	-61.8 ± 2.1 p<0.01
Apathy (NPI)	-1.7 ± 0.4 p<0.01	-2.6 ± 0.3 p<0.01	-4.5 ± 0.1 p<0.01
FAB	3.2 ± 0.7 p<0.01	4.3 ± 0.3 p<0.01	4.9 ±1.0 p<0.01
Barthel Index	8± 9.3 p<0.01	12.3 ± 5.1 p<0.01	28 ± 4 p<0.01
Tinetti score	3.5 ± 0.4 p<0.01	4.1 ± 1.3 p<0.01	6.1 ± 0.2 p<0.01
Hachinski Ischemic Score	0.8 ± 0.3 p<0.01	1.4 ± 0.2 p<0.01	1.4 ± 0.1 p<0.01

Table 4 a. Tests results in the patients observed during follow-up in Group A

Tests	12 months vs baseline	24 months vs baseline	36 months vs baseline
TPCT	0.6 ± 0.1 p<0.05	1.3 ± 0.1 p<0.05	1.5 ± 0.2 p<0.01
NPI	-11 ± 1.2 p<0.05	-41 ± 0.3 p<0.05	-51 ± 2.1 p<0.01
Apathy (NPI)	-0.6 ± 0.2 p<0.05	-1.3 ± 0.2 p<0.05	-3.4 ± 0.3 p<0.01
FAB	3 ± 0.1 p<0.05	3.3 ± 0.2 p<0.05	4 ±0.2 p<0.01
Barthel Index	4 ± 2.8 p<0.05	6 ± 2.1 p<0.05	26 ± 1.5 p<0.01
Tinetti score	0.7 ± 0.2 p<0.05	1.1 ± 0.6 p<0.05	6.4 ± 1.4 p<0.01
Hachinski Ischemic Score	0.2 ± 0.2 p<0.05	1 ± 0.2 p<0.05	1.2 ± 0.3 p<0.01

Table 4 b. Tests results in the patients observed during follow-up in Group B

Tests	baseline	12 months vs baseline	24 months vs baseline	36 months vs baseline
TPCT	-0.3 ±0.2 ns	-0.8 ±0.2 p<0.05	0.6 ±0.3 p <0.01	1.8 ±0.5 p<0.01
NPI	-1 ±0.8 ns	6.9 ±1.1 p <0.05	1.9 ±1.6 p <0.01	-11.38 ±5.9 p <0.01
Apathy (NPI)	-0.4 ±0.2 ns	1.5 ±0.5 p <0.01	2.7 ±0.2 p <0.01	-1.5 ±0.1 p <0.01
FAB	-0.8 ±0.2 p<0.05	-1.2 ±0.6 p <0.05	-1.5 ±0.4 p <0.01	1.7 ±0.5 p <0.01
Barthel Index	-2 ±1.7 ns	-2.1 ±1.2 p <0.05	-4.3 ± 2 p <0.01	8.0 ±3.0 p <0.01
Tinetti score	-0.3 ±0.7 ns	-3.1 ±0.1 p <0.05	3.4 ± 1 p <0.01	4.6 ±0.5 p <0.01
Hachinski Ischemic Score	-0.5 ±0.2 ns	-1.5 ±0.1 p <0.05	-1.1 ±0.2 p <0.01	0.37 ±0.2 p <0.01

Table 4 c. Tests results in the patients observed during follow-up B vs A

In group A, blood pressure mean values are 130/80 ± 6.5 mm Hg at baseline, and then a decrease of 10.4 ± 7.5 mm Hg at twelve months, 15.6 ± 6.7 mm Hg at twenty four months, and

18.7 ± 5.3 mm Hg at thirty six months. In group B, blood pressure mean values are 150/85 ± 10.2 mm Hg at baseline, and then a decrease of 8.4 ± 3.5 mm Hg at twelve months, 7.6 ± 3.5 mm Hg at twenty four months, and 11. 2 ± 5.3 mm Hg at thirty six months. In group A, there was a dramatic decrease of anti-hypertensive drugs prescriptions. In group B, patients maintained their original prescriptions, though under strict medical follow-up. Spearman's rank correlation analyses indicated that there was a significant correlation between NPI scores and Tinetti score over 24 months (NPI= 56.84 ±12.11, $r=0.81$, $p<0.01$), over 36 months (NPI= 66.03 ±8.81, $r=0.87$, $p<0.01$), in both group. Though it has been evidenced a significant decrease of Tinetti score in Group A, with low blood pressure than in Group B (see table 4, 4 1, b and c). We have found a correlation between benzodiazepines and neuroleptics intake and Tinetti score at 12, 24 and 36 months (respectively $r=0.77$, $p<0.05$; $r=0.78$, $p<0.05$; $r=0.67$, $p<0.05$ at 12 months; $r=0.81$, $p<0.01$; $r=0.77$, $p<0.05$; $r=0.84$, $p<0.01$ at 24 months; $r=0.81$, $p<0.01$; $r=0.82$, $p<0.01$; $r=0.89$, $p<0.01$ at 36 months) in both Groups. We have observed a positive correlation between apathy and NPI total scores in both the groups over 12, 24 and 36 months (respectively $r=0.78$, $p<0.05$; $r=0.8$, $p<0.05$ at baseline; $r=0.82$, $p<0.01$; $r=0.67$, $p<0.05$; at 12 months; $r=0.86$, $p<0.01$; $r=0.77$, $p<0.05$ at 24 months; $r=0.91$, $p<0.01$; $r=0.82$, $p<0.01$ at 36 months). Finally, we did observe a positive correlation between apathy scores and FAB scores only in Group A at every session; in Group B at 24 and at 36 months (respectively $r=0.78$, $p<0.05$ at baseline; $r=0.82$, $p<0.01$ at 12 months, only for Group A; $r=0.86$, $p<0.01$; $r=0.77$, $p<0.05$ at 24 months; $r=0.91$, $p<0.01$; $r=0.82$, $p<0.01$ at 36 months, respectively).

4. Discussion

We have studied well selected 864 patients, for three years, suffering from subcortical vascular dementia. Our aim has been to prove if hypotension is a key point in vascular dementia patients, and if this aspect reflects its importance in the daily living assistance. What we have observed are different points. Subcortical vascular dementia is related somehow to hypertension, mainly because) all the patients recruited have been diagnosed hypertension, during their life. Curiously, some of them (n=415; group A), during the follow-up, registered a dramatic decrease of their blood pressure values, constantly during the entire follow-up, even if the anti-hypertensive drugs have been interrupted; some other (n=398; group B), who had a hypertension history, but maintained elevated values of systolic/diastolic pressure during the entire follow-up. These patients have been studied, and what merged is that the two groups did not differ from a neurological, behavioral, and general drug intake at baseline; there was only a significant difference in cognition performance, as far as group A frontal functions (implementation of strategies, executive function, judgment capability, abstract reasoning, go/no go strategies and auto-inhibition) appear significantly worse ($p<0.05$) than those of Group B. During follow-up, both patients did worse, in their life functions, as far as cognition, behavior, gait, functional independence; but, during the entire follow-up, Group A did worse in all the items when compared to Group B. In particular, these patients were referred as more apathic, abulic, with less frontal performances, with major walking impairment and with lower independence. In other words, it seems that given a selected population, in which hypertension has been correctly established and treated, it might have led to a well-defined white-matter deterioration (the previously called Binswanger' disease); then, when dementia has been diagnosed, the sudden modification of blood pressure regulation, changed in hypotension, led to a poorer life expectance, due to a worse performance in cognition (as above mentioned), behavior (more apathy and abulia), walking strategies. All these aspects reflect a functional sufference of frontal subcortical neural pathways: it is not known the reason, but frontal lobes have a metabolism rate under basal condition that is 20% more than that of the other brain areas (Moretti, 2006). And it is also well known that age cognitive modifications are related to frontal dysfunctions (Levine et al., 1997; Esposito, 1999; Kramer et al., 1999), due to a reduction of brain reserve capacity. This brings an aged individual closer to the level of insufficiency where only minor additional lesions may be required to precipitate dementia. The degenerative aging changes, though milder, repeat much of the pathology of Alzheimer's disease. In vascular dementia, especially in subcortical vascular type, there is an accentuate expression of what is found in old age (Moretti, 2006). The complete and incomplete white matter infarction, frequently coexisting, would, by virtue of their high prevalence, be the underlying substrate in the recognition of white matter disease (Capizzano Aristides et al., 2007), leuko-encephalopathy or leuko-araiosis (Hachinski, 1994). Having this point stated, it should be consider another question: why are these patients so sensitive to hypotension? And another major problem is: why do these patients change their historical profile and suddenly have low blood pressure, having a positive history of hypertension and not clear signs of new concomitant pathologies, which can determine, *per se*, low blood pressure? The hypothesis here are suggestive, but not at all conclusive. The small artery vessels of an hypertensive patient show a degeneration of the smooth muscle layer, which is replaced by collagen in a hyaline fibrosis, leading to a subtotal luminal occlusion. These arterioles share traits with non-hypertensive lipohyalinosis (Zhang et al, 1994), as well as with hypertensive arteriolosclerosis, and may concur with hypertensive changes. Anatomically, the smaller resistance blood vessels undergo degenerative changes consisting of thickening and fibrosis of the media (in muscular arteries) and intima, and patchy degeneration of smooth muscle cells producing luminal narrowing and increased vascular resistance. Although the resting CBF is the same in normotensive and hypertensive individuals, these structural changes limit the capacity of the resistance vessels for maximal vasodilatation and impair tolerance of lower blood pressures, while improving tolerance to hypertension through vasoconstriction of these same vessels. Long-term antihypertensive treatment can reverse these adaptive changes and shift the auto-regulation curve back to its normal range, although only limited reversibility occurs in elderly hypertensive patients (Moretti et al., 2008). Moreover, it has been observed that there is another possible explanation which might be related to the sudden dys-regulation observed in these patients. Relatively low blood pressure seems to be correlated with dementia even in a preclinical stage. Different Authors (Guo et al., 1991) started from the speculation that cerebral blood flow is reduced in dementia patients (Brown & Frackowiak, 1991). That was generally thought to be related with reduced metabolic activity of the brain or with a major vascular lesion. The authors hypothesized that the reduction of cerebral blood flow might be related to the impairment of the cerebral autoregulation, secondary to the degenerative disorder. The direct consequence would be a sequential ulterior reduction of blood pressure, due to dys-regulation, which might accelerate the lowering of blood perfusion and therefore the underlying degenerative process (Yamamoto et al., 1998; Bolster et al., 2001; Nilsson et al., 2007; Mehagnoul-Schipper et al., 2002). Moreover, the authors interpreted these results as a potential expression of the frailty and deteriorated vitality of the oldest old, in keeping constantly the auto-regulation capabilities of the normal brain, and expressed their concern, due to this frailty, on the real impact of lowering pressure in oldest age (Nilsson et al., 2007). An age-related impairment of the vascular auto-regulation due to impaired functioning of the autonomic nervous system can lead to symptoms derived from blood pressure altered dysregulation in the elderly. Additionally, age-related arteriolar changes, including endothelial changes, have been suggested to reduce the baroreflex activity and thereby predispose for deleterious blood pressure falls (Salloway, 2003). The prevalence of orthostatic and non-orthostatic hypotension reached 50% in clinically evaluated VaD cases (Salloway et al., 2003; Mirski, 2005). The possible *liaison* that relates lower blood pressure, dysregulation of cerebral blood flow, vascular dementia, (and eventual AD dementia) might be the pivotal role of acetylcholine (Ach). Ach regulates the cerebral blood flow through the parasympathetic innervation of the circle of Willis and of the pial vessels (Vasquez & Purve, 1979), and it causes significant arterial relaxation by promoting the synthesis of vasodilator agents (Vanhoutte, 1989). Preclinical research using the spontaneously hypertensive stroke-prone rat model of VaD has shown a significant reduction in the levels of acetylcholine (ACh) and choline in the cortex, hippocampus and cerebrospinal fluid compared with normal rats (Kimura et al., 2000). When compared with normal rats, spontaneously hypertensive stroke-prone rats have significantly lower levels of acetylcholine in the cerebrospinal fluid (CSF) (Togashi et al., 1994). In the latter study, the differences in CSF levels between normal rats and stroke prone rats increased with age, suggesting progressive deterioration of central cholinergic function in hypertensive stroke prone rats. The cholinesterase inhibitor epistigmine has been shown to improve blood flow in the Sprague-Dawley rat with tandem occlusion of left middle cerebral and common carotid arteries. Epistigmine also enhanced the ischaemia-induced rostral shift of cerebral blood flow maximum in the contralateral hemisphere and the redistribution of cerebral blood flow, a phenomenon possibly related to recovery of function (Scremin et al., 1997). Very recently, to prove the role of acetylcholine in vessel regulation muscarinic receptors, M5, have been studied. The M5 muscarinic receptor is the most recent member of the muscarinic acetylcholine receptor family (M1-M5) to be cloned. Because M5 receptor mRNA has been detected in several blood vessels, Yamada et al. (2001) investigated whether the lack of M5 receptors led to changes in vascular tone by using several in vivo and in vitro vascular preparations in knockout mice. Strikingly, acetylcholine, a powerful dilator of most vascular beds, virtually lost the ability to dilate cerebral arteries and arterioles in M5R_/_ mice. This effect was specific for cerebral blood vessels, because acetylcholine-mediated dilation of extra-cerebral arteries remained fully intact in M5R_/_ mice. Therefore, as often happens in neurological studies, the more hypotheses, the more questions: why should patients with the same pathology (subcortical vascular dementia) respond so differently to blood pressure regulation? What is the role of blood pressure dysregulation in sVAD patients, without a previous history of hypertension? Should we consider the possibility to treat differently patients with dementia and hypertension? More studies should consider these fundamental points, in order to implement knowledge and eventfully ameliorate treatment options for vascular dementia.

5. Conclusions

In conclusion, we could state:

1. low flow states are critical to the pathogenesis of ischemic leuko-encephalopathy; in particular this is particularly true in subcortical vascular dementia, where the cerebral frontal subcortical regions are particularly sensitive to hypo-perfusion
2. We do not know several points: is hypotension a primary event in vascular dementia or is it secondary to the degeneration of brain structure? What is the role of acetylcholine in blood flow dys-regulation? Why do patients with dementia have such different response to blood pressure control?
3. Taking into considerations all these points, we strictly recommend to the clinicians who face every day these patients that they should check strictly blood pressure, and that they should taper anti-hypertensive medications according to aging-associated declines in BP and tendency toward orthostasis? The neurological concept of "tailored therapy" should begin with the most huge and wide-spread diffused drugs, such as hypertensive drugs
4. In frail patients, such as the old patients with dementia, clinicians should consider the concept of the minimization of ancillary drugs, e.g. anti-diabetes, bronchodilators, diuretics, anty-arythmics, and so on. The entire drug set should be reconsidered at every visit, taking into account the real state of the patients, updated at the moment
5. Benzodiazepines and other meds that could lower BP in the elderly should be prescribed when necessary, without doubts, but the prescriptions should be followed during the time course of the life span of the demented patients.

6. References

American Psychiatric Association. 2000. *Diagnostic and Statistical Manual of Mental Disorders-R*. 4th edition. American Psychiatric Association. ISBN: 0890420246. Washington DC

Blennow K, Wallin A, Uhlemann C, Gottfries CG. 1991. White matter lesions on CT in Alzheimer patients: relation to clinical symptomatologic and vascular factors. *Acta Neurol Scand.* 83, pp 187-193. ISSN 0065-1427

Bolster BD, Serfaty JM, Atalar E. 2001. In vivo measurements of pulse wave in small vessels using intravenous MR. *Magn. Resonance Med.* 45, pp 53-60. ISSN: 1522-2594

Brookmeyer, R., S. Gray, Kawas C. 1998. Projections of Alzheimer's disease in the United States and the public health impact of delaying disease onset. *Am J Public Health.* 88, (9), pp 1337-1342. ISSN: 0090-0036

Brown WD, Frackowiak RSJ. 1991. Cerebral blood flow and metabolism studies in multi-infarct dementia. *Alzh Dis Assoc Dis.* 5,pp 131-143. ISSN:0893-0341

Burke WJ, Coronado PG, Schmitt CA, Gillespie KM, Chung HD. 1994. Blood pressure regulation in Alzheimer's disease. *J. Auton. Nerv. Syst.* 48, pp 65-71. ISSN: 0165-1838

Capizzano Aristides A, Schuff Norbert, Amend Diane L, Tanabe Jody L, Norman David, Maudsley Andrew A, Jagust William, Chui Helena C, Fein George, Segal Mark R, Weiner Michael W. 2007. Subcortical Ischemic Vascular Dementia: Assessment with Quantitative MR Imaging and 1H MR Spectroscopy. *AJNR Am J Neuroradiol.* 16, 21(4), pp 621–630. ISSN: 0195-6108

Chamorro A, Pujol J, Saiz A, Vila N, Vilanova JC, Alday M, Blanc R. 1997. Periventricular white matter lucencies in patients with lacunar stroke: a marker of too high or too low blood pressure? *Arch Neurol.* 54, pp 1284–1288. ISSN: 0003-9942

Chui HC. Dementia. 1989. A review emphasizing clinico-pathologic correlation and brain-behaviour relationships. *Arch. Neurol.* 46, ,7, pp 806-814. ISSN: 0003-9942

Cummings JL, Mega M, Gray K. 1994. The Neuropsychiatric Inventory: comprehensive assessment of psychopathology in dementia. *Neurology* 44, pp 2308–2314. ISSN: 10158618

De Buyzere M, Clement DL, Duprez D. 1998. Chronic Low Blood Pressure: A Review. *Cardiovascular Drugs and Therapy* 12, pp 29–35. ISSN: 1573-7241

Dubois B, Pillon B, Slachevsky A, Litvan I. 1997. *Frontal Assessment Battery (FAB).* Retrieved from: Documents and Settings\UK\Documenti\PSICO\Test-Scales\FAB.doc

Erkinjuntti T, Inzitari D, Pantoni L, Wallin A, Scheltens P, Rockwood K, Desmond DW. 2000. Limitations of clinical criteria for the diagnosis of vascular dementia in clinical trials. Is a focus on subcortical vascular dementia a solution? *Ann NY Acad Sci* 903, pp 262–272. ISSN: 0077-8923

Erkinjuntti T. 1997. Vascular dementia: challenge of clinical diagnosis. *Int Psychogeriatr.* 9, 77–83. ISSN: 1041-6102

Esposito G. 1999. Context-dependent, neural system-specific neuropsychological concomitants of aging: mapping PET correlates during cognitive activation. *Brain,* 122: 963-979. ISSN 0006-8950

Ferrer I, Kaste M, Kalimo H. Vascular diseases.2008. In: *Greenfield's Neuropathology* Love S, Louis D, Ellison D, (eds.). pp 121–240. Oxford University Press. ISBN: 978-0-0340906820 Oxford

Fletcher AE, Bulpitt CJ. 1992. How far should blood pressure be lowered? *N Engl J Med* 326, 251–254. ISSN 0028-4793

Folstein M, Folstein S, McHugh P. 1975. Mini-Mental state. A practical method for grading the cognitive state of patients for the clinician. *J Psychiatr Res.* 12, 189–198. ISSN: 1049-8931

Forette, F., Seux M.L., Staessen J.A., Thijs L., Birkenhager W.H., Babarskiene M.R., et al. 1998. Prevention of dementia in randomised double-blind placebo-controlled Systolic Hypertension in Europe (Syst-Eur) trial. *Lancet* 352, 9137, pp. 1347-1351. ISSN: 0140-6736

Glynn RJ, Field TS, Rosner B, Hebert PR, Taylor JO, Hennekens CH. 1995. Evidence for a positive linear relation between blood pressure and mortality in elderly people. *Lancet* 345, pp. 825–829. ISSN: 0140-6736

Gorelick PB. 1997. Status risk factors for dementia associated with stroke. Stroke. 28, pp 459-463. ISSN: 00392499

Guo Z, Vintanen M, Winblad B, Fratiglioni L.1999. Low blood pressure and incidence of dementia in a very old sample: dependent on initial cognition. *J. Am. Ger. Soc.* 47, pp 723-726. ISSN: 0002-8614

Hachinski V. 1994. Vascular dementia: a radical redefinition. *Dementia* 5, pp. 130-132. ISSN: 1471-3012

Hachinski VC, Iliff LD, Zhilka E. 1975. Cerebral blood flow in dementia. *Arch. Neurol.* 32, pp. 632-637. ISSN 0003-9942

Hebert R, Lindsay J, Verreault R, Rockwood K, Hill G, Dubois MF. 2000. Vascular dementia : incidence and risk factors in the Canadian study of health and aging. *Stroke* 31, pp 1487-1493. ISSN: 00392499

Hebert LE, Scherr PA, Bienias JL, Bennett DA, Evans DA. 2003. Alzheimer disease in the US population: prevalence estimates using the 2000 census. *Arch Neurol* 60, 8, pp. 1119-22. ISSN 0003-9942

Kalaria RN. 2010. Vascular basis for brain degeneration: faltering controls and risk factors for dementia *Nutrition Reviews*. 68 (Suppl. 2), pp S74–S87. ISSN 0029-6643

Kalaria RN. 1996. Cerebral vessels in ageing and Alzheimer's disease. *Pharmacol Ther.* 72, pp 193–214. ISSN: 0163-7258

Kario K, Matsuo T, Kobayashi H, Imiya M, Mastuo M, Shimada K. 1996. Nocturnal fall of blood pressure and silent cerebrovascular damage in elderly hypertensive patients: advanced silent cerebrovascular damage in extreme dippers. *Hypertension.* 27, pp 130–135. ISSN: 1062-4821.

Kimura S, Saito H, Minami M. 2000. Pathogenesis of vascular dementia in stroke-prone spontaneously hypertensive rats. *Toxicology* 153, pp 167–87. ISSN: 0378-4274

Kohara K, Jiang Y, Igase M, Takata Y, Fukuoka T, Okura T, Kitami Y, Hiwada K. 1999. Postprandial hypotension is associated with asymptomatic cerebrovascular damage in essential hypertensive patients. *Hypertension.* 33, pp 565–568. ISSN: 1062-4821.

Kramer AE, Hahn S., Gopher D. 1999. Task coordination and aging: explorations of executive control processes in the task switching paradigm. *Acta Psychol.*, 101, pp 339-378. ISSN: 0439-755X

Langer RD, Ganiato TG, Barrett-Conner E. 1989. Paradoxical survival of elderly men with high blood pressure. *Br Med J* 298, pp 1356–1358. ISSN: 09598138

Launer LJ, Masaki K, Petrovitch H, Foley D, Havlik RJ. 1995. The association between midlife blood pressure levels and late-life cognitive function. The Honolulu-Asia Aging Study. *JAMA* 274, pp 1846-1851. ISSN 0098-7484

Lawton MP, Brody EM. 1969. Assessment of older people: self-maintaining and instrumental activities of daily living. *Gerontologist* 9, pp 179-186. ISSN: 0016-9013

Levine B, Stuss DT, Milberg WP. 1997. Effects of aging on conditional associative learning: process analyses and comparison with focal frontal lesions. *Neuropsychology* 11, pp 367-381. ISSN: 1380-3395

Manos PJ. 1997. The utility of the ten-point clock test as a screen for cognitive impairment in general hospital patients. *Gen Hosp Psych* 8, pp 469–476. ISSN: 0163-8343

Matsubayashi K, Okumiya K, Wada T, Osaki Y, Fujisawa M, Doi Y, Ozawa T.1997. Postural dysregulation in systolic blood pressure is associated with worsened scoring on neurobehavioral function tests and leukoaraiosis in the older elderly living in a community. *Stroke* 28, pp 2169–2173. ISSN: 00392499

Mattila K, Haavisto M, Rajala S, Heikinheimo R. 1988. Blood pressure and five years survival in the very old. *Br Med J* 296:887–889. ISSN: 09598138

Mehagnoul-Schipper DJ, Colier WN, Hoefnagels WH, Verheugt FW, JANser RW. 2002. Effects of furosemide versus captopril on post-prandial and orthostatic blood pressure and on cerebral oxygenation in patients ≥ 70 years old of age with heart failure. *Am. J. Cardiol.* 90, pp 596-600, ISSN 0002-9149

Mielke MM, Rosenberg PB, Tschanz J, Cook L, Corcoran C, Hayden KM, Norton M, Rabins PV, Green RC, Welsh-Bohmer KA, Breitner JC, Munger R, Lyketsos CG. 2007. Vascular factors predict rate of progression in Alzheimer disease. *Neurology* 6, 69, 19, pp 1850-1858. ISSN: 10158618

Mirski MA. 2005. *Pharmacology of blood pressure management during cerebral ischemia.* American Academy of Neurology lecture collections (AAN) on CD-ROM. Miami, 5PC-004, pp. 456-469.

Moretti R. (Ed.) 2006. *Subcortical vascular dementia*, NovaPublisher Editorials. New York. ISBN 1-59454-996-6.

Moretti R, Torre P, Antonello RM. 2008. Alzheimer's Dementia and Vascular Risk Factors. In: *Alzheimer's Disease: New Research.* Visser AM (Ed). Pp. 193-209. NovaPublishers Editorials. ISBN: 978-1-60456-481-5. New York.

Morris MC, Scherr PA, Hebert LE, Glynn RJ, Bennett DA, Evans DA. 2001. Association of incident Alzheimer disease and blood pressure measured from 13 years before to 2 years after diagnosis in a large community study. *Arch Neurol* , 58, pp 1640-1646. ISSN 0003-9942

Nakamura K, Oita J, Yamaguchi T. 1995. Nocturnal blood pressure dip in stroke survivors: a pilot study. *Stroke,* 26, pp 1373–1378. ISSN: 00392499

Nilsson SE, Read S, Berg S, Johansson B, Melander A, Lindblad V. 2007. Low systolic blood pressure is associated with impaired cognitive function in the oldest old: longitudinal observations in a population-based sample 80 years and older. *Aging Clin. Exp. Res.* 19, pp 41-47. ISSN: 1594-0667

Pantoni L, Rossi R, Inzitari D. 2000. Efficacy and safety of nimodipine in subcortical vascular dementia: a subgroup analysis of the Scandinavian Multi-Infarct Dementia Trial. *J Neurol Sci* 175:124–34. ISSN: 0022-510X

Posner HB, Tang MX, Luchsinger J, Lantigua R, Stern Y, Mayeux R. 2002. The relationship of hypertension in the elderly to AD, vascular dementia, and cognitive function. *Neurology* 58, pp 1175-1181. ISSN: 10158618

Roman GC, Tatemichi TK, Erkinjuntti T. 1993. Vascular dementia: diagnostic criteria for research studies. Report of the NINDS-AIREN international work group. *Neurology* 43, pp 250-260. ISSN: 10158618

Ruitenberg A, Skoog I, Ott Am Aevarsson O, Witteman JCM, Lernfelt B, vanHarskamp F, Hofman A, Bretler MMB. 2001. Blood pressure and risk of dementia: results from the Rotterdam Study and the Gothenburg H-70 study. *Dem.Ger. Cog. Dis.* 12, pp 33-39. ISSN: 1420-8008

Salloway S. *Subcortical vascular dementia: Binswanger's and CADASIL.* American Academy of Neurology (AAN) lecture collections on CD-ROM. 2003; Honolulu: 8AC.006-2, pp. 1-29.

Scheltens Ph., Barkhof F, Leys D. 1993. A semiquantitative rating scale for the assessment of signal hyperintensities on magnetic resonance imaging. *J. Neurol. Sci.* 114, pp 7-12. ISSN: 0022-510X

Schmidt R, Fazekas F, Kappeller P, Schmidt H, Hartung HP. 1999. MRI white matter hyperintensities: three-year follow up of the Austrian Stroke Prevention Study. *Neurology* 53, pp 132–139. ISSN: 10158618

Scremin OU, Li MG, Scremin AM, Jenden DJ.1997. Cholinesterase inhibition improves blood flow in the ischemic cerebral cortex. *Brain Res Bull* 42, pp 59–70. ISSN: 0361-9230

Skoog I, Nilsson L, Palmertz B. 1993. A population-based study of dementia in 85-year olds. *NEJM* 328, pp 153–158. ISSN 1533-4406

Tinetti ME.1986. Performance-oriented assessment of mobility problems in elderly patients. *J. Am. Ger. Soc.* 34, pp 119-126. ISSN: 0002-8614.

Togashi H, Matsumoto M, Yoshioka M, Hirokami M, Minami M, Saito H. 1994. Neurochemical profiles in cerebrospinal fluid of stroke-prone spontaneously hypertensive rats. *Neurosci Lett.* 17, 166,1, pp 117-20. ISSN 0304-3940

Tzourio C. 2007. Hypertension, cognitive decline, and dementia: an epidemiological perspective. *Dialog. Clin Neurosci.* 9, 1, pp 61-70. ISSN:1294-8322

van Dijck EJ, Breteler M, Schmidt R, Berger K, Nilsson LG, Oudkerk M, Pajak A, Sans S, de Ridder M. 2004. The association between blood pressure, hypertension, and cerebral white matter lesions. *Hypertension* 44, pp 625- 650, ISSN: 0194911X.

Vanhoutte PM. 1989. Endothelium and control of vascular function. State of the art. *Hypertension* 13, pp 658–667. ISSN: 0194911X.

Vasquez J, Purve MJ. 1979. The cholinergic pathway to cerebral blood vessels. I. Morphological studies. *Pflugers Arch* 379, pp 157–163. ISSN: 1432-2013

Vermeer SE, Prins ND, den Heijer T, Hofman A, Koudstaal PJ, Breteler MM. 2003. Silent brain infarcts and the risk of dementia and cognitive decline. *NEJM*, 348, 13, pp 1215-22. ISSN 1533-4406

Watanabe N, Imai Y, Nagai K, Tsuji I, Satoh H, Sakuma M, Sakuma H, Kato J, Onodera-Kikuchi H, Yamada M, Abe F, Hisamichi S, Abe K.1996. Nocturnal blood pressure and silent cerebrovascular lesions in elderly Japanese. *Stroke* 27, pp 1319–1327. ISSN: 00392499.

Wolf PA, D'Agostino RB, Belanger AJ, Kannel WB. 1991. Probability of stroke: a risk profile from the Framingham Study. Stroke, 1991. 22(3): p. 312-8. ISSN: 00392499

Wu CC, Mungas D, Petkov CI, Eberling JL, Zrelak PA, Buonocore MH, Brunberg JA, Haan MN, Jagust WJ. 2002. Brain structure and cognition in a community sample of elderly Latinos. *Neurology* 59, 3, pp. 383-391. ISSN: 10158618

Yamada M, Lamping KG., Duttaroy A , Zhang W , Cui Y , Bymaster FP. , McKinzie DL., Felder CC, Deng CX, Faraci FM, Wess J. 2001. Cholinergic dilation of cerebral blood vessels is abolished in M5 muscarinic acetylcholine receptor knockout mice. *PNAS*, 98, 24, pp 14096–14101. ISSN: 1091-6490

Yamamoto Y, Akiguchi I, Oiwa K, Hayashi M, Kimura J. 1998. Adverse effect of nighttime blood pressure on the outcome of lacunar infarct patients. *Stroke* 29, pp 570–576 . ISSN: 00392499

Zhang WW, Badonic T, Höög A, Jiang MH, Ma KC, Nie JX, Olsson Y, Sourander P. 1994. Structural and vasoactive factors influencing intracerebral arterioles in cases of vascular dementia and other cerebrovascular disease: a review. *Dementia* 5, pp 153-62. ISSN: 1471-3012

Zhu L, Viitanen M, Guo Z, Winblad B, Fratiglioni L. 1998. Blood pressure reduction, cardiovascular disease, and cognitive decline in the Mini-Mental State Examination in a community population of normal very old people: a three year follow-up. J. Clin Epidem. 51, 5, pp 385-391. ISSN: 0895-4356

3

The Relations Between the Vitamins and Alzheimer Dementia

Emel Koseoglu
Erciyes University, Medicine Faculty, Neurology Department, Kayseri Turkey

1. Introduction

The number of people suffering from dementia might triple over the next 50 years, measures for treatment and prevention of dementia are crucial. As vitamins are involved in many biochemical processes, they are essential for good health. They can possibly take role more probably in the prevention and treatment of dementia. For this reason, the relations between the vitamins and dementia, especially Alzheimer Dementia (AD) have been studied for many years.

Until the 1900s, vitamins were obtained solely through food intake, and changes in diet can alter the types and amounts of vitamins ingested. Vitamins have been produced as commodity chemicals and made widely available as inexpensive pills for several decades, allowing supplementation of dietary intake.

There are many observational studies indicating associations of vitamin deficiencies with cognitive dysfunction. Most of the studies in the subject are cross sectional studies. Nevertheless, these type of studies can not prove whether a nutritional deficit is the cause or the result of an impaired cognitive status. Longitudinal prospective observational studies and interventional studies are more suitable to releave causal relationships. Interventional studies with long follow up periods are preferred, since short follow up time can not be enough to evaluate the effects. There are some individual studies reporting promising, positive results about vitamin supplementation in prevention and treatment of dementia.

Vitamin A, C and E have antioxidant activity, which have been investigated for its prevention from neuronal death and improving neuronal function through maintaining mitochondrial homeostasis. Vitamin E may modulate signal transduction pathways and participate in the synthesis pathways of neurotransmitters. Several epidemiological studies have indicated a relationship between blood concentrations of antioxidant micronutrients and cognitive impairment. Though not sufficient, there are some prospective longitudinal and interventional studies indicating the useful effects of antioxidant vitamins in prevention and treatment of dementia.

Deficiencies of several B vitamins, including thiamine (B1), riboflavin (B2), niacin (B3), pyridoxine (B6), folate (B9) and cobalamin (B12) have been reported to be associated with cognitive dysfunction in many studies. In some studies, pathophysiological models have been formulated, including the association of B vitamin deficiencies with metabolic disturbances in the structural constituents of cerebral tissue, such as phospholipids and myelin, as well as in signaling molecules, such as neurotransmitters. More recently, the association between the deficiency of B vitamins, particularly folate and cobalamin, and cognitive impairment has been investigated in relation to hyperhomocysteinemia. It was shown that plasma homocysteine is a better correlate of cognitive function than the serum folate or cobalamin concentrations themselves. Homocysteine is a well established risk factor for vascular disease, but some epidemiological and cross sectional studies have also suggested that it may play a role in cognitive performance and pathophysiology of dementia in older people, possibly as the metabolic link between micro-vascular disease and Alzheimer dementia. Some prospective longitudinal and interventional studies have reported the useful effects of some B vitamins, though there existed contradictory results also. Furthermore, there was a large heterogenity among present vitamin B interventional studies with cognitive assessments in terms of dosage, routes of intervention (for vitamin B12), age and cognitive function assessments. It seems that it will be worthwhile to perform new larger studies, especially considering the results of the studies reporting recovering effect of folate supplementation on cognition.

The most recent reported vitamins related to cognitive functioning are vitamin D and vitamin K. Vitamin D has been reported to be critical to healthy brain development and function. Vitamin D in sufficient amounts seemed to protect brain cells and reduce inflammation according to some biological evidence. Some epidemiological and cross-sectional studies showed the association of vitamin D deficiency with Alzheimer disease and dementia. To disclose if there is a causal relationship between them, prospective longitudinal studies are needed in the subject. Vitamin K is also required for normal brain development and function. Some authors proposed a possible role of vitamin K deficiency in the pathogenesis of Alzheimer disease. It is obviously useful to do experimental animal and case controlled human studies in the first step to clarify the role of vitamin K in the pathogenesis of dementia.

In this section, we will try to discuss the relations of AD with the antioxidant vitamins, B vitamins and lastly vitamin D and K with the help of cross-sectional or longitudinal prospective observational studies, and interventional studies. Nevertheless, the subject has many aspects. As vitamin deficiencies can cause cognitive impairment, cognitive impairment can also determine changes in dietary habits and consequently cause vitamin deficiencies. Vitamin intake through food or supplementation forms can have different effects. There is also a possibility that vitamins have useful effects in different subgroups of people, based on age, nutritional status or vitamin level. Multivitamin supplementation may be more useful. Detailed investigations about these aspects will be informative.

2. Antioxidant vitamins

2.1 Pathophysiological mechanisms

Brain tissue is particularly vulnerable to free-radical damage because of its low level of endogenous antioxidants (Reiter, 1995). Neuropathological studies documented typical lesions from exposure to free radicals in the brains of patients with AD (Behl, 1997; Christen, 2000; Pratico & Delanty, 2000; Varadarajan et al., 2000). Lipid peroxidation seems to be especially susceptible to oxidative stress (Knopman, 1998; Pitchumoni et al., 1998; Sinclair et al., 1998). Increasing evidence also implicates neuronal membrane associated oxidative stress (for example, consequent to deposition of amyloid β-peptide (Aβ)) and alteration of membrane lipid metabolism (and consequent accumulation of ceramides and cholesterol) as pathogenetic factors of synaptic dysfunction and neuronal degeneration (Cutler et al., 2004; Hyun et al., 2010; L.J. Miller & Chacko, 2004). Antioxidant treatment improved neuronal function through maintaining mitochondrial homeostasis. In a canine model of human aging, it was shown that aged canine mitochondria showed significant increases in reactive oxygen species production and a reduction in NADH-linked respiration. Mitochondrial function was improved selectively in aged dogs treated with antioxidant diet (Head et al., 2009).

Vitamin A levels in brain decline with age and lower still in individuals with AD (Goodman, 2006).A metabolic product of vitamin A, retinoic acid, is known to slow cell death and offer protection from Aβ (Sahin et al., 2005). In addition to its antioxidant activity, vitamin E may modulate signal transduction pathways and participate in the synthesis pathways of neurotransmitters (Azzi et al., 1992; Martin et al., 1997; Meydani et al., 1997). Plasma vitamin C level was decreased in AD in addition to vitamin A and E (Foy et al., 1999). Vitamin C enhances the effect of medications used to treat dementia allowing the drugs to pass more easily into the brain and therefore to cause a greater effect. As a conflicting result, in the analysis of the association between the level of serum antioxidants and memory performance in an elderly, multiethnic sample of 4809 subjects; Perkins et al (Perkins et al., 1999) found a decreased serum level of vitamin E consistently associated with memory deficit after adjustment for age, education, income and vascular risk factors. Serum levels of other antioxidants (vitamins A and C, β-carotene and selenium) did not correlate with memory performance.

2.2 Studies

SENECA study reported a positive, although weak, correlation between plasma concentrations of lycopene, α- carotene, β-carotene, total carotenes, β-cryptoxanthin, α-tocopherol and Mini Mental State Examination (MMSE) scores (Haller et al., 1996). In the elderly population studied by Ortega et al., dietary intake of vitamin C, β-carotene and vitamin E were associated with a better cognitive function (Ortega et al., 2002). Perrig et al. (Perrig et al., 1997) showed that higher plasma ascorbic acid and β-carotene concentrations were associated with better memory performance in older people, both cross-sectionally and longitudinally over a 22 year period. In another cohort study performed on 455 elderly people with a duration of 7 year, high β-carotene levels were associated with less cognitive decline in APOE4 carriers but not in APOE4 negatives (Hu et al., 2006). Rats given dietary supplements of fruit and vegetable extracts for 8 months, beginning at 6 months of age, slowed age-related declines in neuronal and cognitive functions (Joseph et al., 1998). More importantly, these rats were able to reverse age-related deficits in several neuronal and behavioral parameters when administration was started at 19 months of age (Joseph et al., 1999). In another study investigating the effects of acute, short and long term pre-training administration of ascorbic acid on passive avoidance learning and memory in rats, it was concluded that short- and long-term supplementation with ascorbic acid (vitamin C) had facilitatory effects on acquisition and retrieval processes of passive avoidance learning and memory in rats (Shadidi et al., 2008).

Vitamin C supplements were shown to protect against cognitive decline in a 4 year follow up study (Paleologos et al., 1998). In Rotterdam Study (Engelhart et al., 2002), the cohort study of dietary antioxidants with a duration of 6 years, high intakes of vitamin C and E were found to be associated with lower risk of AD. In a recent study on 5395 participants older than 54 years of age and free of dementia with a mean follow up period of 9.6 years, it was shown that participants in the highest tertile of vitamin E intake were 25% less likely to develop dementia compared with those in the lowest tertile of the intake. Dietary intake levels of vitamin C, beta carotene, and flavonoids were not related with dementia risk after multivariate adjustments. Results were similar when risk for AD was specifically assessed (Devore et al., 2010). In CHAP cohort study, on 815 elderly residents free of AD at baseline with a follow up period of 3.9 years, it was found that dietary vitamin E was associated with decreased risk for AD, while intakes of vitamin C, β-carotene and vitamin E from supplements were not associated at all (M.C. Morris et al., 2002). In another study investigating the effects of high dietary intake of vitamin E on prevention from AD, it was found that α-tocopherol alone may not be as protective as the combined tocopherols (M.C. Morris et al., 2005a). In addition, the risk of AD was inversely related to the intake of α, γ and δ but not β tocopherol. It was found that higher levels of dietary vitamin E lowered the risk of AD and slowed cognitive decline over the six-year course of the investigation.

In Cache County study, performed on 3227 subjects older than 64 years of age with a follow-up period of 3 years, vitamin E and C supplements in combination were associated with reduction in AD incidence, but not in users of those supplements alone (Zandii et al., 2004). Likewise, in another cohort study with a 5 year follow-up period, conducted on 894 elderly subjects, combined use of vitamins E and C supplements were associated with less cognitive decline (Maxwell et al., 2005); while in another study performed on 2969 elderly participants without cognitive impairment at baseline, the use of supplemental vitamin E and C, alone or in combination, did not reduce risk of AD or overall dementia over 5.5 years of follow-up period (Gray et al., 2008). In spite of the successful results of dietary intake of vitamin E on the prevention, supplemental use of it alone (2000 IU/day) was not shown to have an effect on progression of minimal cognitive impairment to AD and on mean cognitive change in randomised controlled studies respectively (Kang et al., 2006; Petersen et al., 2005). In a randomised controlled study performed on 341 patients with moderate AD, the patients treated with selegiline, α-tocopherol supplement or combination of them had longer time to institutionalization (Sano et al., 1997). However, no significant benefit was shown in cognitive tests.

About the role of vitamin E in treatment, there is a safety problem other than analying its effectiveness. Recent meta-analyses of randomized trials involving vitamin E in cardiac patients and other patient groups suggest a slightly higher mortality risk associated with vitamin E treatment (Bjelokovic et al., 2007; E.R. Miller et al., 2005; Vivekananthan et al., 2003). One meta -analysis (E.R. Miller, 2005) concluded that the mortality rate associated with vitamin E treatment increased in a nonlinear dose-dependent manner, with the relative risk beginning to rise above 1 at doses ≥ 400 IU/day. In a study about this subject performed on 847 probable or mixed AD patients with a follow up period up to 15 years, there was no evidence that treatment with high doses of vitamin E (2000 IU/day)had an adverse effect on survival. In fact, patients whose regimens included vitamin E tended to survive longer than those taking no drug or a choline esterase inhibitor alone. It is noteworthy that the survival benefit to those taking vitamin E did not become apparent until after 4 or more years of follow up. In light of the potential for beneficial effects on vitamin E and mixed clinical trial evidence, these results emphasize the need for additional research on vitamin E supplementation in AD using a dose range that extends above 400 IU per day.

2.3 Comments

In conclusion, there are positive results about the use of antioxidant vitamins on mostly prevention of AD and mostly through diet. There is not sufficient evidence about their use in the treatment. In recent years, it seems that the researches on vitamin E and C have dominated. This can be due to the relation of these vitamins to the structure and physiology of brain and, more consistent finding of association between serum levels of vitamin E and memory performance in the studies. However, vitamin A is also a good candidate for more future studies.

The intake of vitamins through diet or supplementation forms and the number or quantity of different vitamins and presence of other ingredients in the supplementation forms can change the effect. For example, in the manufactured capsules of vitamin E, only α-tocopherol is present. But at real, vitamin E is composed of 4 different tocopherol forms and 4 corresponding tocotrienols. This may cause ineffectiveness of vitamin E supplementation found in some studies. Also, the interaction of antioxidant vitamins with other antioxidants like flavonoids and other chemicals present in fruits and vegetables can provide benefit in the dietary intake of vitamins.

3. B vitamins

3.1 Pathophysiological mechanisms

Deficiencies of several B vitamins, including thiamine (B1), riboflavin (B2), niasin (B3), pyridoxine (B6), folate (B9) and cobalamin (B12), have been related with cognitive dysfunction in many observational study (Riedel et al., 1998). In some studies, pathophysiological models have been formulated, including the association of B vitamin deficiencies with metabolic disturbances in the structural constituents of cerebral tissue, such as phospholipids and myelin, as well as in signaling molecules, such as neurotransmitters (Rampersaud et al., 2003). In particular, thiamine deficiency has been associated with lactic acid accumulation, reduction in oxygen uptake, decrease in transketolase activity, and an impairment in cholinergic activity, leading to the loss of memory and other cognitive functions (Micheau et al., 1985). Cobalamin is essential for neuronal generation and its deficiency can cause degeneration of the nervous system (Herrmann & Obeid, 2007). Various cobalamines were shown to have intracellular antioxidant activity in vitro. The compounds inhibited intracellular peroxide production, maintained intracellular glutathione levels, and prevented apoptotic and necrotic cell death (Birch et al., 2009). Folic acid plays an important role in neuroplasticity and in the maintenance of neuronal integrity (Kronenberg et al., 2009). It enhances the plasma concentrations of docosahexaenoic acid (DHA) and eicosapentaenoic acid (EPA). EPA, DHA, and arachidonic acid are of benefit in dementia by up-regulating gene expression concerned with neurogenesis, neurotransmission and connectivity, improving endothelial nitric oxide (eNO) generation, enhancing brain acetylcholine levels, suppressing the production of proinflammatory cytokines and precursing to anti-inflammatory compounds that protect neurons from cytotoxic action of various noxious stimuli, oxidative stress and neuronal apoptosis (Das, 2008).

Recently, the association between the deficiency of B vitamins, particularly folate and cobalamin, and cognitive impairment has been investigated in relation to hyperhomocysteinemia (hHcy). Several epidemiological studies have also suggested that hHcy may play a role in the cognitive performance (Prins ND, 2002) and pathophysiology of dementia in older people (Bell et al, 1992; Nilsson et al., 1996; Wahlin et al., 1996), possibly as the metabolic link between micro-vascular disease and old-age dementia (M.S. Morris et al., 2001; Parnetti et al., 1997). Feeding mice with a B-vitamin deficient diet for 10 weeks induced hHcy, significantly impaired learning and memory, and caused a significant rarefaction of hippocampal microvasculature unrelated to gliosis and neurodegeneration (Troen et al., 2008).

Homocystein (Hcy) is an aminoacid entirely derived from the body's intermediary metabolism (Fekkes et al., 1998; Pietrzik & Bronstrup, 1997), which can be converted to either methionine or cysteine. Both folate and cobalamin participate in the methylation of Hcy to methionine and in the remethylation and synthesis of S-adenosylmethionine (Bottiglieri, 1996; Parnetti et al., 1997). The other metabolic pathway, which converts Hcy to cysteine requires the active form of vitamin B6 (pyridoxal phosphate) (Pietrzik & Bronstrup, 1997). The most common cause of hHcy is accepted to be a deficiency of folate or cobalamin (Selhub, 2000). Almost two-thirds of the prevalance of hHcy is attributable to low vitamin B status or intake (Selhub J, 2008). Although the catabolic rate of Hcy results from the interaction between genetic make-up and B vitamin status, it is generally accepted that elevated plasma Hcy concentrations are a sensitive marker for folate and cobalamin tissue deficiency (Bottiglieri, 1996; Joosten et al., 1993; Lokk, 2003; McCaddon et al., 1998; Nilsson et al., 1996; Nilsson et al., 1999; Parnetti et al., 1997).

Folate and vitamin B12 are essential cofactors for the methionine/Hcy cycle in the brain. These vitamins mediate the remethylation of Hcy, which affects the production of the universal methyl donor, S-adenosylmethionine, in the brain among other organs. Hypomethylation, caused by low B-vitamin and hHcy, is linked to key pathomechanisms of dementia (Obeid et al., 2007). Also, Hcy is recognised to be proatherogenic and protrombotic (Hassan et al., 2004) and accepted to be an independent risk for developing occlusive arterial diseases (Refsum et al., 1998; Ueland & Refsum, 1989). hHcy exerts an inhibitory effect on adult mouse brain neurogenesis (Rabaneda et al., 2008). Low folate status and elevated Hcy increase the generation of reactive oxygen species and contribute to excitotoxicity and mitochondrial dysfunction which may lead to apoptosis (Kronenberg et al., 2009). hHcy is also proposed to be one of the effects of the oxidation of vitamin B12, as a result of oxidative stress (McCaddon et al., 2002). Furthermore, experimental studies in cell cultures have shown that Hcy is neurotoxic, possibly by activating N-methyl-D-aspartate receptors (Lipton et al., 1997) or DNA damage and consequent apoptosis (Kruman et al., 2000). In a population based study on 1779 subjects, hHcy has been reported to be an independent risk factor for dementia and cognitive impairment without dementia (Haan et al., 2007).

Depending on the used marker, 3-60 % of the elderly are classified as vitamin B12 deficient and about 29 % as folate deficient. Predominantly, the high prevalance of poor cobalamin status is caused by the increasing prevalance of atrophic gastritis type B, which occurs with a frequency of approximately 20-50% in elderly subjects (Wolters et al., 2004). Another cause of atropfic gastritis is long term treatment with proton pump inhibitors (Kuipers et al., 1995,1996; Lundell et al., 2006). Atrophic gastritis results in declining gastric acid and pepsinogen secretion, and hence decreasing intestinal digestion and absorption of both B vitamins. Such patients with atrophic gastritis require parenteral supplements. Folic acid intake among elderly subjects is generally well below the recommended dietary reference values (Wolters et al., 2004). So, folic acid deficiency is primarily caused by dietary deficiency. Meanwhile, vitamin B12 deficiency is due to two main causes, food cobalamin malabsorption and pernicious anemia (Andres et al., 2004).

3.2 Studies

Many epidemiological, cross-sectional and case control studies reported the association of dementia with low blood levels of vitamin B12 and folate or hHcy. Hovewer, these studies are unable to exclude the possibility that such associations of hHcy or vitamin B deficiencies are rather a result than a cause of the disease.

Kivipelto M et al (Kivipelto et al., 2009), in their prospective study found that persons with high Hcy had more than twice as high a risk of developing AD than persons with low Hcy, even after adjusting for confounding or mediating factors, suggesting that Hcy is involved in the development of dementia and AD. Vitamin B12 itself seemed not to be directly involved, because holo-transcobalamin showed no association with dementia. In some cohort studies, hHcy was found to be correlated with decline in constructional praxis and recall memory (Tucker et al., 2005) and increased risk for dementia (Dufoil et al., 2003; Haan et al., 2007; Ravaglia et al., 2005; Seshadri et al., 2002; McCaddon et al., 2001), while in some others it was not correlated with cognitive decline (Clarke et al., 2007; Kalmijn et al., 1999; Luchsinger et al., 2004; Mooijaart et al., 2005; Teunissen et al., 2003). In the cohort studies, low plasma level of folate was found to be associated with decline in constructional praxis and lower cognitive function regardless of Hcy respectively (de Lau et al., 2007; Tucker et al., 2005). In another cohort study performed on 370 non demented persons older than 74 years of age, persons with low serum level of vitamin B12 or folate had the risk of developing AD (Wang et al., 2001). In addition to low folate and high Hcy plasma levels, low plasma concentration of vitamin B12 was also associated with decline of constructional praxis in a 3 year cohort study (Tucker et al., 2005).

Cohort studies of dietary intake of B vitamins in healthy elderly persons revealed conflicting results. In one of them, dietary intake was found to be not related with the risk of developing AD (MC Morris, 2006a). In another, the highest quartile of total folate intake was related to lower risk of AD (Luchsinger et al., 2007), while the other reported that rate of cognitive decline among persons in the top folate intake was more than twice that of those in the lowest fifth of intake (MC Morris et al., 2005b).

Despite potential benefits of vitamin B supplementation for lowering Hcy, the positive contribution of this supplementation to cognitive function among demented and non-demented persons remains debatable. There was a large heterogeneity among present vitamin B interventional studies with cognitive assessments in terms of dosage, routes of intervention (for vitamin B12), age and cognitive function assessments.

It has been proven that folate supplementation reduces plasma Hcy levels. This was observed by Jacques et al. in the Framingham Offspring Study cohort, after the folate fortification of grain in the Unites States started in January 1998 (Jacques et al., 1999). Nevertheless, the relationship between dietary folic acid intakes and plasma Hcy concentrations seems to be characterized by a threshold effect (Selhub, 1993): above a certain dosage of folate supplementation, there is no additional effect on lowering circulating Hcy. It is not clear where this threshold stands: a metanalysis of 12 randomized controlled trials assessed that the minimum dosage of folate capable of determining a maximum reduction (about %25) of circulating Hcy was 0.5 mg/day. More recent randomized trials determined this threshold at 0.8 mg/day (Wald et al., 2001) or 0.4 mg/day (van Oort et al., 2003). The differences are possibly explained by population selection biases (van Oort et al., 2003).

Some randomised controlled trials, including persons with normal cognitive function, cognitive impairment and dementia, evaluated the effect of folate supplementation on cognitive function. Among cognitively impaired subjects (n=30) with low folate serum levels, Fioravanti et al (Fioravanti et al., 1998) observed a significant improvement of some scores of the Randt Memory Test in the folate treated group compared with the placebo group after 60 days of treatment. In another trial using a mixed factorial design in normal subjects (n=211), the authors observed that folate-treated older women's cognitive test scores (Rey Auditory-Verbal Learning Test) improved (Bryan et al., 2002). Controversially, in another small study including 7 subjects with dementia reported no statistically significant differences between the supplemented group and the control group, and noted a negative trend in specific test scores of the supplemented group (Sommer et al., 2003). Because of the small number of subjects, study results need to be interpreted cautiously. Finally, the 3-year randomised controlled FACIT trial included 818 older subjects (older than 60 years) with augmented plasma total Hcy and normal serum vitamin B12 levels. The effect of folic acid supplementation on cognition was the secondary end point. The 3-year change in memory, information processing speed and sensorimotor speed were significantly improved in the folic acid group in comparison to the placebo group (Durga et al., 2007). Folic acid potentiated the effect of memantine on spatial learning and neuronal protection in an AD transgenic model (Chen et al., 2010).

Some other randomised controlled studies assessed the effect of vitamin B12 intervention on cognitive functions in humans. There is a large heterogeneity among trials regarding the cognitive status of participants, the doses and administration routes of vitamin B12, the duration of supplementation and the applied cognitive function assessment instruments. Sample sizes ranged from 18 to 78 subjects receiving vitamin B12, and the duration of supplementation ranged from 4 weeks to 6 months. For most cognitive tests, there was no significant improvement in vitamin B12 supplemented patients as compared with the placebo group (Eussen et al., 2006; Hvas et al., 2004; Stoot et al., 2008). However, Bryan J et al found that healthy younger, middle-aged and older women (n=211) who took vitamin B12 (or either of folate and vitamin B6) for 35 days showed better performance on some measures of memory performance compared to placebo (Bryan et al., 2002). Interestingly, a statistically significant worsening of cognitive tests was reported in two studies. In 195 vitamin B12 deficient subjects of normal and impaired cognition, Eussen et al (Eussen et al., 2006) observed that improvement of the cognitive test score in the placebo group was significantly more marked than that of the vitamin B12 group. Similarly, another study reported a significant worsening of the '12 words learning test' score in a vitamin B12 treated population of 140 old patients with cognitive impairment and methylmalonic acidemia, in comparison to the placebo group (Hvas et al., 2004). For reasons of heterogeneity of these controlled trials, no reasonable conclusion can be drawn regarding the effects of vitamin B12 on cognition. In addition, several uncontrolled cohort studies assessed the effects of vitamin B12 intervention on cognitive function in humans with conflicting results.

A few studies (Lewerin et al., 2005; McMahon et al., 2006; Stott et al., 2005; van Uffelen et al., 2007) reported data of combined B vitamin intervention on cognition, in subjects with normal cognition, dementia or vascular disease (17-409 participants). Trial durations ranged from 12 weeks to 2 years. One study found a significant improvement in one of eight cognitive tests (Reitan trail-making test, part B) (McMahon et al., 2006). In a recent randomized, double-blind controlled study in 271 individuals over 70 years old with mild cognitive deficit, high dose B vitamins lowering Hcy level slowed the rate of accelerated brain atrophy, which was found to be major determinant of cognitive decline in this population (Smith et al., 2010). It was reported that trials were needed to see if the same treatment will delay the development of AD (Smith et al., 2010).

3.3 Comments

Most studies reporting associations between cognitive function and Hcy or B vitamins have used a cross-sectional or case-control design and have been unable to exclude the possibility that such associations are a result of the disease rather than being causal. The prospective study indicating that persons with high Hcy have more than twice as high as developing AD than persons with low Hcy, even after adjusting for confounding or mediating factors, is an important one. The Hcy hypothesis of dementia has attracted considerable interest, as Hcy can be easily lowered by folic acid and vitamin B12, raising the prospect that B-vitamin supplementation could lower the risk of dementia (Clarke et al., 2008). While some trials assessing effects on cognitive function have used folic acid alone, vitamin B12 alone or a combination, few trials have included a sufficient number of participants to provide reliable evidence. Among these studies, FACIT Trial (Durga et al., 2007) is an outstanding one. This large, randomised and controlled trial on elderly participants with high plasma Hcy and normal vitamin B12 serum level have showed that folic acid supplementation improved several cognitive domains that tend to decline with advancing age. Therefore, folate supplementation may be an interesting approach to prevent cognitive decline in elderly people. New trials with larger number of participants are needed to test the importance of vitamin B intake through diet or supplementation forms in the prevention and treatment of AD.

4. Vitamin D

Vitamin D exhibits functional attributes that may prove neuroprotective through antioxidative mechanisms, neuronal calcium regulation, immunomodulation, enhanced nerve conduction and detoxification mechanisms. Compelling evidence supports a beneficial role for the active form of vitamin D in developing brain as well as in adult brain function. The vitamin D receptor and, biosynthetic and degredative pathways for the hydroxylation of vitamin D have been found in the rodent brain; more recently these findings have been confirmed in humans. The vitamin D receptor and catalytic enzymes are colocalized in the areas of the brain involved in complex planning, processing, and the formation of new memories. These findings potentially implicate vitamin D in neurocognitive function (Buell & Dawson-Hughes, 2008).

Treatment with 1,25 $(OH)_2D_3$ attenuated hippocampal atrophy and protected neuron density (a marker for neuronal death) in aging rats (Landfield & Cadwalleder-Neal, 1998). Data in human subjects with AD revealed a reduction in VDR mRNA in specific regions of the hippocampus (CA1 and CA2) compared to controls (Sutherland et al., 1992) and a higher frequency of VDR polymorphisms were found in Alzheimer's brains than age-matched controls (Gezen-Ak et al., 2007).

Low serum levels of 25(OH)D have been associated with increased risk for cardiovascular diseases, diabetes mellitus, depression, dental caries, osteoporosis, and periodontal disease, all of which are either considered risk factors for dementia or have preceded incidence of dementia. There is a higher prevalence of falls and fractures in patients with AD (Buchner & Larson, 1987) and community studies have shown that residents with AD and dementia had lower serum concentrations of 25(OH)D (Kipen et al., 1995). While the temporal associations of these findings remains unclear, in a study in patients with AD, 25(OH)D concentrations were significantly elevated after year-round sun exposure. Additionally, the sun- exposed cohort had a reduced risk of falls and fractures compared to the unexposed (Sato et al., 2005).

Data from the Nutrition and Memory in Elderly study (NAME) (Scott et al., 2004) supported these findings. In subjects (n=318) who completed a full neurological and psychiatric examination, in addition to magnetic resonance imaging, it was observed that vitamin D concentrations were lower in patients with dementia than those without. Additionally, vitamin D concentrations lesser than 50 nmol/L were associated with a higher prevalence of a diagnosis of possible or probable AD. In a recent cross-sectional investigation of vitamin D, dementia and MRI measures of cerebrovascular disease among 318 participants, mean vitamin D concentrations were lower in subjects with dementia. There was a higher prevalence of dementia, large vessel infarcts and increased white matter hyperintensity volume among participants with vitamin D insufficiency. After adjustment for age, race, sex, bodymass index, and education, vitamin D insufficiency was associated with more than twice the odds of all cause dementia, AD and stroke (Buell et al., 2010). Based on increasing number of studies linking the risk factors of AD with vitamin D deficiency, Grant WB (Grant, 2009) states that there are established criteria for causality in a biological system. The important criteria include strength of association, consistency of findings, determination of the dose-response relation, an understanding of the mechanisms, and experimental verification. Grant WB (Grant, 2009) suggests that further investigation of possible direct or indirect linkages between vitamin D and dementia is needed. Studies of incidence of dementia with respect to prediagnostic serum 25(OH)D or of vitamin D supplementation are warranted. In addition, since the elderly are generally vitamin D deficient and since vitamin D has so many health benefits, those over the age of 60 years should consider having their serum 25(OH)D tested, looking for a level of at least 30 ng/ml but preferably over 40 ng/ml, and supplementing with 1000-2000 IU/day of vitamin D3 or increased time in the sun spring, summer, and fall if below those values (Grant, 2009).

5. Vitamin K

Vitamin K is necessary for the liver functioning. Vitamin K dependent γ-carboxylation of glutamate takes part in formation of the coagulation factors 2, 7, 9 and 10. More recently, it has been established that vitamin K dependent γ-carboxylation of glutamate occurs also in extrahepatic sites and modifies proteins with other functions. One of these sites is brain. Allison AC (Allison, 2001) proposed a possible role of vitamin K deficiency in the pathogenesis of AD and in augmenting brain damage associated with cerebrovascular disease, based on the potential actions of vitamin K in the brain and through a link to the apolipoprotein E genotype. The apolipoprotein E4 allele, an established risk factor for AD (Mattson, 2004), strongly influences plasma vitamin K levels (Kohlmeier M, 1996; Saupe J, 1993). Thus, carriers of apolipoprotein E4 allele could also those with the lowest vitamin K concentrations, an association that has not yet been investigated. Vitamin K is required for normal brain development and function. The maternal exposure to coumarin derivatives is associated with abnormalities of the central nervous system (Pauli & Haun, 1979). Vitamin K deficiency is associated with decrased sulfation in the brain. Keratan sulfate is dramatically decreased in cerebral cortex of AD patients (Lindahl, 1996). Considering keratan sulfate proteoglycan being the major protein of synaptic vesicles (Scranton et al., 1993), one manifestation of decreased sulfation can be abnormal structure and function of the major protein of synaptic vesicles (Allison, 2001). Likewise, addition of vitamin K to the chick embriyo increases tyrosine phosphorylation in the brain adhesion and cytoskletal proteins (Saxena et al., 1997), suggesting that vitamin K plays an role in the development of the central nervous system. Another vitamin K dependent protein in the brain is Gas 6, a product of growth arrest specific gene 6. Both Gas 6 and its tyrosine kinase receptor are widely distributed throughout the central nervous system (Prieto et al., 1999). Interaction of these plays an important role in preventing neurons from apoptosis (Allen et al., 1999). Cell culture studies have shown that Gas 6 can rescue cortical neurons from Aβ induced apoptosis (Yagami et al., 2002) and provided evidence that vitamin K can have a protective role against oxidative injury in developing oligodendrocytes and neurons (Denisova & Booth, 2005).

Considering that a relative deficiency of vitamin K, affecting the extrahepatic functions of the vitamin, is common in aging men and women; Allison AC (Allison, 2001) suggests that it is obviously useful to do experimental animal and case controlled human studies in the first step to clarify the role of vitamin K in the pathogenesis of dementia. In a likely study, low vitamin K intakes in 31 community-dwelling elders at an early stage of AD was detected in comparison to 31 age and sex matched cognitively intact control subjects (Presse et al., 2008).

6. Multi-intervention

Due to the fact that the interventional trials with antioxidants and B-vitamins did not hold the expectations, studies combining micronutriens are of particular interest. To date, a few prospective studies estimating the effect of nutrition and vitamin supplementation exist. One of these studies (Wolters et al., 2005) was performed on 220 healthy, free living women older than 60 years of age. After taking multivitamins (containing 8 vitamins and 4 minerals) for 6 months daily, no change on cognitive performance was observed as compared to placebo. The intervention period of only 6 months may be too short for improving cognitive performance in well-educated elderly women without dementia. Another study (McNeill et al., 2007) was performed on 910 healthy men and women aged 65 years and over. Four hundred and fifty six of them were on active daily treatment with 11 vitamins and 5 minerals for 12 months, while the remaining ones took placebo. Benefit was detected only on verbal fluency tests in the subgroups of participants aged over 74 years or those with increased risk of micronutrient deficiency. In a 12 month, open label trial with 14 mild AD patients, the efficacy of a multi-component formulation showed promising results regarding neuropsychiatric inventory and activities of daily living (Chan et al., 2008). This was confirmed by placebo-controlled data from 12 institutionalized patients with moderate to severe AD showing improvement in cognition, mood, and daily function (Remington et al., 2009). As a result, to draw any conclusion, larger randomized controlled studies with combined supplements are needed, especially in the context that multi-component dietary approaches such as Mediterranean diet or fruit and vegetable (or juice) consumption have been shown to be successful (Barberger-Gateau et al, 2007; Dai et al., 2006; MC Morris et al., 2006b; Scarmeas et al., 2006, 2009).

7. Conclusion

There is a relationship of levels of antioxidant vitamins and B vitamins to vascular dementia. Nevertheless, if this relationship is based on causality, it is not so clear after performed longitudinal and interventional studies. New trials with larger number of participants will be more clarifying. Recently, vitamin D deficiency has been found to be related with AD. Longitudinal and interventional studies, especially with long follow up

period, will be informative about its role. Additionally, vitamin K is thought to have a possible role in the pathogenesis of dementia.
The subject has multiple aspects. As vitamin deficiencies can cause cognitive impairment, cognitive impairment can also determine changes in dietary habits and consequently cause vitamin deficiencies. Vitamin intake through diet or supplementation forms can have different effects. There is also a possibility that vitamins have useful effects in different subgroups of people, based on age, nutritional status or vitamin level. Multivitamin supplementation may be more useful. The roles of vitamins in dementia are not clear yet as those of macronutrients in spite of the reports expressing the benefits of caloric restriction and intake of higher unsaturated fatty acids on cognitive functions. Presence of relationships between macronutrients and vitamins is also possible. Detailed investigations about these aspects will be informative.

8. References

Allen MP, Zeng C, Schneider K, Xiong X, Meintzer MK, Bellosta P, Basilico C, Varnum B, Heidenreich KA & Wierman ME. (1999). Growth arrest-specific gene 6 (gas6)/adhesion related kinase (Ark) signaling promotes gonadotropin-releasing hormone neuronal survival via extracellular signal related kinase (ERK) and Akt. *Mol Endocrinol,* Vol.13, No.2, (February 1999), pp. 191-201, ISSN 0888-8809.

Allison AC. (2001). The possible role of vitamin K deficiency in the pathogenesis of Alzheimer's disease and in augmenting brain damage associated with cardiovascular disease. *Medical Hypothesis,* Vol.57, No.2, (August 2001), pp. 151-5, ISSN 0306-9877.

Andres E, Loukili NH, Noel E, Kaltenbach G, Abdelgheni MB, Perrin AE, Noblet-Dick M, Maloisel F, Schlienger JL & Blickle JF. (2004). Vitamin B12 (cobalamin) deficiency in elderly patients. *CMAJ,* Vol.171, No.3, (August 2004), pp. 251-9, ISSN 0820-3946.

Azzi A, Boscoboinik D & Hensey C. (1992). The protein kinase C family. *Eur J Biochem,* Vol.208, No.3, (September 1992), pp. 547-57, ISSN 0014-2956.

Barberger-Gateau P, Raffaitin C, Letenneur L, Berr C, Tzourio C, Dartigues JF & Alperovitch A. (2007). Dietary patterns and risk of dementia: the three-city cohort study. *Neurology,* Vol.69, No.20, (November 2007), pp. 1921-30, ISSN 0028-3878.

Behl C. (1997). Amyloid beta-protein toxicity and oxidative stres in Alzheimer's disease. *Cell Tissue Res,* Vol.290, No.3, (December 1997), pp. 471-80, ISSN 0302-766X.

Bell IR, Edman JS, Selhub J, Morrow FD, Marby DW, Kayne HL & Cole JO. (1992). Plasma homocysteine in vascular disease and in non-vascular dementia of depressed elderly people. *Acta Psychiatr Scand,* Vol.86, No.5, (November 1992), pp. 386-90, ISSN 0001-690X.

Birch CS, Brach NE, McCaddon A & Williams JH. (2009). A novel role for vitamin B(12): Cobalamins are intracellular antioxidants in vitro. *Free Radic Biol Med,* Vol.47, No.2, (July 2009), pp.184-8, ISSN 0891-5849.

Bjelakovic G, Nikolova D, Gluud LL, Simonetti RG & Gluud C. (2007). Mortality in randomized trials of antioxidant supplements for primary and secondary prevention: systematic review and meta-analysis. *JAMA,* Vol.297, No.8, (February 2007), pp. 842-57, ISSN 0098-7484.

Bottiglieri T. (1996). Folate, vitamin B12, and neuropsychiatric disorders. *Nutr Rev,* Vol.54, No.12, (December 1996), pp. 382-90, ISSN 0029-6643.

Bryan J, Calvaresi E & Hughes D. (2002). Short-term folate, vitamin B-12 or vitamin B-6 supplementation slightly affects memory performance but not mood in women of various ages. *J Nutr*, Vol.132, No.6, (June 2002), pp. 1345-56, ISSN 0022-3166.

Buchner DM & Larson EB. (1987). Falls and fractures in patients with Alzheimer-type dementia. *JAMA*, Vol.257, No.11, (March 1987), pp. 1492-5, ISSN 0098-7484.

Buell JS & Dawson-Hughes B. (2008). Vitamin D and neurocognitive dysfunction: Preventing Decline? *Molecular Aspects of Medicine*, Vol.29, No.6, (December 2008), pp. 415-22, ISSN 0098-2997.

Buell JS, Dawson-Hughes B, ScottTM, Weiner DE, Dallal GE, Qui WQ, Bergethon P, Rosenberg IH, Folstein MF, Patz S, Bhadelia RA & Tucker KL. (2010). 25-Hydroxyvitamin D, dementia, and cerebrovascular pathology in elders receiving home services. *Neurology*, Vol.74, No.1, (January 2010), pp. 18-26, ISSN 0028-3878.

Chen TF, Huang RF, Lin SE, Lu JF, Tang MC & Chiu MJ. (2010). Folic acid potentiates the effect of memantine on spatial learning and neuronal protection in an Alzheimer's disease transgenic model. *J Alzheimers Dis*, Vol.20, No.2, pp.607-15, ISSN 1387-2877.

Christen Y. (2000). Oxidative stress and Alzheimer disease. *Am J Clin Nutr*, Vol.71, No.2, (February 2000), pp.S621-9, ISSN 0002-9165.

Clarke R, Birks J, Nexo E, Ueland PM, Schneede J, Scott J, Molloy A & Evans JG. (2007). Low vitamin B-12 status and risk of cognitive decline in older adults. *Am J Clin Nutr*, Vol.86, No.5, (November 2007),pp. 1384-91, ISSN 0002-9165.

Cutler RG, Kelly J, Storie K, Pedersen WA, Tammara A, Hatanpaa K, Troncoso JC, Mattson MP. (2004). Involvement of oxidative stres-induced abnormalities in ceramide and cholesterol metabolism in brain aging and Alzheimer's disease. *Proc Natl Acad Sci USA*, Vol.101, No.9, (February 2009), pp. 2070-5, ISSN 0027-8424.

Dai Q, Borenstein AR, Wu Y, Jackson JC & Larson EB. (2006). Fruit and vegetable juices and Alzheimer's disease: the Kame Project. *Am J Med*, Vol.119, No.9, (September 2006), pp. 751-9, ISSN 0002-9343.

Das UN. (2008). Folic acid and polyunsaturated fatty acids improve cognitive function and prevent depression, dementia, and Alzheimer's disease-but how and why? *Prostaglandins Leukot Essent Fatty Acids*, Vol.78, No.1, (January 2008), pp. 11-9, ISSN 0952-3278.

de Lau LM, Refsum H, Smith AD, Johnston C & Breteler MM. (2007). Plasma folate concentration and cognitive performance: Rotterdam Scan Study. *Am J Clin Nutr*, Vol.86, No.3, (September 2007), pp. 728-34, ISSN 0002-9165.

Denisova NA, Booth SL. (2005). Vitamin K and sphingolipid metabolism: Evidence to date. *Nutr Rev*, Vol.63, No.4, (July 2010), pp. 111-21, ISSN 0029-6643.

Devore EE, Grodstein F, van Rooij FJA & Hofman A. (2010). Dietary antioxidants and long term risk of dementia. *Arch Neurol*, Vol.67, No.7, (July 2010), pp. 819-25, ISSN 0002-9262.

Dufouil C, Alperovitch A, Ducros V & Tzourio C. (2003). Homocysteine, white matter hyperintensities, and cognition in healthy elderly people. *Ann Neurol*, Vol.53, No.2, (February 2003), pp. 214-21, ISSN 0364-5134.

Durga J, van Boxtel MP, Schouten EG, Kok FJ, Jolles J, Katan MB & Verhoef P. (2007). Effect of 3-year folic acid supplementation on cognitive function in older adults in the FACIT trial: a randomised, double blind, controlled trial. *Lancet*, Vol.369, No.9557, (January 2007), pp. 208-16, ISSN 0140-6736.

Engelhart MJ, Geerlings MI, Ruitenberg A, van Switen JC, Hofman A, Witteman JC & Breteler MM. (2002). Dietary intake of antioxidants and risk of Alzheimer disease. *JAMA*, Vol.287, No.24, (June 2002), pp. 3223-9, ISSN 0098-7484.

Eussen SJ, de Groot LC, Joosted LW, Bloo RJ, Clarke R, Ueland PM, Schneede J, Blom HJ, Hoefnagels WH & van Staveren WA. (2006). Effect of oral vitamin B-12 with or without folic acid on cognitive function in older people with mild vitamin B-12 deficiency: a randomised, placebo controlled trial. *Am J Clin Nutr*, Vol.84, No.2, (August 2006), pp. 361-70, ISSN 0002-9165.

Fekkes D, van der Cammen TJ, Van Loon CP, Verschoor C, van Harskamp F, de KI, Schudel WJ & Pepplinkhuizen L. (1998). Abnormal amino acid metabolism in patients with early stage Alzheimer dementia. *J Neural Transm*, Vol.105, No.2-3, pp. 287-94, ISSN 0300-9564.

Fioravanti M, Ferrario E, Massaia M, Cappa G, Rivolta G, Grossi E & Buckley AE. (1998). Low folate levels in the cognitive decline of elderly patients and the efficacy of folate as a treatment for imprpving memory deficits. *Arch Gerontol Geriatr*, Vol.26, No.1, (January-February 1998), pp. 1-13, ISSN 0167-4943.

Foy CJ, Passmore AP, Vahidassr MD, Young IS & Lawson JT. (1999). Plasma chain-breaking antioxidants in Alzheimer's disease, vascular dementia and Parkinson's disease. *Q J Med*, Vol.92, No.1, (January 1999), pp. 39-45, ISSN 0033-5622.

Gezen-Ak D, Dursun E, Ertan T, Hanagasi H, Gürvit H, Emre M, Eker E, Ozturk M, Engin F & Yilmazer S. (2007). Association between vitamin D receptor gene polymorphism and Alzheimer's disease. *Tohoku J Exp Med*, Vol.212, No.3, (July 2007), pp. 275-82, ISSN 0040-8727.

Goodman AB. (2006). Retinoid receptors, transporters, and metabolizers as therapeutic targets in late onset Alzheimer disease. *J Cell Physiol*, Vol.209, No.3, (December 2006), pp. 598-603, ISSN 0021-9541.

Grant WB. (2009). Does vitamin D reduce the risk of dementia? *J Alzheimers Dis*, Vol.17, No.1, pp. 151-9, ISSN 1387-2877.

Gray SL, Anderson ML, Crane PK, Breitner JC, McCormick W, Bowen JD, Teri L & Larson E. (2008). Antioxidant vitamin supplement use and risk of dementia or Alzheimer's disease in older adults. *J Am Geriatr Soc*, Vol.56, No.2, (February 2008), pp. 291-5, ISSN 0002-8614.

Haan MN, Miller JW, Aiello AE, Whitmer RA, Jagust WJ, Mungas DM, Allen LH & Green R. (2007). Homocysteine, B vitamins, and the incidence of dementia and cognitive impairment: results from the Sacramento Area Latino Study on Aging. *Am J Clin Nutr*, Vol.85, No.2, (February 2007), pp. 511-7, ISSN 0002-9165.

Haller J, Weggemans RM, Lammi-Keefe CJ & Ferry M. (1996). Changes in the vitamin status of elderly Europeans: plasma vitamins A, E, B-6, B-12, folic acid and carotenoids. *Eur J Clin Nutr*, Vol.50, No. Suppl 2, (July 1996), pp. S32-36, ISSN 0954-3007.

Hassan A, Hunt BJ, O'Sullivan M, Bell R, D'Souza R, Jeffery S, Bamford JM, Markus HS. (2004). Homocysteine is a risk factor for cerebral small vessel disease acting via endothelial function. *Brain*, Vol.127, No.1, (January 2004), pp. 212-9, ISSN 0006-8950.

Head E, Nukala VN, Fenoglio KA, Muggenburg BA, Cotman CW & Sullivan PG. (2009). Effects of age, dietary, and behavioral enrichment on brain mitochondria in a canine model of human aging. *Exp Neurol,* Vol.220, No.1, (November 2009), pp. 171-6, ISSN 0014-4886.

Herrmann W, Obeid R. (2007). Biomarkers of folate and vitamin B(12) status in cerebrospinal fluid. *Clin Chem Lab Med,* Vol.45, No.12, pp. 1614-20, ISSN 1434-6621.

Hu P, Bretsky P, Crimmins EM, Guralnik JM, Reuben DM & Seeman TE. (2006). Association between serum beta-carotene levels and decline of cognitive function in high-functioning older persons with or without apolipoprotein E4 alleles: MacArthur studies of successful aging. *J Gerontol A Biol Sci Med Sci,* Vol.61, No.6, (June 2006), pp. 616-20, ISSN 1079-5006.

Hvas AM, Juul S, Lauritzen L, Nexo E & Ellegaard J. (2004). No effect of vitamin B-12 treatment on cognitive function and depression: a randomized placebo controlled study. *J Affect Disord,* Vol.81, No.3, (September 2004), pp. 269-73, ISSN 0165-0327.

Hyun DH, Mughal MR, Yang H, Lee JH, Ko EJ, Hunt ND, de Cabo R, Mattson MP. (2010). The plasma membrane redox system is impaired by amyloid β-peptide in the hippocampus and cerebral cortex of 3xTgAD mice. *Exp Neurol,* Vol.225, No.2, (October 2010), pp. 423-9, ISSN 0014-4886.

Jacques PF, Selhub J, Bostom AG, Wilson PW & Rosenberg IH. (1999). The effect of folic acid fortification on plasma folate and total homocysteine concentrations. *N Eng J Med,* Vol.340, No.19, (May 1999), pp. 1449-54, ISSN 0028-4793.

Joosten E, van den BA, Riezler R, Naurath HJ, Lindenbaum J, Stabler SP & Allen RH. (1993). Metabolic evidence that deficiencies of vitamin B-12 (cobalamin), folate, and vitamin B-& occur commonly in elderly people. *Am J Clin Nutr,* Vol.58, No.4, (October 1993), pp. 468-76, ISSN 0002-9165.

Joseph JA, Shukitt-Hale B, Denisova NA, Prior RL, Cao G, Martin A, Taglialatela G & Bickford PC. (1998). Long- term dietary strawberry, spinach, or vitamin E supplementation retards the onset of age- related neuronal signal transduction and cognitive behavioral deficits. *J Neurosci,* Vol.18, No.19, (October 1998), pp. 8047-55, ISSN 0270-6474.

Joseph JA, Shukitt-Hale B, Denisova NA, Bielinski D, Martin A, McEwen JJ & Bickford PC. (1999). Reversals of age-related declines in neuronal signal transduction, cognitive, and motor behavioral deficits with blueberry, spinach, or strawberry dietary supplementation. *J Neurosci,* Vol.19, No.18, (September 1999), pp. 8114-21, ISSN 0270-6474.

Kalmijn S, Launer LJ, Lindemans J, Bots ML, Hofman A & Breteler MM. (1999). Total homocysteine and cognitive decline in a community-based sample of elderly subjects: the Rotterdam study. *Am J Epidemiol,* Vol.150, No.3, (August 1999), pp. 283-9, ISSN 0002-9262.

Kang JH, Cook N, Manson J, Buring JE & Grodstein F. (2006). A randomized trial of vitamin E supplementation and cognitive function in women. *Arch Intern Med,* Vol.166, No.22, (December 2006), pp. 2462-8, ISSN 0003-9926.

Kipen E, Helme RD, Wark JD & Flicker L. (1995). Bone density, vitamin D nutrition, and parathyroid hormone levels in women with dementia. *J Am Geriatr Soc,* Vol.43, No.10, (October 1995), pp. 1088-91, ISSN 0002-8614.

Kivipelto M, Annerbo S, Hultdin J, Backman L, Viitanen M, Fratiglioni L & Lokk J. (2009). Homocysteine and holo-transcobalamin and the risk of dementia and Alzheimers disease: a prospective study. *Eur J Neurol,* Vol.16, No.7, (July 2009), pp. 808-13, ISSN 1351-5101.

Knopman DS. (1998). Current pharmacotherapies for Alzheimer's disease. *Geriatrics,* Vol.53, No. Suppl.1, (September 1998), pp. S31-4, ISSN 0016-867X.

Kohlmeier M, Solomon A, Saupe J & Shearer MJ. (1996). Transport of vitamin K to bones in humans. *J Nutr,*Vol. 126, No.4 Suppl1, (April 1996), pp. S1192-6, ISSN 0022-3166.

Kronenberg G, Colla M & Endres M. (2009). Folic acid, neurodegenerative and neuropsychiatric disease. *Curr Mol Med,* Vol.9, No.3, (April 2009), pp. 315-23, ISSN 1566-5240.

Kruman II, Culmsee C, Chan SL, Kruman Y, Guo Z, Penix L & Mattson MP. (2000). Homocysteine elicits a DNA damage response in neurons that promotes apoptosis and hypersensitivity to excitotoxicity. *J Neurosci,* Vol.20, No.18, (September 2000), pp. 6920-6, ISSN 0270-6474.

Kuipers EJ, Uyterlinde AM, Pena AS, Hazenberg HJ, Bloemena E, Lindeman J, Klinkenberg-Knol EC & Meuwissen SG. (1995). Increase of Helicobacter pylori-associated corpus gastritis during acid suppressive therapy: implications for long term safety. *Am J Gastroenterol,* Vol.90, No.9, (September 1995), pp. 1401-6, ISSN 0002-9270.

Kuipers EJ, Lundell L, Klinkenberg-Knol EC, Havu N, Festen HP, Liedman B, Lamers CB, Jansen JB, Dalenback J, Snel P, Nelis GF &Meuwissen SG. (1996). Atrophic gastritis and Helicobacter pylori infection in patients with reflux esophagitis treated with omeprazol or fundoplication. *N Engl J Med,* Vol.334, No.16, (April 1996), pp. 1018-22, ISSN 0028-4793.

Landfield PW & Cadwallader-Neal L. (1998). Long term treatment with calcitriol (1,25 (OH)2 vit D3) retardsa biomarker of hippocampal aging in rats. *Neurobiol Aging,* Vol.19, No.5, (September-October 1998), pp. 469-77, ISSN 0197-4580.

Lewerin C, Matousek M, Steen G, Johansson B, Steen B & Nilsson-Ehle H. (2005). Significant correlations of plasma homocysteine and serum methylmalonic acid with movement and cognitive performance in elderly subjects but no improvement from short-term vitamin therapy: a placebo-controlled randomized study. *Am J Clin Nutr,* Vol.81, No.5, (May 2005), pp. 1155-62, ISSN 0002-9165.

Lindahl B, Eriksson L, Spillmann D, Caterson B & Lindahl U. (1996). Selective loss of cerebral keratan sulfate in Azheimer's disease. *J Biol Chem,* Vol.271, No.29, (July 1996), pp. 16991-4, ISSN 0021-9258.

Lokk J. (2003). News and views on folate and elderly persons. *J Gerontol A Biol Sci Med Sci,* Vol.58, No.4, (April 2003), pp. 354-61, ISSN 1079-5006.

Luchsinger JA, Tang MX, Shea S, Miller J, Green R & Mayeux R. (2004). Plasma homocysteine levels and risk of Alzheimer disease. *Neurology,* Vol.62, No.11, (June 2004), pp. 1972-6, ISSN 0028-3878.

Lundell L, Havu N, Miettinen P, Myrvold HE, Wallin L, Julkunen R, Levander K, Hatlebakk JG,

Liedmann B, Lamm M, Malm A & Walan A: Nordic Gerd Study Group. (2006). Changes of gastric mucosal architecture during long-term omeprazole therapy: results of a randomized clinical trial. *Aliment Pharmacol Ther,* Vol.23, No.5, (March 2006), pp. 639-47, ISSN 0269-2813.

Martin A, Foxall T, Blumberg JB & Meydani M. (1997). Vitamin E inhibits low-density lipoprotein-induced adhesion of monocytes to human aortic endothelial cells in vitro. *Arterioscler Thromb Vasc Biol,* Vol.17, No.3, (March 1997), pp. 429-36, ISSN 1079-5642.

Mattson MP. (2004). Pathways towards and away from Alzheimer's disease. *Nature,* Vol.430, No.7000, (August 2004), pp. 631-9, ISSN 0028-0836.

Maxwell CJ, Hicks MS, Hogan DB, Basran J & Ebly EM. (2005). Supplemental use of antioxidant vitamins and subsequent risk of cognitive decline and dementia. *Dement Geriatr Cogn Disord,* Vol.20, No.1, pp. 45-51, ISSN 1420-8008.

McCaddon A, Davies G, Hudson P, Tandy S & Cattell H. (1998). Total serum homocysteine in senile dementia of Alzheimer type. *Int J Geriatr Psychiatry,* Vol.13, No.4, (April 1998), pp. 235-9, ISSN : 0885-6230.

McCaddon A, Hudson P, Davies G, Hughes A, Williams JH & Wilkinson C. (2001). Homocysteine and cognitive decline in healthy elderly. *Dement Geriatr Cogn Disord,* Vol.12, No.5, (September-October 2001), pp. 309-13, ISSN 1420-8008.

McCaddon A, Regland B, Hudson P & Davies G. (2002). Functional vitamin B (12) deficiency and Alzheimer disease. *Neurology,* Vol.58, No.9, (May 2002), pp. 1395-9, ISSN 0028-3878

McMahon JA, Green TJ, Skeaff CM, Knight RG, Mann JI & Williams SM. (2006). A controlled trial of homocysteine lowering and cognitive performance. *N Eng J Med,* Vol.354, No.26, (June 2006), pp. 2764-72, ISSN 0028-4793.

McNeill G, Avenell A, Campbell MK, Cook JA, Hannaford PC, Kilonzo MM, Mile AC, Ramsay CR, Seymour DG, Stephen AI & Vale LD. (2007). Effect of multivitamin and multimineral supplementation on cognitive function in men and women aged 65 years and over: a randomised controlled trial. *Nutr J,* Vol.2, No.1, (May 2007), pp. 6-10, ISSN 1475-2891.

Meydani SN, Meydani M, Blumberg JB, Leka LS, Siber G, Loszewski R, Thompson C, Pedrosa MC, Diamond RD & Stollar BD. (1997). Vitamin E supplementation and in vivo immune response in healthy elderly subjects. A randomised controlled trial. *J Am Med Assoc,* Vol.277, No.17, (May 1997), pp. 1380-6, ISSN 0002-9955.

Micheau J, Durkin TP, Destrade C, Rolland Y & Jaffard R. (1985). Chronic administration of sulbutiamine improves long term memory formation in mice: possible cholinergic mediation. *Pharmacol Biochem Behav,* Vol.23, No.2, (August 1985), pp. 195-8, ISSN 0091-3057.

Miller ER 3rd, Pastor-Barriuso R, Dala D, Riemersma RA, Appel LJ & Guallar E. (2005). Meta-analysis: high- dosage vitamin E supplementation may increase all-cause mortality. *Ann Intern Med,* Vol.142, No.1, (January 2005), pp. 37-46, ISSN 0003-4819.

Miller LJ & Chacko R. (2004). The role of cholesterol and statins in Alzheimer's disease. *Ann Pharmacother,* Vol.38, No.1, (January 2004), pp. 91-8, ISSN 1060-0280.

Mooijaart SP, Gussekloo J, Frölich M, Jolles J, Stott DJ, Westendorp RG & de Craen AJ. (2005). Homocysteine, vitamin B-12, and folic acid and the risk of cognitive decline in old age: the Leiden 85-Plus study. *Am J Clin Nutr,* Vol.82, No.4, (October 2005), pp. 627-35, ISSN 0002-9165.

Morris MS, Jacques PF, Rosenberg IH & Selhub J. (2001). Hyperhomocysteinemia associated with poor recall in the third National Health and Nutrition Examination Survey. *Am J Clin Nutr,* Vol.73, No.5, (May 2001), pp. 927-33, ISSN 0002-9165.

Morris MC, Evans DA, Bienias JL, Tangney CC & Wilson RS. (2002). Vitamin E and cognitive decline in older persons. *Arch Neurol,* Vol.59, No.7, (July 2007), pp. 1125-32, ISSN 0003-9942.

Morris MC, Evans DA, Tangney CC, Bienias JL, Wilson RS, Aggarwal NT & Scherr PA. (2005a). Relation of tocopherol forms to incident Alzheimer disease and to cognitive change. *Am J Clin Nutr,* Vol.81, No.2, (February 2005), pp. 508-14, ISSN 0002-9165.

Morris MC, Evans DA, Bienias JL, Tangney CC, Hebert LE, Scherr PA & Schneider JA. (2005b). Dietary folate and vitamin B12 intake and cognitive decline among community-dwelling older persons. *Arch Neurol,* Vol.62, No.4, (April 2005), pp. 641-5, ISSN 0003-9942.

Morris MC, Evans DA, Schneider JA, Tangney CC, Bienias JL & Aggarwal NT. (2006a). Dietary folate and vitamins B-12 and B-6 not associated with incident Alzheimer's disease. *J Alzheimers Dis,* Vol.9, No.4, (August 2006), pp. 435-43, ISSN 1387-2877.

Morris MC, Evans DA, Tangney CC, Bienias JL & Wilson RS. (2006b). Associations of vegetable and fruit consumption with age-related cognitive change. *Neurology,* Vol.67, No.8, (October 2006), pp. 1370-6, ISSN 0028-3878.

Nilsson K, Gustafson L, Faldt R, Andersson A, Brattstrom L, Lindgren A, Israelson B & Hultberg B. (1996). Hyperhomocysteinaemia- a common finding in psychogeriatric population. *Eur J Clin Invest,* Vol.26, No.10, (October 1996), pp. 8534-9, ISSN 0014-2972.

Nilsson K, Gustafson L & Hultberg B. (1999). Plasma homocysteine is a sensitive marker for tissue deficiency of both cobalamines and folates in a psychogeriatric population. *Dement Geriatr Cogn Disord,* Vol.10, No.6, (November-December 1999), pp. 476-82, ISSN 1420-8008.

Obeid R, McCaddon A & Herrman W. (2007). The role of hyperhomocysteinemia and B-vitamin deficieny in neurological and psychiatric diseases. *Clin Chem Lab Med,* Vol.45, No.12, pp. 1590-606, ISSN 1434-6621.

Ortega RM, Requejo AM, Lopez-Sobaler AM, Andres P, Navia B, Perea JM & Robles F. (2002). Cognitive function in elderly people is influenced by Vitamin E status. *J Nutr,* Vol.132, No.7, (July 2002), pp. 2065-8, ISSN 0022-3166.

Paleologos M, Cumming RG & Lazarus R. (1998). Cohort study of Vitamin C intake and cognitive impairment. *Am J Epidemiol,* Vol.148, No.1, (July 1998), pp. 45-50, ISSN 0002-9262.

Parnetti L, Bottiglieri T & Lowenthal D. (1997). Role of homocysteine in age related vascular and non-vascular disease. *Aging (Milano),* Vol.9, No.4, (August 1997), pp. 241-57, ISSN 0011-3662.

Pauli RM & Haun JM. (1979). Warfarin embryopathy. *Lancet,* Vol.2, No.8134, (July 1999), pp. 144, ISSN 0140-6736.

Perkins AJ, Hendrie HC, Callahan CM, Gao S, Unverzagt FW, Xu Y, Hall KS & Hui SL. (1999). Association of antioxidants with memory in a multiethnic elderly sample using the Third National Health and Nutrition Examination Survey. *Am J Epidemiol,* Vol.150, No.1, (July 1999), pp. 37-44, ISSN 0002-9262.

Perrig WJ, Perrig P & Stahelin HB. (1997). The relation between antioxidants and memory performence in the old and very old. *J Am Geriatr Soc,* Vol.45, No.6, (June 1997), pp. 718-24, ISSN 0002-8614.

Petersen RC, Thomas RG, Grundman M, Bennett D, Doody R, Ferris S, Galasko D, Jin S, Kaye J, Levey A, Pfeiffer E, Sano M, van Dyck CH & Thal LJ. (2005). Vitamin E and donepezil for the treatment of mild cognitive impairment. *N Eng J Med,* Vol.352, No.23, (June 2005), pp. 2379-88, ISSN 0028-4793.

Pietrzik K & Bronstrup A. (1997). Causes and consequences of hyperhomocyst(e)inemia. *Int J Vitam Nutr Res,* Vol.67, No.5, pp. 389-95, ISSN 0300-9831.

Pitchumoni SS & Doraisway PM. (1998). Current status of antioxidant therapy for Alzheimer's Disease. *J Am Geriatr Soc,* Vol.46, No.12, (December 1998), pp. 1566-72, ISSN 0002-8614.

Pratico D & Delanty N. (2000). Oxidative injury in diseases of the central nervous system: focus on Alzheimer's disease. *Am J Med,* Vol.109, No.7, (November 2000), pp. 577-85, ISSN 0002-9343.

Presse N, Shatenstein B, Kergoat MJ & Ferland G. (2008). Low vitamin K intakes in community-dwelling elders at an early stage of Alzheimer's disease. *J Am Diet Assoc,* Vol.108, No.12, (December 2008), pp.2095-9, ISSN 0002-8223.

Prieto AL, Weber JL, Tracy S, Heeb MJ & Lai C. (1999). Gas 6, a ligand for the receptor tyrosine kinase tyro 3, is widely expressed in the central nervous system. *Brain Res,* Vol.816, No.2, (January 1999), pp. 646-61, ISSN 0006-8993.

Prins ND, Den Heijer T, Hofman A, Koudstaal PJ, Jolles J, Clarke R & Breteler MM. (2002). Homocysteine and cognitive function in the elderly: Rotterdam Scan Study. *Neurology,* Vol.59, No.9, (November 2002), pp. 1375-80, ISSN 028-3878.

Rabaneda LG, Carrasco M, Lopez-Toledano MA, Murillo-Carretero M, Ruiz FA, Estrada C & Castro C. (2008). Homocysteine inhibits proliferation of neuronal precursors in the mouse adult brain by impairing the basic fibroblast growth factor signaling cascade and reducing extracellular regulated kinase-dependent cyclin E expression. *FASEB J,* Vol.22, No.11, (November 2008), pp. 3823-35, ISSN 0892-6638.

Rampersaud GC, Kauwell GP & Bailey LB. (2003). Folate: a key to optimizing health and reducing disease risk in the elderly. *J Am Coll Nutr,* Vol.22, No.1, (February 2003), pp. 1-8, ISSN 0731-5724.

Ravaglia G, Forti P, Maioli F, Martelli M, Servadei L, Brunatti N, Porcellini E & Licastro F. (2005). Homocysteine and folate as risk factors for dementia and Alzheimer disease. *Am J Clin Nutr,* Vol.82, No.3, (September 2005), pp. 636-43, ISSN 0002-9165.

Refsum H, Ueland PM, Nygard O & Vollset SE. (1998). Homocysteine and cardiovascular disease. *Annu Rev Med,* Vol.49, No.1, pp. 31-62, ISSN 0066-4219.

Reiter R.J. (1995). Oxidative processes and antioxidative defence mechanisms in the aging brain. *FASEB J,* Vol.9, No.7, (April 1995), pp. 526-33, ISSN 0892-6638.

Remington R, Chan A, Paskavitz J & Shea TB. (2009). Efficacy of a vitamin/nutriceutical formulation for moderate-stage to later stage Alzheimer's disease: a placebo-controlled pilot study. *Am J Alzheimers Dis Other Demen,* Vol.24, No.1, (February-March 2009), pp. 27-33, ISSN 1533-3175.

Riedel WJ, Jorissen B & Nutrients L. (1998). Age and cognitive function. *Curr Opin Clin Nutr Metab Care,* Vol.1, No.6, (November 1998), pp. 579-85, ISSN 163-1950.

Sahin M, Karauzum SB, Perry G, Smith MA & Aliciguzel Y. (2005). Retinoic acid isomers protect hippocampal neurons from amyloid-beta induced neurodegeneration. *Neurotox Res,* Vol.7, No.3, pp. 243-50, ISSN 1029-8428.

Sano M, Ernesto C, Thomas RG, Klauber MR, Schafer K, Grundman M, Woodbury P, Growdon J, Cotman CW, Pfeiffer E, Schneider LS & Thal LJ. (1997). A controlled trial of selegiline, alpha-tocopherol, or both as treatment for Alzheimer's disease. The Alzheimer's Disease Cooperative Study. *N Eng J Med,* Vol.336, No.17, (April 1997), pp. 1216-22, ISSN 0028-4793.

Sato Y, Iwamoto J, Kanoko T & Satoh K. (2005). Amelioration of osteoporosis and hypovitaminosis D by sunlight exposure in hospitalized, elderly women with Alzheimer's disease: a randomized controlled trial. *Journal of Bone&Mineral Research,* Vol.20, No.8, (August 2005), pp. 1327-33, ISSN 0884-0431.

Saupe J, Shearer MJ & Kohlmeier M. (1993). Phylloquinone transport and its influence on y-carboxyglutamate residues of osteocalcin in patients on hemodialysis. *Am J Clin Nutr,* Vol.58, No.2, (August 1993), pp. 204-8, ISSN 0002-9165.

Saxena SP, Fan T, Li M, Israels ED & Israels LG. (1997). A novel role for vitamin K, in a tyrosine phosphorylation cascade during chick embryogenesis. *J Clin Invest,* Vol.99, No.4, (February 1997), pp. 602-7, ISSN 0021-9738.

Scarmeas N, Stern Y, Tang MX, Mayeux R & Luchsinger JA. (2006). Mediterranean diet and risk for Alzheimer's disease. *Ann Neurol,* Vol.59, No.6, (June 2006), pp. 912-21, ISSN 0364-5134.

Scarmeas N, Stern Y, Mayeux R, Manly JJ, Schupf N & Luchsinger JA. (2009). Mediterranean diet and mild cognitive impairment. *Arch Neurol,* Vol.66, No.2, (February 2009), pp. 216-25, ISSN 0003-9942.

Scott TM, Peter I, Tucker KL, Arsenault L, Bergethon P, Bhadelia R, Buell J, Collins L, Dashe JF, Griffith J, Hibberd P, Leins D, Liu T, Ordovas JM, Patz S, Price LL, Qiu WQ, Sarnak M, Selhub J, Smaldone L, Wagner C, Wang L, Weiner D, Yee J, Rosenberg I & Folstein M. (2006). The Nutrition, Aging, and Memory in Elders (NAME) study: design and methods for a study of micronutrients and cognitive function in a homebound elderly population. *Int J Geriatr Psychiatr,* Vol.21, No.6, (June 2006), pp. 519-28, ISSN 0885-6230.

Scranton TW, Iwata M & Carlson SS. (1993). The SV-2 protein of synaptic vesicles is a keratan sulfate proteoglycan. *J Neurochem,* Vol.61, No.1, (July 1993), pp. 29-44, ISSN 0022-3042.

Selhub J, Jacques PF, Wilson PW, Rush D & Rosenberg IH. (1993). Vitamin status and intake as primary determinants of homocysteinemia in an elderly population. *J Am Med Assoc,* Vol.270, No.22, (December 1993), pp. 2693-8, ISSN 0002-9955.

Selhub J, Bagley LC, Miller J & Rosenberg IH. (2000). B vitamins, homocysteine, and neurocognitive function in the elderly. *Am J Clin Nutr,* Vol.71, No.2, (February 2000), S614-20, ISSN 0002-9165.

Selhub J. (2008). Public health significance of elevated homocysteine. *Food Nutr Bull,* Vol.29, No.2 Suppl), pp. S116-25, ISSN 0379-6721.

Seshadri S, Beiser A, Selhub J, Jacques PF, Rosenberg IH, D'Agostino RB, Wilson PW & Wolf PA. (2002). Plasma homocysteine as a risk factor for dementia and Alzheimer's disease. *N Eng J Med,* Vol.346, No.7, (February 2002), pp. 476-83, ISSN 0028-4793.

Shahidi S, Komaki A, Mahmoodi M, Atrvash H & Ghodrati M. (2008). Ascorbic acid supplementation could affect passive avoidance learning and memory in rats. *Brain Res Bull,* Vol.76, No.1-2, (May 2008), pp.109-13, ISSN 0361-9230.

Sinclair AJ, Bayer AJ, Johnston J, Warner C & Maxwell SR. (1998). Altered plasma antioxidant status in subjects with Alzheimer's disease and vascular dementia. *Int J Geriatr Psychiatry,* Vol.13, No.12, (December 1998), pp. 840-5, ISSN 0885-6230.

Smith AD, Stephen MS, de Jager CA, Whitbread P, Johnston C, Agacinski G, Oulhaj A, Bradley KM, Jacoby R & Refsum H. (2010). Homocysteine-lowering by B vitamins slows the rate of accelerated brain atrophy in mild cognitive impairment: a randomized controlled trial. In: *PLoS ONE,* 5(9), 17.05.2011, Available from e12244. doi:10.1371/journal.pone.0012244.

Sommer BR, Hoff AL & Costa M. (2003). Folic acid supplementation in dementia: a preliminary report. *J Geriatr Psychiatry Neurol,* Vol.16, No.3, (September 2003), pp. 156-9, ISSN 0891-9887.

Stott DJ, MacIntosh G, Lowe GD, Rumley A, McMahon AD, Langhorne P, Tait RC, O'Reilly DS, Spilg EG, MacDonald JB, MacFarlane PW, Westendorp RG. (2005). Randomized controlled trial of homocysteine-lowering vitamin treatment in elderly patients with vascular disease. *Am J Clin Nutr,* Vol.82, No.6, (December 2006), pp. 1320-6, ISSN 0002-9165.

Sutherland MK, Somerville MJ, Yoong LK, Bengeron C, Haussler MR & McLachlan DR. (1992). Reduction of vitamin D hormone receptor mRNA levels in Alzheimer as compared to Huntington hippocampus: correlation with calbindin -28k mRNA levels. *Brain Res Mol Brain Res,* Vol.13, No.3, (April 1992), pp. 239-50, ISSN 0169-328X.

Teunissen CE, Blom AH, Van Boxtel MP, Bosma H, de Bruijn C, Jolles J, Wauters BA, Steinbusch HW & de Vente J. (2003). Homocysteine: a marker for cognitive performance? A longitudinal follow-up study. *J Nutr Health Aging,* Vol.7, No.3, pp. 153-9, ISSN 1279-7707.

Troen AM, Shea-Budgell M, Shukitt-Hale B, Smith DE, Selhub J & Rosenberg IH. (2008). B-vitamin deficiency causes hyperhomocysteinemia and vascular cognitive impairment in mice. *Proc Natl Acad Sci USA,* Vol.105, No.34, (August 2008), pp. 12474-9, ISSN 0027-8424.

Tucker KL, Qiao N, Scott T, Rosenberg I & Spiro A 3rd. (2005). High homocysteine and low B vitamins predict cognitive decline in aging men: the Veterans Affairs Normative Aging Study. *Am J Clin Nutr,* Vol.82, No.3, (November 2005), pp. 627-35, ISSN 0002-9165.

Ueland PM & Refsum H. (1989). Plasma homocysteine, a risk factor for vascular disease: plasma levels in health, disease, and drug therapy. *J Lab Clin Med,* Vol.114, No.5, (November 1989), pp. 473-501, ISSN 0022-2143.

van Oort FV, Melse-Boonstra A, Brouwer IA, Clarke R, West CE, Katan MB & Verhoef P. (2003). Folic acid and reduction of plasma homocysteine concentrations in older adults: a dose-response study. *Am J Clin Nutr,* Vol.77, No.5, (May 2003), pp. 1318-23, ISSN 0002-9165.

van Uffelen JG, Chin A, Paw MJ, Hopman-Rock M & van Mechelen W. (2007). The effect of walking and vitamin B supplementation on quality of life in community-dwelling adults with mild cognitive impairment: a randomized, controlled trial. *Qual Life Res,* Vol.16, No.7, (September 2007), pp. 1137-46, ISSN 0962-9343.

Varadarajan S, Yatin S, Aksenova M & Butterfield DA. (2000). Review: Alzheimer's amyloid beta-peptide-associated free radical oxidative stress and neurotoxicity. *J Struct Biol*, Vol.130, No.2-3, (June 2000), pp. 184-208, ISSN 1047-8477.

Vivekananthan DP, Penn MS, Sapp SK, Hsu A & Topol EJ. (2003). Use of antioxidant vitamins for the prevention of cardiovascular disease: meta-analysis of randomised trials. *Lancet*, Vol.361, No.9374), pp. 2017-23, ISSN 0140-6736.

Wahlin A, Hill RD, Winblad B & Backman L. (1996). Effects of serum vitamin B12 and folate status on episodic memory performance in very old age: a population- based study. *Psychol Aging*, Vol.11, No.3, (September 1996), pp. 487-96, ISSN 0882-7974.

Wald DS, Bishop L, Wald NJ, Law M, Hennessy E, Weir D, McPartlin J & Scott J. (2001). Randomized trial of folic acid supplementation and serum homocysteine levels. *Arch Intern Med*, Vol.161, No.5, (March 2001), pp. 695-700, ISSN 0003-9926.

Wang HX, Wahlin A, Basun H, Fastbom J, Winblad B & Fratiglioni L. (2001). Vitamin B(12) and folate in relation to the development of Alzheimer's disease. *Neurology*, Vol.56, No.9, (May 2001), pp. 1188-94, ISSN 0028-3878.

Wolters M, Strohle A & Hahn A. (2004). Age-associated changes in the metabolism of vitamin B (12) and folic acid: prevalance, aetiopathogenesis and pathophysiological consequences. *Z Gerontol Geriatr*, Vol.37, No.2, (April 2004), pp. 109-35, ISSN 0948-6704.

Wolters M, Hickstein M, Flintermann A, Tewes U & Hahn A. (2005). Cognitive performance in relation to vitamin status in healthy elderly German women-the effect of 6-month multivitamin supplementation. *Prev Med*, Vol.41, No.1, (July 2005), pp. 253-9, ISSN 0091-7435.

Yagami T, Ueda K, Asakura K, Sakaeda T, Nakazato H, Huroda T, Hata S, Sakaguchi G, Itoh N, Nakano T, Kambayashi Y & Tsuzuki H. (2002). Gas6 rescues cortical neurons from amyloid β protein-induced apoptosis. *Neuropharmacology*, Vol.43, No.8, (December 2002), pp. 1289-96, ISSN 0028-3908.

Zandi PP, Anthony JC, Khachaturian AS, Stone SV, Gustafson D, Tschanz JT, Norton MC, Weish-Bohmer KA, Breitner JC. (2004). Reduced risk of Alzheimer disease in users of antioxidant vitamin supplements. *Arch Neurol*, Vol.61, No.1, (January 2004), pp. 82-8, ISSN 0003-9942.

4

Alzheimer's Disease and Metal Contamination: Aspects on Genotoxicity

Lima, P.D.L.[1], Vasconcellos, M.C.[2], Montenegro, R.C.[3] and Burbano, R.R.[3]
[1]*Molecular Biology Laboratory, Center of Biological and Health Sciences, State University of Pará*
[2]*Biological Activities Laboratory, Federal University of Amazonas*
[3]*Human Cytogenetics Laboratory, Institute Biological Institute of Biological Science, Federal University of Pará, Brazil*

1. Introduction

Despite the genetic and environmental factors and the aging process itself, multiple evidence from experimental models and postmortem studies in Alzheimer's disease (AD) brain tissue demonstrate that neurodegeneration is associated with morphological and biochemical features. Considerable evidence suggests a role for oxidative stress/damage (amyloid beta peptide, iron/hydrogen peroxide) or neurotoxic by-products of lipid peroxidation (4-hydroxy-2-nonenal, acrolein) and inflammation, in the pathogenesis of neuron degeneration, which, in turns, are known to cause cell death.

Recently, several reports indicate that, among factors, metal ions (Al, Zn, Cu, Fe, etc) could specifically impair protein aggregation and their oligomeric toxicity. Also, metal-induced (direct) and metal-amyloid-β (indirect) linked neuronal cell death through the formation of reactive oxygen species (ROS) being critical to the understanding of the mechanisms which metal-induced cell death, and thus its role in neurodegenerative disorders.

Some metals are essential for humans and for all forms of life. Even though metals are necessary in biological systems, they are usually required only in trace amounts; in excess, it can be toxic, if not fatal. Environmental metal exposure has been suggested to be a risk factor for AD. High-term exposure to certain metals like manganese (Mn), iron (Fe), aluminum (Al) and many others like copper (Cu), mercury (Hg), zinc (Zn), lead (Pb), arsenic (As), alone or in combination, can increase neurodegenerative process, especially to Alzheimer's disease (AD).

Aluminum is the most widely distributed metal in the environment and is extensively used in daily life that provides easy exposure to human beings. No biological function of the element has been identified, whereas some aspects of its toxicity have been described. It has been suggested that there might be a relationship between high levels of Al and increased risk of a number of pathogenic disorders, such as microcytic anemia, osteomalacia and, possibly, neurodegenerative disorders including dialysis encephalopathy, Parkinson's disease and Alzheimer's disease.

This metal is known to be extremely neurotoxic and in high levels is capable to inhibit the prenatal and post-natal development of the brain. Evidence from clinical and animal studies demonstrated that brain Al content increases with age and that Al generates reactive oxygen species (ROS) that activates signaling pathways which leads to degeneration of neuronal cells. Together with ROS or alone, Al is biochemically attracted to the DNA reveling its genotoxic and mutagenic potential.

Furthermore, high level of Al has been found in brain lesions, such as plaques and tangles, in patients with AD. Several studies demonstrated that among others, Al appears to be the most efficient cation in promoting Aβ aggregation, increasing dramatically cellular neurotoxicity. According to the "amyloid cascade hypothesis", accumulation of Aβ in the brain is the primary event driving AD pathogenesis, increasing the evidences by which Al is involved in AD.

Iron is an essential trace element used by almost all living organisms, being often incorporated into the heme complex, which mediate redox reactions. Disturbances of brain iron homeostasis have been linked to acute neuronal injury. Moreover, iron is toxic to neural tissue, leading to neurodegenerative disorders.

Organic iron (Fe) may increase the genotoxic effects of other compounds when they are combined. Together with aluminum sulfate, at nanomolar concentrations, iron trigger the release of reactive oxygen species (ROS). In high levels, iron can be mutagenic and genotoxic. In AD, iron is an important cause of oxidative stress because of its over-accumulation in the brain and colocalizes with AD lesions, senile plaques and neurofibrillary tangles.

Recent studies also show that homeostasis of essential metals such as copper, iron, selenium and zinc may be altered in the brain of subjects with Alzheimer's disease. It is demonstrated that the plasma concentrations of manganese and total mercury were significantly higher in subjects with AD than in controls, however the concentrations of vanadium, manganese, rubidium, antimony, cesium and lead were significantly lower among subjects with AD cerebrospinal fluid.

The influence of metal ions such as Fe, Cu, and Zn in stimulating Aβ aggregation have been widely studied where they appears to vary depending on tissue pH. It should be noticed that, although there is co-localization of metal ions in the pathological markers of AD, this does not indicate a causative role for these elements in the pathogenesis of the disease. Independently of metals being a primary cause or consequence of the disease mechanism, a change in a single metal ion can cause a significant imbalance on homeostasis in elemental levels in the body (serum, CSF and brain) leading to as a sort of "domino effect". It is clear the need to understand the fundamental biochemical mechanisms linking brain biometal metabolism, environmental metal exposure, genotoxicity and AD pathophysiology. In this review, we discuss the role of metals in Alzheimer disease and its involvement in genotoxicity.

2. Source of metal exposure

Metals have been used throughout human history to make several utensils, machines, jewelry, and so on, where many of then were obtained through mining and smelting, activities that increases their distribution throughout the environment. Furthermore, the use of metals in industry, medicine, agriculture have been increased over the years, which increase the exposure, not only for those workers involved directly in working with metals but also consumers of the products and the general public through environmental contamination (Ferrer, 2003; Ansari *et al.*, 2004).

Metals are among the oldest toxic agents known by humans. Its history starts prior to 2000 BC when it became available as a byproduct of silver smelting. The early Greeks and Romans documented both the toxic as well as the potential healing effects of metals. Theophrastus of Erebus (370-287 BC) and Pliny the Elder (23-79 AD) described the pernicious effects of arsenic and mercury on miners and smelters (Hollenberg, 2010).

In an industrialized world, there are thousands of types of metals in use, and humans are exposed to them at work, or as a result of contamination of food, water and environment. There is abundant evidence indicating an increase of neurodegenerative disorders like AD in industrialized countries (Veldman et al., 1998; Butterworth, 2010). The chronic exposure to metals from several years together with the advance of medical tools may explain why the diagnosis of AD and so its epidemic starts around 1980.

Aluminum is the most widely distributed metal in the environment and is extensively used in a wide variety of products: cans, foils and kitchen utensils, as well as parts of airplanes, rockets and other items that require a strong, light material. It can be deposited on the surface of glass to make mirrors, and also to make synthetic rubies and sapphires for lasers. Al is found in the environment in its natural forms or as a source of human contamination resulting from mining and smelting, activities that increase their distribution throughout the environment. Al occurs naturally only in compounds, never as a pure metal. Because of its strong affinity to oxygen, it is almost never found in the elemental state; instead it is found in oxides or silicates (WHO, 1997; Nayak, 2002).

In nature, this trace element is found in its oxidized state Al^{3+} (soluble toxic form of Al), which binds to others molecules like chloride, forming Aluminum chloride ($AlCl_3$) (Smith, 1996; WHO, 1997). Aluminum chloride ($AlCl_3$) is an important coagulant used in water treatment and purification (WHO, 1997; Zhang e Zhou, 2005) being another source for exposure. Two of the most common compounds are potassium aluminum sulfate ($KAl(SO_4)_2 \cdot 12H_2O$), and aluminum oxide (Al_2O_3).

Although aluminum is a widespread element, almost all metallic aluminium is produced from the ore bauxite ($AlO_x(OH)_{3-2x}$). Bauxite is a complicated mixture of compounds consisting of 55% of aluminum, oxygen, and other elements (WHO, 1997; Nayak, 2002). Large reserves of bauxite are found in Australia, Brazil, Guinea, Jamaica, Russia, and the United States.

No biological function of the element has been identified, whereas some aspects of its toxicity have been described (Berthon, 1996; Corain *et al.*, 1996; Suwalsky *et al.*, 2001). The exposure to this toxic metal occurs through air, food, water and it is also present in medical, cosmetic and environmental products (Berthon, 2002).

Daily consumed of Al by food and beverages is 2.5 to 13 mg, where drinking water can contributes to 0.2 to 0.4 mg of Al daily. Drugs can contribute with increase levels of Al; antiacid drugs (2 tablets) can contribute up to 500 mg of Al (WHO, 1997). As the world becomes more industrialize, the chronic exposure to Al increases, increasing the risk for the development of neurodegenerative disorders like AD and PD.

The period in human history beginning in about 1200 B.C. is called the Iron Age. Iron is a transition metal and normally does not occur as a free element (Meteoric origen) (O´Neil, 1994). The most common ores of iron are hematite, or ferric oxide (Fe_2O_3); limonite, or ferric oxide (Fe_2O_3); magnetite, or iron oxide (Fe_3O_4); and siderite, or iron carbonate ($FeCO_3$). An increasingly important source of iron is taconite. Taconite is a mixture of hematite and silica (sand). The largest iron resources in the world are in China, Russia, Brazil, Canada,

Australia, and Índia. Furthermore, almost all rocks and soils contains at least trace amounts of iron (Sienko, 1977).

Iron is a very reactive metal. Most of then are found as Fe^{2+} which are oxidize to Fe^{3+}. Combines with oxygen in moist air and the product of this reaction is iron oxide (Fe_2O_3) (Cox, 1995). Iron also reacts with very hot water and steam to produce hydrogen gas. It also dissolves in most acids and reacts with many other elements. All of this reaction can be a source for contamination.

Iron is a silvery-white or grayish metal. It is ductile and malleable, very high tensile strength and workable. In general, iron products can be found in automotive, construction, containers, machinery and industrial equipment, railroad tracks, oil and gas industries, electrical tools, appliances and utensils (Ilo, 1997). Furthermore, the fastest growing use of iron compounds is in water treatment systems.

Populations are exposed to iron mainly through foods and beverages. It is available in a number of foods, including meat, milk, eggs, nuts, coffee, tea, fish, grain, soil and raisins. Iron can also be found in fresh water, where recommended levels can not exceed 0.3 mg of iron in 1 liter of water (WHO, 1996). The United State Recommended Daily Allowance (USRDA) for iron is 18 milligrams, being the amount of iron that a person needs to stay healthy. Also, daily recommended doses of Fe varies among age; for children up to 3 months, 1.7 mg/kg/daily are recommended, whereas for adults this is 10 times more (18 mg/kg/daily)(WHO, 1996).

An iron deficiency can cause serious health problems in humans. Also, several alterations have been related to high iron intake where iron is toxic to neural tissue, leading to neurodegenerative disorders like AD (Montgomery, 1995; Campbell & Bondy, 2000; Stankiewicz & Brass, 2009).

Manganese is a transition metal and it took several years to discover the difference between manganese and iron, mainly because it oftens occurs together in the Earth's crust and its similarity properties.

Manganese is a moderately active metal and never occurs as a pure element in nature. It always combines with oxygen in the air to form manganese dioxide (MnO_2) or other elements. It also combines with fluorine and chloride to make manganese difluoride (MnF_2) and manganese dichloride ($MnCl_2$) (WHO, 1999). The most common ores of manganese are pyrolusite (MnO_2), manganite, psilomelane, and rhodochrosite. Manganese is also found mixed with iron ores. The largest producers of manganese ore in the world are China, South Africa, the Ukraine, Brazil, Australia, Gabon, and Kazakstan.

Early artists were familiar with pyrolusite and they used the mineral to give glass a beautiful purple color, and/or to remove color from a glass. By the middle 1700s, chemists proved that pyrolusite contained manganese dioxide. Until now, coloring agents (textiles, paints, inks, glass, and ceramics) still contains manganous chloride.

The most common alloy of manganese is ferromanganese, containing about 48 percent manganese combined with iron and carbon, being the source for making a very large variety steel products, including tools, heavy-duty machinery, railroad tracks, bank vaults, construction components, and automotive parts. Also, manganous chloride ($MnCl_2$), is an additive in animal food for cows, horses, goats, and other domestic animals. In agriculture, manganous chloride are present in fertilizers (Barceloux, 1999).

Manganese is one of the chemical elements that has both positive and negative effects on living organisms because manganese is used by many enzymes in an organism. A very small amount of the element is needed to maintain good health. The absortion of Mn is only

3 to 5%, being food the primary source of this metal. Mn is found in green vegetables, nut, raisins, and also in teas, its main source for human consumption. Low concentrations are found in Milk, meat, fish, eggs and fruits (Barceloux, 1999). Taking all together, soil, fertilizer and food, one can say that humans are exposed to Mn and that excess of manganese can create health problems. Also, a variety of drugs and supplements have Mn in its composition (WHO, 1999).

Human exposure can be also by inhalation. Workers may inhale manganese dust in the air in a factory or mine. Also, human can be exposed by the ingestion of contaminated water with fertilizers and pesticides (WHO, 1999). Exposures to high levels of manganese by ingestion or inhalation can damage the central nervous system. Daily-recommended doses of Mn for children are 0.3 mg/Kg/daily, being 3 times more for adults (10 mg/Kg/daily) (WHO, 1999).

3. Metal neurotoxicity

Abnormal production or clearance of a small peptide, the amyloid β-peptide (Aβ), which is the major constituent of the senile plaques, is a widely accepted causative agent in degenerative disorders like AD (Hardy & Selkoe, 2002; LaFerla et al., 2007; Qiu & Folstein, 2006; Rauk, 2009; Sayre et al., 1997; Selkoe, 2000). Aβ is a 39- to 43-residue peptide cleaved from the C-terminal region of a much larger protein, the amyloid precursor protein (APP), where the most abundant fragments are Aβ (1–40) and Aβ (1–42), being the latter the most neurotoxic (Rauk, 2009).

Several studies have shown that Aβ exerts its toxicity by generating reactive oxidative stress (ROS) molecules, leading to peroxidation of membrane lipids and lipoproteins, induction of H_2O_2 and hydroxynonenal (HNE) in neurons, damages DNA and transport enzymes inactivation (Behl et al., 1994; Kontush et al., 2001; Mark et al., 1997; Mark et al., 1997; Varadarajan et al., 2000; Xu et al., 2001). In addition to a high metabolically levels of ROS, there are other sources that are thought to play an important role in the AD progression. Among them, mitochondrial and metal abnormalities are the major sources of oxidative stress (Su et al., 2008).

Increasing evidences suggest that altered metal homeostasis may contribute to neuronal loss in neurodegenerative diseases (Gerlach et al., 2006; Sayre et al., 2005; Wright, 2008). Given a likely role for metal-associated oxidative stress, herein it is discuss the involvement of metals, such as Al(III), Fe(III) and Mg(II) in neurotoxicity.

3.1 Aluminum and neurotoxicity

Aluminum (Al) is the third most abundant element in the earth's crust and is not an essential trace metal for mammals. However, the concentrations found in the body can be sufficient to modify the activity of several key enzymes and second messenger pathways (Bondy, 2010).

Aluminum is known to be extremely neurotoxic and in high levels is capable to inhibit the prenatal and post-natal development of the brain (Yumoto et al., 2001). Several studies correlated the risk of developing Alzheimer's disease with residing in areas where aluminum concentrations in the drinking water are 100 mg/L or greater (McLachlan et al., 1996; Rondeau et al., 2000).

The hypothesis that there is a link between aluminum and Alzheimer's disease (AD) was first brought out in the 1960s by Terry and Pena (1965) and by Klatzo and colaborators in

1965 (Terry et al., 1969). Early on 1976, high levels of aluminum have been found in brain lesions, such as plaques and tangles, in patients with AD (Crapper et al., 1976), and also in other conditions such as Parkinson's disease (PD), pre-senile dementia, amiotrofic lateral esclerosis, neurofibrilar degeneration, dialysis encephalopathy syndrome and nigroestriatal sindrome (Altschuler, 1999; Gupta et al., 2005; Nayak, 2002; Yasui et al., 1992; Zatta et al., 1991). Elevated aluminum levels have also been reported in other less common neurological disorders such as the Guamanian Parkinsonian-ALS constellation and Hallervorden-Spatz disease (Eidelberg et al., 1987; Garruto et al., 1989).

The most common neurostrutural alterations induced by high levels of aluminum in the brain is: brain ventricle dilatation and thinning of the corpus callosum (Lapresie et al., 1975), reduce neural cell density, degenerative changings like picnosis, vacuolization, chromatin condensation (Varner et al., 1998), increase neural filaments in neuron from the spinal cord and brainstem (Terry et al., 1969), axonal intumescence (Troncoso et al., 1985) and cerebellar disorder with degeneration of the Purkinje cells (Ghetti et al., 1985; Yokel, 1994).

There is some experimental evidence that Al exposure can adversely affect the dopaminergic system. Extended exposure to 100mM Al lactate increased striatal levels of the dopamine metabolite (Li et al., 2008), what, in turns, suggests that exposure to Al may cause increased turnover of dopamine. The development of an encephalopathy, characterized by cognitive deficits, in-coordination, tremor and spinocerebellar degeneration, among workers in the aluminum industry also indicates that exposure to the metal can be profoundly deleterious. Abnormal neurological symptoms have been observed in several patients receiving intramuscular injections of Al-containing vaccines.

There have been many experimental studies on animals and on isolated cells showing that aluminum has toxic effects on the nervous system. In 1991, Guy and colaborators showed that the uptake of aluminum by human neuroblastoma cells display an epitope associated with Alzheimer's diseases. Chronic exposure of animals to aluminum is associated with behavioural, neuropathological and neurochemical changes. Among them, deficits of learning and behavioural functions are most evident (Kummar et al., 2009; Ribes et al., 2010; Sethi et al., 2008). Also, when mice were injected with adjuvants containing aluminum in amounts equivalent to those given to US military service personnel, neuroinflammation and cell loss were found in spinal cord and motor cortex, together with memorial deficits (Petrik et al., 2007).

Several metals interact with β-amyloid (Aβ) in senile plaques. It is interesting to note that, compared to other Aβ-metal complexes (Aβ-Fe, Aβ-Zn, Aβ-Cu), Aβ-Al is unique in promoting a specific form of Aβ oligomerization that has marked neurotoxic effects (Drago et al., 2008).

There are a lot of ways which Al can damage neural cells: (i) interfering with glucose metabolism, leading to low amounts of Acetilcholine (Ach) precursors; (ii) interacting to ATPase Na^+/K^+ and Ca^{2+}/Mg^{2+} -depending, altering excitatory aminoacid release; (iii) inhibition the binding of Ca^{++}; (iv) incresing the production of AMPc; (v) causing changes in the cytoskeleton protein, leading to phosphorilation, proteolysis, transport and synthesis disruption; (vi) interacting directly to genomic structures, and most importantly (vii) inducing oxidative damage by lipid peroxidation (Nayak & Chatterjee, 1999).

Being involved in the production of reactive oxygen species (ROS), aluminum may cause impairments in mitochondrial bioenergetics and may lead to the generation of oxidative stress which may lead to a gradual accumulation of oxidatively modified cellular proteins, lipids and affects endogenous antioxidant enzyme activity, leading to degeneration of neuronal cells (Kummar et al., 2009; Sethi et al., 2008; Wu et al., 2010). In this way, aluminum is a strong candidate for consideration as a subtle promoter of events typically associated with brain aging and neurodegenerative disorders.

3.2 Iron and neurotoxicity

Metal ion homeostasis is maintained through highly regulated mechanisms of uptake, storage, and secretion (Mills et al., 2010). Iron plays a role in oxygen transportation, myelin synthesis, neurotransmitter production, and electron transfers, being a crucial cofactor in normal central nervous (CNS) metabolism. Iron is also abundantly in substantia nigra and globus palladium when compared with other regions and is found to increase with age in humans (Bartzokis et al., 1994; Lee et al., 2010; Zecca et al., 2001). Normally, under healthy conditions, these metal ions are bound to ligands (e.g., transferrin), however when they are found nonbound, iron are potentially harmful mainly due to their redox activities in the synaptic cleft (Salvador et al., 2011).

Free iron catalyzes the conversion of superoxide and hydrogen peroxide into hydroxyl radicals, which promote oxidative stress by the Fenton reaction (Berg et al., 2001). Furthermore, ROS interacts with a variety of molecules, including unsaturated fatty acids, proteins and DNA leading to subsequent cell death/apoptosis, especially on CNS tissue, whereas the antioxidant defenses are rare (Demougeot et al., 2003; Stankiewicz & Brass, 2009; Willmore & Rubin, 1984). Thus, disturbances of brain iron homeostasis have been linked to acute neuronal injury leading to neurodegenerative disorders (Campbell & Bondy, 2000; Montgomery, 1995) such as Alzheimer's (AD), Parkinson's (PD), and Huntington's (HD) diseases as well as amyotrophic lateral sclerosis (ALS) (Connor & Benkovic, 1992; Kell, 2010; Liu et al., 2006; Rouault, 2001; Youdim et al., 2005).

Degradation of the dopaminergic system, where catechols molecules should be produced, may play a role in the extrapyramidal symptoms in PD (Prikhojan et al, 2002; Santiago et al., 2000). *In vitro* studies have shown that iron is accumulated in microglia and astrocytes in the cerebral cortex, cerebellum, substantia nigra, and hippocampus, and it is believed that this metal would be involved in the neuroinflammation observed in AD and PD (Ong & Farooqui, 2005).

Postmortem studies in PD subjects, suggests that accumulation of iron in the substantia nigra stimulates lipid peroxidation, which can lead to cell damage (Nakano, 1993; Riederer et al., 1989). Studies conducted with PD subjects demonstrated that in mild PD, there were no significant differences in the content of total iron between the PD group and control, whereas there was an increase in total iron and iron (III) in substantia nigra of severely affected patients (Riederer et al., 1989). Indeed, lateral substantia nigra pars compacta abnormalities were observed in early PD together with increased iron content.

Within the reduction on glutathione and the change of the iron (II)/iron (III) ratio in favor of iron (III), it is suggest that these changes might contribute to pathophysiological processes underlying PD (Griffiths et al., 1999; Lan & Jiang, 1997; Martin & Wiler, 2008). Interestingly, the increase in iron in the degenerating substantia nigra (SN) occurs only in the advanced stages of the disease, suggesting that these phenomena may be a secondary event, rather than a primary (Double et al., 2000). Patients with diagnosed AD and in normal elderly patients, iron concentrations have been found to be increased in the bilateral hippocampus, parietal cortex, frontal white matter, putamen, caudate nucleus, thalamus, red nucleus, substantia nigra, and dentate nucleus subregions. Particularly in the parietal cortex, at the early stages of AD, studies have been found to positively correlate with the severity of patients' cognitive impairment (Sullivan et al., 2009; Zhu et al., 2009).

Although extensive evidence links the iron metabolism, aging, and neurodegenerative disorders, relatively little is known about the resulting forms of iron that accumulate in the brain. Numerous techniques have been developed in order to characterize, locate, and quantify iron species and iron- containing compounds in the brain, however, more studies are needed to understand the role of this transition metal in the onset and progression of neurodegenerative diseases and neurological age-related disorders.

3.3 Manganese and neurotoxicity

Manganese is an essential element for many living organisms, especially humans, where some enzymes require (e.g., manganese superoxide dismutase), and some are activated, by manganese (Hurley & Keen, 1987). Excess accumulation of these metal by ingestion or inhalation (mostly in working place) (Agency for Toxic Substances and Disease Registry [ATSDR], 2000) can damage the central nervous system (Winder et al., 2010) most likely due to impaired transport or failure of hepatic detoxification mechanisms, what have deleterious effects on cell function and integrity (Butterworth, 2010).

It is known that astrocytes have a much higher affinity and capacity for manganese uptake compared to neurons and that exposure to manganese results primarily in alterations of astrocyte morphology and function (Aschner et al., 1992). Excessive exposure to Mn can also lead to neural lesion, primarily on the dopaminergic pathway (globus pallidus and substantia nigra pars reticulata), inhibiting dopamine metabolism (Vidal et al., 2005).

Short-term repeated pulmonary exposure to manual metal arc-hard surfacing or gas metal arc-mild steel fumes resulted in selective deposition of Mn in the brain, particularly in dopaminergic brain areas. It is interesting to note that, other constituents of the fumes like Fe, Cr, Ni or Cu did not appear to translocate to the brain despite their large accumulation in the lungs and its associated lymph nodes. Molecular markers of dopaminergic neurotoxicity and injury response can be found in the brain of welding fumes, extended beyond the globus pallidus, considered the primary site of damage in manganism, to broader dopaminergic areas (Sriram et al., 2010).

Neurotoxic effect of Mn can be due to its interaction with detoxification enzymes that protects the cells, and/or its interaction with the redox system. In this way, Mn^{2+} (necessary in the brain) can be oxidize to Mn^{3+}, a toxic compound that enhances the oxidation of dopamine leading to a lots of neurotoxic products (Donaldson et al., 1982). Recent studies reveal that repeated exposure to Mn or Mn-containing welding fumes can cause mitochondrial dysfunction and alterations in the expression of proteins in dopaminergic brain areas, also, events that contribute to dopaminergic neurotoxicity (Sriram et al., 2010).

Some evidences indicate that the neurological abnormalities can be found on the striatum and on subthalamic nucleus in the CNS of the monkey receiving $MnCl_2$ by inhalation (Newland et al., 1999). Also, undesirable neurological effects were observed in children who were exposed to excess manganese (Zheng et al., 1998), what can explain the enhanced incidence of neurological symptoms in isolated populations (Florence & Stauber, 1989; Iwami et al., 1994).

Adverse health effects can be caused by inadequate intake or overexposure to manganese. Chronic exposure to high levels of Mn induces a syndrome known as "manganism", characterized by extrapyramidal dysfunction (bradykinesia, rigidity and dystonia) and neuropsychiatric symptoms that resemble idiopathic Parkinson's disease (Santamaria & Sulsky, 2010).

Although is not completely clear the relationship between Mn and PD patogenesis, or neurodegenerative disorders, it is suggest that this metal accelerates neuronal death and increase the risk of its development (Zheng et al., 1998).

4. Metal contamination and AD developing

Metal are essential for humans and for all forms of life. Even though metals are necessary in biological systems, they are usually required only in trace amounts. As regard to the brain, metals are essential for neuronal activities. However, if not correctly regulated, redox-active can react with molecular oxygen to generate ROS thus causing brain lipid peroxidation and protein oxidation (Salvador et al., 2011; Sayre et al., 1997; Smith et al., 1996; Smith et al., 1997). Also, metal imbalance can lead to aberrant interactions between metals and AD-related proteins, being a potential source of oxidative stress, which is evolved into the "metal hypothesis" of AD (Iqbal et al., 2005).

Protein misfolding associated with Aβ aggregation, is significantly affected by various biological, biophysical and chemical factors including metal ions such as Al, Cu, Zn, and Fe, which have been found in high concentration in the AD brain (Beauchemin et al., 1998; Dong et al., 2003; Lovell et al., 1993; 1998; Miu et al., 2006; Suh et al., 2000;). Also, some metals are able to accelerate the dynamic of Aβ aggregation, thus increasing the neurotoxic effects on neuronal cells (Bush, 2003; House et al., 2004; Maynard et al., 2005; Miu et al., 2006; Morgan et al., 2002; Ricchelli et al., 2005). Kawahara et al. (2001) showed that aluminum induces neuronal apoptosis in vivo as well as in vitro and causes the accumulation of hyperphosphorylated tau protein and Aβ protein in in vivo model.

Several studies have focused on the role of metal ions including Al on the Aβ aggregation properties (House et al., 2004; Kawahara et al., 1994; Pratico et al., 2002; Ricchelli et al., 2005), suggesting that, among various metal ions assessed, Al seems to be the most efficient in promoting Aβ aggregation in vitro, increasing cellular neurotoxicity (Kawahara et al., 2001; Kawahara, 2005; Ricchelli et al., 2005). Also, Al induces the spontaneous increase of Aβ1-42 surface hydrophobicity compared to Aβ alone, which in turns, the complex Aβ1-42-Al reduced the capillary sequestration increasing its permeability through the blood brain barrier resulting intracerebral accumulation as demonstrated by Banks et al. (2006).

Environmental metal exposure has been suggested to be a risk factor for AD. High-term exposure to certain metals like manganese (Mn), iron (Fe), aluminum (Al) and many others, alone or in combination, can increase neurodegenerative process, especially to Alzheimer's disease (AD).

Aluminum (Al) is the most abundant neurotoxic metal on earth, widely bioavailable to humans and repeatedly shown to accumulate in AD-susceptible neuronal foci. Furthermore, several groups reported an increased amounts of Al in neurofibrillary tangles (NFT)-bearing neurons of AD brains, suggesting the association of Al with NFTs (Good et al., 1992; Lovell et al., 1993). Evidence from clinical and animal model studies demonstrated that brain Al content increases with age, suggesting an increased exposure or a decreased ability to remove Al from brain with age (Savory et al., 1999). Furthermore, high levels of Al has been found in brain lesions, such as plaques and tangles, in patients with AD and could be involved in the aggregation of Aβ peptides to form toxic fibrils (Sakae et al., 2009).

Iron is an essential trace element used by almost all living organisms. However, disturbances of brain iron homeostasis have been linked to acute neuronal injury. Increased iron levels were found both in the cortex and cerebellum from the preclinical AD cases (Sullivan et al., 2009; Zhu et al., 2009). Cellular studies have shown that iron is particular accumulated in microglia and astrocytes in the cerebral cortex, cerebellum, substantia nigra, and hippocampus, and it is believed that this metal would be involved in the neuroinflammation found in AD and PD (Ong & Farooqui, 2005; Sullivan et al., 2009; Zhu et al., 2009). It is important to note that these brain iron concentrations, especially in the parietal cortex at the early stages of AD, have been found to positively correlate with the severity of patients' cognitive impairment (Zhu et al., 2009). Interestingly, Aβ insoluble aggregates have been demonstrated to be dissolved by metal chelators (Cherny et al., 1999). Iron itself has been related neurotoxicity, and its accumulation, has been observed to before AD lesions are measurable. In AD, iron is an important cause of oxidative stress because of its over-accumulation in the brain and colocalizes with AD lesions, senile plaques and neurofibrillary tangles. Interestingly, iron has been involved in lipid and protein oxidation and also in DNA damage. Iron is able to oxidize DNA bases, and it has been suggested that the accumulation of this transition metal in some neurodegenerative disorders could act by both increasing oxidative genome damage and also preventing its repair (Hegde et al., 2010).

Manganese (Mn) is an essential element for humans, animals, and plants and is required for growth, development, and maintenance of health, although it has been recognized as a neurotoxic metal for over 150 years (Weiss, 2010). Unbalance of Mn homeostasis has show cognitive deficiencies features that include diminished attention, reduced scores on tests of working memory, lower scores on intelligence tests, impaired learning, and slowed response speed. Also, Weiss (2010) reports that signs of Mn poisoning are impaired coordination, abnormal gait, abnormal laughter, expressionless face, weakness, bradykinesia, somnolence, dysarthria, difficulty walking, clumsiness, lack of balance, muscle pains, and diminished leg power. Furthermore, exposure to high levels of inhaled manganese, as in miners working leads to motor symptoms.

Nonhuman primates can be the most appropriate animal models for studies of manganese neurotoxicity because of their similarities to humans in brain anatomy and neurobehavioral function (Schneider et al., 2009). A recent study by Schneider et al. (2009) demonstrated that trained Cynomologous monkeys for memory test followed by a regimen of intravenous manganese sulfate injections over a period of about 230 days, displayed mild deficits in spatial memory, greater deficits in nonspatial memory, and no deficits in reference memory on animals treated. By analyzing Mn concentrations, the study showed a significant inverse relationship between working memory task performance and Mn levels.

The relationship by Mn exposure and Alzheimer's disease has also been investigated by gene array analysis of frontal cortex from Cynomologous monkeys after Schneider et al. (2009) studies (Guilarte et al., 2010). Amyloid-β Precursor-like Protein 1 (APLP1), a member of the Amyloid Precursor Protein (APP) family was the most expressed out of the 61 upregulated genes. Along with this finding, immunochemistry revealed the presence of Amyloid-β plaques in the brain of subjects with only 6–8 years of age. Thus, these findings links the Mn-induced β-amyloid deposits to impaired memory function what may be extrapolated to human brain and so the features of AD pathogenesis.

5. Metal genotoxicity

Cellular stresses, including DNA damage, have been linked to cell cycle deregulation in neurons (Park et al., 1998; Kruman et al., 2004). Studies on the biological causes of neuronal death in AD have been guided by observations of cell cycle reentry in cellular populations that degenerate in human disease (Busser et al., 1998; Yang et al., 2003). In addition to ectopic cell cycling, AD is also linked to DNA damage; accumulation of DNA damage in neurons is associated with aging (Lu et al., 2004) and is exacerbated in neurodegenerative disorders including AD (Rass et al., 2007). The occurrance of DNA damage was related in astrocytes of AD hippocampus (Myung et al., 2008) and in neurons within the cerebellar dentate nucleus that show the robust DNA damage response (Chen et al., 2010).

The appearance of DNA damage during the course of lateonset neurodegenerative disease has been attributed in part to the fact that neurons exhibit high mitochondrial respiration, which is known to lead to the production of reactive oxygen-species. Over time this oxidative stress results in the accumulated damage of mitochondrial and nuclear DNA (Rass et al., 2007). These findings emphasize the value of using direct markers of neuronal distress, like DNA damage, as neuropathological markers in AD. They augment the classical histopathological picture achieved by staining for amyloid plaques and tau inclusions by providing an early neuronal vulnerability marker (Chen et al., 2010).

As a consequence of industrial production, a large quantity of toxic material is released in the ambient. Due to the elevated concentrations of metals present in different environments, metals are ubiquitous contaminants of ecosystems; therefore, they are among the most intensely studied contaminants. They do not only deteriorate the physicochemical equilibrium of the ecosystems, but they also disrupt the food web and bring about morphological, physiological and cytogenetic changes in the inhabitants (Boge & Roche, 1996). Genotoxic studies have shown that exposure to some metals causes adverse effects to different organisms, especially to humans, and these DNA damages may be implicated in the pathogenesis of some types of cancer and neurodegenerative diseases.

5.1 Genotoxicity of aluminum

Metal-induced genotoxicity is an important pathogenic mechanism whereby toxic metals that riches the nucleus affect the normal structure and function of the genome (Alexandrov et al., 2005; Lukiw, 2001; Sarkander et al., 1983).

There are only few studies in the literature about the genotoxic activities of Al, both in vitro and in vivo. Aluminum is biochemically attracted to interact to the phosphates that form an active part of the DNA. Its mutagenic potential has been studied by micronucleus assay, sister chromatid exchange, Ames and chromosomal aberration analysis, showing a significant genotoxicity in vitro (Banasik et al., 2005; Lankoff et al., 2006). Also, in vivo studies revealed that aluminum could induce in a dose-dependent manner an increase chromosomal aberrations (Roy et al., 1991).

In vitro chromosomal aberrations induction, mostly numeric (anaphasic), was shown first by Moreno et al., (1997), in the Balb c 3T3 cell line exposed to atmospheric dust (20–80 mg/mL), a mixture of particles of potassium aluminum silicates (98%) and sodium dioxide (2%), from Mexicali, Mexico. Other studies (Dovgaliuk et al., 2001a, 2001b) also demonstrated the cytogenetic effects of toxic metal salts including aluminum (Al[NO3]3) in meristematic cells from Allium cepa and the clastogenic and aneugenic effects (disturbances in mitosis and cytokinesis) in these cells.

More recently, the genotoxic potencial of AlCl3 on Vicia faba was investigated using cytogenetic tests, demonstrating that aluminum causes significant increase in the frequencies of micronuclei and anaphase chromosome aberrations in the root cells of Vicia faba (Yi et al., 2009).

Iron and aluminum-sulfate together, at nanomolar concentrations, trigger the release of reactive oxygen species (ROS) in cultures of human brain cells, up-regulating pro-inflammatory and pro-apoptotic genes that redirect cellular fate toward cytoplasmic dysfunction, nuclear DNA fragmentation and cell death (Alexandrov et al., 2005; Lukiw, 2001; Sarkander et al., 1983).

On neural cells from Parkinson´s disease patients, Al treatment did not increase the micronucleus frequency, indicating that Al had no amplified mutagenic effect on these patients (Trippi et al., 2001). Also, chromosome breaks were observed in V79-4 Chinese hamster cells irradiated with low-energy aluminum ions (Botchway et al., 1997). Furthermore, no teratogenic effects on the mouse fetus or genotoxic effects as detected by the Ames assay was observed for aluminum-containing cosmetic formulations (Elmore, 2003).

Lukim & Pogue (2007) first described the neurotoxic effects of aluminum-sulfate and aluminum- plus iron-sulfate on miRNA expression patterns in untransformed human brain cells in primary co-cultures of neurons and glia. Low doses of aluminum have been found to disturb RNA Pol II-directed gene transcription in isolated human brain cell nuclei (Alexandrov et al., 2005; Lukiw, 2001) suggesting an involvement of soluble aluminum- and iron-sulfate in several different aspects of human brain gene expression, specially associated with transcriptional and post-transcriptional control. Synapsin mRNA has been found to be down-regulated in both AD brain and in iron- plus aluminum-sulfate treated primary cell culture (Alexandrov et al., 2005; Lukiw, 2007; Yumei et al., 1998).

On the other hand, studies have demonstrated the mutagenic potential of Al in human cells. For example, genotoxicity of the dust derived from an electrolytic Al plant was evaluated using the Ames assay, unscheduled DNA synthesis test, sister chromatid exchange and micronuclei frequencies in human lymphocytes. The results of these four experiments indicated a high genotoxicity potential of the dust organic extract (Varella et al., 2007). The mutagenic activity of waste material originating from an Al products factory was determined by the Salmonella/microsome assay, where all extracts from the factory had mutagenic activity, especially in the YG1024 yeast strain, suggesting the presence of aromatic amines (WHO, 1997).

Scalon et al (2011) assessed the genotoxic effects in fish exposed to samples from the Sinos River (Rio Grande do Sul - Brazil), and evaluated DNA damage from aluminum, lead, chromium, copper, nickel, iron and zinc contamination. They collected samples of different sites and on differente seasons in the Sinos River, and chemical analysis of the water showed presence of Al and Fe, exceeding the accepted limits in most of the water samples. The index of DNA damage assessed by the comet assay in the peripheral blood of a native fish species demonstrated no significant differences in different seasons or at the different sampling sites. Only the frequency of cells with higher level of DNA damage showed significant difference in comparison to the sampling period. However, the increase in that parameter of genotoxicity does not seem to be related to differences between sampling periods regarding the presence or concentration of the heavy metals analysed.

Garcia-Medina et al (2011) evaluated de genotoxic and cytotoxic effects of Aluminum sulphate on common carp (Cyprinus carpio). They exposed the fishes to 0.05, 120, and 239 mg/L $Al_2 (SO_4)_3 \cdot 7H_2O$ and analysed the cells with the comet assay, flow cytometry, and the TUNEL method. The analyzed cells showed significant increase in the amount of DNA, damage, DNA content increase and ploidy modifications, as well as apoptosis and disturbances of the cell cycle progression and an increase in the amount of apoptotic cells. These results suggests, in a contrary way to the study of Scalon et al (2011), that Al caused deleterious DNA and cellular effects in aquatic organisms.

Recently our research group published a study on the genotoxic, clastogenic and cytotoxic effects of AlCl3 in different phases of the cell cycle using in vitro temporary cultures of human lymphocytes (Lima et al., 2007). Moreover, the mitotic index (MI), chromosomal aberrations (CAs) and DNA damage index were analyzed by the comet assay. The study indicated that AlCl3 induces DNA damage and is cytotoxic during all phases of the cell cycle. Also, the treatment of the cells at G1 phase resulted in polyploidy and endoreduplication, consistent with AlCl3 interacting with the mitotic spindle apparatus (Lima et al., 2007). These data, along with the results of other studies reported in the literature, indicates that AlCl3 is genotoxic and should be used with caution.

More research is needed on this topic, since the use of aluminum cookware, aluminum-containing deodorants and other products are increasing in general population. Moreover, environmental metal contamination contributes with the increase levels of metal exposure (Ansari et al., 2004).

5.2 Genotoxicity of iron

Several studies have been conducted to demonstrate the potential induction of DNA aberrations by iron (Fe) and also by drugs and compounds containing this metal. However, the results are inconclusive, and its toxicity and mutagenic effect is still incompletely understood.

Organic Fe may increase the genotoxic effects of other compounds when they are combined (WHO, 1998). For example, the mutagenic activity by doxorubicin is significantly increased within this metal, as evaluated by the Ames test (Kostoryz & Yourtee, 2001). Furthermore, Jurkat cells simultaneously treated with hydrogen peroxide and desferrioxamine (Fe chelator) significantly inhibit DNA damage, indicating that intracellular Fe, which is a redoxactive metal, plays a role in the induction of DNA strand breaks induced by hydrogen peroxide (Barbouti et al., 2001).

High levels of chromosome and chromatid aberrations were found in human lymphocytes and TK6 lymphoblast cells exposed to high-energy iron ions (56Fe) (Durante et al., 2002; Evans et al., 2001, 2003). Significant DNA damage was detected, by microgel electrophoresis, in differentiated human colon tumor cells (HT29 clone 19A) treated with ferric-nitrilotriacetate (Fe-NTA) (Glei et al., 2002). Mutagenic activity was also found in elemental and salt forms of Fe, evaluated by mutagenicity tests in Salmonella typhimurium and L5178Y mouse lymphoma cells (Dunkel et al., 1999).

Iron compounds have also been reported to be mutagenic in mammalian cells, as detected by the Syrian hamster embryo cell transformation/viral enhancement assay (Heidelberger et al., 1983), sister chromatid exchange (SCE) in hamster cells (Tucker et al., 1993) and base tautomerization in rat hepatocyte cultures (Abalea et al., 1999).

Few or no DNA damage (detected by the comet assay) occurred after treatment of human lymphocytes with ferric chloride (FeCl3) and ferrous chloride (FeCl2), all of them known to be iron compounds (Anderson et al., 2000a, 2000b). Also, low concentrations of either Fe2+ or Fe3+ were not mutagenic in Chinese hamster ovary cells (CHO-9) treated in vitro, and the mitotic index was also unaffected when compared to negative control. In the other hand, high concentrations of ferrous sulfate, induces significant DNA damage, probably as a consequence of chemical contamination of the metal salt (Antunes et al., 2005).

Mutagenic potential of metallic agents used in dietary supplementation, including iron sulfate, was also investigated by means of the comet assay. The authors reported a genotoxic effect of this metal in mouse blood cells after 24 h of treatment, at all tested concentrations (Franke et al., 2006). Genotoxic effects of Fe were also reported by Garry et al. (2003) in rats treated with iron oxide (Fe_2O_5) for 24 h. They observed that this metal only showed mutagenic potential when the animals were simultaneously treated with benzopyrene.

Furthermore, Hasan et al. (2005) reported that ferritin, an ubiquitously distributed iron storage protein, interacts with microtubules in vitro. In a study conducted by Maenosono et al. (2007) the bacterial reverse mutation assay using S. typhimurium was weakly positive for water-soluble FePt nanoparticles capped with tetramethylammonium hydroxide. Mice subchronically exposed to 33.2 mg/Kg Fe displayed genotoxic effects in whole blood in the alkaline version of the comet assay, with a significant increase in the hepatic level of Fe (Prá et al., 2008).

High-energy iron ions (LET=151 keV/microM) could induce chromosomal aberrations (measured using the fluorescence whole-chromosome painting technique) in normal and repair-deficient human fibroblasts cell lines (George et al., 2009).

Park & Park (2011) screened the potential toxicity of various iron-overloads on human leukocytes using comet assay. Ferric-nitrilotriacetate (Fe-NTA), FeSO(4), hemoglobin and myoglobin were not cytotoxic in the range of 10-1000 microM by trypan blue exclusion assay. The exposure of leukocytes to Fe-NTA (500 and 1000 microM), $FeSO_4$ (250-1000 microM), hemoglobin (10 microM) and myoglobin (250 microM) for 30 min induced significant DNA damage. Iron-overloads generated DNA strand break were rejoined from the first 1h, but no genotoxic effect was observed at 24h.

Recently, our research group conducted an in vitro study aiming to investigate the genotoxic, clastogenic and cytotoxic effects of FeSO4 in different phases of the cell cycle, using short-term cultures of human lymphocytes. The bioactivity parameters tested were the mitotic index, chromosomal aberrations and DNA damage index as detected by the comet assay. Our results showed that Fe induces alterations and inhibition of DNA synthesis, which together explains the concomitant occurrence of mutagenicity and cytotoxicity (Lima et al., 2008).

5.3 Genotoxicity of manganese

Manganese displays an interestingly behavior with regard to its toxicity, since it is relatively non-toxic to the adult organism with an exception to the brain. Even at moderate amounts in a long period of time, when inhaleted can causes Parkinson-like symptoms. Those findings were also observed in animal studies which repeated intravenous Mn administration to monkeys (Olanow et al., 1996) produced a Parkinson-like syndrome characterized by bradykinesia, rigidity, and facial grimacing.

The association of Mn with the risk of developing neurodegenerative processes can be related to DNA damage. Relatively high doses of Mn can disrupt DNA integrity and DNA replication (Beckman et al., 1985; De Meo et al., 1991; Van de Sande et al., 1982) and causes mutations in microorganism (Orgel & Orgel 1965; Rossman et al., 1984; Rossman & Molina, 1986) and mammalian cells although the Ames test does not appear to be particularly responsive to manganese or no suitable to detect toxicity of metal salts (Léonard, 1988).

There are few studies in the literature on the genotoxic action of Mn. Its toxic potential has been studied by in vitro tests in bacteria and by in vivo/in vitro tests in insect and mammalian cells, showing that some chemical forms of this metal have mutagenic potential. Gerber et al. (2002) demonstrated that high doses (0.05 M) of various Mn compounds could affect DNA replication and repair in bacteria. As for mammalian cells, high doses of Mn (compared to the Mn doses recommended for daily consumption) can affect fertilization and are toxic to the embryo and fetus, demonstrating the teratogenic potential of this metal.

Dutta et al. (2006) suggests the manganese dioxide as an established genotoxicant and clastogenic metal that can induce DNA strand breaks, chromosomal aberration and micronucleus in human peripheral lymphocytes. Manganese chloride ($MnCl_2$) was also subjected to the wing spot test of Drosophila melanogaster and was shown to be clearly effective in inducing spots with one or two mutant hairs (small spots) at concentrations over 12 μM (Ogawa et al., 1994).

Concentrations of manganese in the general environment and manufacture products vary widely. Brega et al. (1998) demonstrated that farm workers exposed to pesticides containing Mn, even at a low levels, revealed an increased in the mutagenic potential of those pesticides, as evidenced by an increased number of CAs. It is possible that, at low doses, Mn has genotoxic effects only with long-term exposure, and this may be the reason why Timchenko et al. (1991) did not find CAs in the nasal mucosa of mammals exposed to Mn dioxide aerosol (40–12,000 Hz, 80–100 dB). Furthermore, it is possible that chronic exposure to low doses of Mn can induces CAs over the years.

Studies on eukaryotic cell, revealed that manganese sulfate ($MnSO_4$) did not display mutagenic potential in different strains of Salmonella typhimurium, while, manganese chloride, showed mutagenicity in the TA1537 strain of S. typhimurium as well as in the T7 strain of Saccharomyces cerevisiae (doses over 0.5 mM) (WHO, 1999). In vivo studies have demonstrated that oral doses of manganese sulfate or potassium permanganate (KMnO4) induce CAs in the bone marrow of animals, whereas no CAs have been seemed after oral doses of manganese chloride, even at concentrations over 12 μM (WHO, 1999). These results show that the mutagenic potential of compounds of Mn may be different in permanganate salts and in manganese salts, depending on its chemical formulation, and thus being able to altering their biological availability, activity, and consequently, their toxicity.

De Meo et al. (1991) evaluated the genotoxicity of potassium permanganate ($KMnO_4$), manganese sulfate and manganese chloride using the Ames test within TA97, TA98, TA100 and TA102 strains, with and without metabolic activation. The presence of direct-acting mutagens was detected in all Mn samples in TA102 strain without metabolic activation. Only manganese chloride induced DNA damage in human lymphocytes with a dose-dependent response, as determined by the comet assay.

Animal studies, demonstrated that acute lethality of manganese appears to vary depending on the chemical species. The central nervous system is the chief target of manganese toxicity. Oral doses produced a number of neurological effects in rats and mice, mainly involving alterations in neurotransmitter and enzyme levels in the brain (ATSDR, 2000; Deskin et al., 1980), which can be accompanied to changes in activity level (ATSDR, 2000). Chronic ingestion of manganese (1–2 mg/kg/day) changes appetite and reduces haemoglobin synthesis in different animals (Hurley & Keen, 1987).

Long-term exposure to manganese can cause transient effects on biogenic amine levels and activities of dopamine β-hydroxylase and monoamine oxidase in rat brain (Eriksson et al., 1987; Lai et al., 1984; Nachtman et al., 1986; Subhash & Padmashree, 1990). Also, high doses (1800–2250 mg/kg/day as manganese (II) sulfate) in mice induce hyperplasia, erosion and inflammation in the stomach. Also, number of chromosomal aberrations and micronuclei were observed in rat bone marrow (ATSRD, 2000).
According to WHO (1999) data, other chemical forms of Mn have mutagenic potential, both in vitro and in vivo. Thus, more studies are necessary in order to elucidate the probable mutagenicity of Mn and its chemical forms and their effects on human health.
Erbe et al. (2011) evaluated damage to the genetic material of fish (Astyanax sp. B) exposed to samples of water from a river and a lake located near a hospital waste landfill. Among other parameters, aluminum and manganese were above acceptable levels that have been established in environmental legislation. The comet assay detected significant damage to genetic material in fish that were acutely exposed in the laboratory to these water samples.
Bomhorst et al (2010) evaluated the cytotoxicity and genotoxicity potencial of $MnCl_2$, as well as its impact on the DNA damage response in human cells (HeLa S3) in culture. Whereas up to 10 μM $MnCl_2$ showed no induction of DNA strand breaks after 24 h incubation, manganese strongly inhibited H_2O_2-stimulated poly(ADP-ribosyl)ation at low, completely non-cytotoxic, for certain human exposure, relevant concentrations starting at 1 μM. These results indicate that manganese, under conditions of either overload due to high exposure or disturbed homeostasis can disturb the cellular response to DNA strand breaks, which has been shown before to result in neurological diseases.
Our research group also conducted an in vitro study on the genotoxic, clastogenic and cytotoxic potential of $MnCl_2$-$4H_2O$ (one of the most common forms of Mn) in different phases of the cell cycle, using short-term cultures of human lymphocytes. These effects were determined by the mitotic index (MI), chromosomal aberrations (CAs) and DNA damage index as detected by the comet assay. $MnCl_2$-$4H_2O$ displayed a strong cytotoxicity in all phases of the cell cycle. Genotoxicity was observed at G2 phase of the cell cycle and also in the comet assay, what may be related to the lack of time for the cellular repair system to act. The absence of CAs in the other phases of the cell cycle suggests that Mn-mediated damage may be repaired in vitro (Lima et al., 2008).

6. Conclusion

Metal are essential for humans and for all forms of life. Even though metals are necessary in biological systems, they are usually required only in trace amounts. As regard to the brain, metals are essential for neuronal activities. However, if not correctly regulated, redox-active can react with molecular oxygen to generate ROS thus causing brain tissue damage.
In this chapter, the authors compile several studies that allow to propose that environmental metal exposure are a risk factor for neurodegenerative process. A large quantity of toxic material is released in the ambient as a consequence of industrial production. High-term exposure to certain metals like manganese (Mn), iron (Fe), aluminum (Al) and many others, alone or in combination, can lead to neuronal losts and increase Alzheimer's disease (AD).
In the cellular neurotoxicity, the Al seems to be the most efficient in promoting Aβ aggregation leading to a specific form of Aβ oligomerization that has marked neurotoxic effects. Iron has been found to be accumulated in the substantia nigra and is more related with neurodegenerative disorders, such as Alzheimer's (AD) and Huntington's (HD)

diseases and its severity on cognitive impairment aspect (parietal cortex). As for Mn its toxicity has been associated with dopamine metabolism leading to neuropsychiatric symptoms that resemble idiopathic Parkinson's disease.

Our research group published studies on the genotoxic, clastogenic and cytotoxic effects of Al, MN and Fe in different phases of the cell cycle using in vitro temporary cultures of human lymphocytes. The study indicated that these metals induce DNA damage and is cytotoxic during all phases of the cell cycle. Genotoxic studies have shown that exposure to some metals cause adverse effects to humans and may be implicated in the pathogenesis of some types of neurodegenerative diseases as the AD.

Although is not completely clear the relationship between some metals and neurodegenerative disorders, this chapter suggest that Al, Mn and Fe metals can accelerates neuronal death and increase the risk of its development.

7. References

Abalea, V., Cillard, J., Dubos, M.P., Sergent, O., Cillard, P. & Morel, I. (1999). Repair of iron-induced DNA oxidation by the flavonoid myricetin in primary rat hepatocyte cultures. *Free Radical Biology & Medicine*, Vol. 26, No. 11-12, (Jun. 1999), pp. 1457–1466, ISSN 0891-5849.

Aschner, M., Gannon, M., Kimelberg, H.K. (1992). Manganese uptake and efflux in cultured rat astrocytes. *Journal of Neurochemistry*, Vol. 58, No. 2, (Feb. 1992), pp. 730-735, ISSN 0022-3042.

Alexandrov, P.N., Zhao, Y., Pogue, A.I., Tarr, M.A., Kruck, T.P.A., Percy, M.E., Cui, J.G. & Lukiw, W.J. (2005). Synergistic effects of iron and aluminum on stress-related gene expression in primary neural cells. *Journal of Alzheimer's Disease*, Vol. 8, No. 2, (Nov. 2005), pp. 117–127, ISSN 1387-2877.

Altschuler, E. (1999). Aluminum-containing antacids as a cause of idiopathic Parkinson´s disease. *Medical Hypotheses*, 53, 22-23. Vol. 53, No.1 , (Jul. 1999), pp. 22-23, ISSN 0306-9877.

Anderson, D., Yardley-Jones, A., Hambly, R.J., Vives-Bauza, C., Smykatz-Kloss, V., Chua-Anusorn, W. & Webb, J. (2000). Effects of iron salts and haemosiderin from a thalassaemia patient on oxygen radical damage as measured in the comet assay. *Teratogenesis, Carcinogenesis and Mutagenesis*, Vol. 20, No. 1, (Sep. 2000), pp. 11–26, ISSN 0270-3211.

Anderson, D., Yardley-Jones, A., Vives-Bauza, C., Chua-Anusorn, W., Cole, C. & Webb, J. (2000). Effect of iron salts, haemosiderins, and chelating agents on the lymphocytes of a thalassaemia patient without chelation therapy as measured in the comet assay. *Teratogenesis, Carcinogenesis and Mutagenesis*, Vol. 20, No. 5, (May 2000), pp. 251–264, ISSN 0270-3211.

Ansari, T.M., Marr, I.L. & Tariq, N. (2004). Heavy metals in marine pollution perspective - a mini review. *Journal of Applied Sciences*, Vol. 4, No. 1, (Jan. 2004), pp. 1-20, ISSN 1812-5662.

Antunes, L.M.G., Araújo, M.C.P., Dias, F.L. & Takahashi, C.S. (2005). Effects of H_2O_2, Fe^{2+}, and Fe^{3+} on curcumin-induced chromosoma aberrations in CHO cells. *Genetics and Molecular Biology*, Vol. 28, No. 1, (Jan.-Mar. 2005), pp. 161-164, ISSN 1415-4757.

ATSDR. Toxicological profile for manganese. 2000. Atlanta, GA, US Department of Health and Human Services, Public Health Service, Agency for Toxic Substances and Disease Registry.

Banasik, A., Lankoff, A., Piskulak, A., Adamowska, K., Lisowska, H. & Wojcik, A. (2005). Aluminium-induced micronuclei and apoptosis in human peripheral blood lymphocytes treated during different phases of the cell cycle. *Environmental Toxicology* , Vol. 20, No. 4, (Aug. 2005), pp. 402–406, ISSN 1520-4081.

Banks, W.A., Niehoff, M.L., Drago, D. & Zatta, P. (2006). Aluminum complexing enhances amyloid beta protein penetration of blood–brain barrier. *Brain Research,* Vol. 1116, No.1 , (Oct. 2006), pp. 215-221, ISSN 0006-8993.

Barbouti, A., Doulias, P.T., Zhu, B.Z., Frei, B. & Galaris, D. (2001). Intracellular iron, but not copper, plays a critical role in hydrogen peroxide-induced DNA damage. *Free Radical Biology & Medicine,* Vol., 31, No. 4, (Aug. 2001), pp. 490–498, ISSN 0891-5849.

Barceloux, D.G., (1999). Manganese. *Journal of toxicology. Clinical toxicology,* Vol. 37, No, 2, (1999), pp. 293-307, ISSN 0731-3810.

Bartzokis, G., Mintz, J., Sultzer, D., Marx, P., Herzberg, J.S., Phelan, C.K. & Marder, S.R. (1994). In vivo MR evaluation of age-related increases in brain iron. *American Journal of Neuroradiology,* 15, 1129–1138; Vol. 15, No. 6, (Jun. 1994), pp. 1129-1138, ISSN 0306-9877.

Beauchemin, D., Kisilevsky, R. (1998). A method based on ICP-MS for the analysis of Alzheimer's amyloid plaques. *Analytical Chemistry,* Vol. 70, No.5, (Mar. 1998), pp. 026-1029, ISSN 0003-2700.

Beckman, R.A., Mildvan, A.S. & Loeb, L.A. (1985). On the fidelity of DNA replication: manganese mutagenesis in vitro. *Biochemistry,* Vol. 24, No. 21, (Oct. 1985), pp. 5810–17, ISSN 0006-2960.

Behl, C., Davis, J.B., Lesley, R., Schubert, D. (1994). Hydrogen peroxide mediates amyloid beta protein toxicity. *Cell,* Vol. 17, No. 6, (Jun 1994), pp. 817-827, ISSN 0092-8674.

Berg, D., Gerlach, M., Youdim, M.B., Double, K.L., Zecca, L., Riederer, P. & Becker, G. (2001). Brain iron pathways and their relevance to Parkinson's disease. *Journal of Neurochemistry,* Vol.79 , No. 2, (Oct. 2001), pp. 225-236, ISSN 0022-3042.

Berthon G (1996) Chemical speciation studies in relation to aluminium metabolism and toxicity. *Coordination Chemistry Reviews,* Vol. 149, (1996), pp. 241-280, ISSN 0010-8545.

Berthon, G., (2002). Aluminium speciation in relation to aluminium bioavailability, metabolism and toxicity. *Coordination Chemistry Reviews,* Vol. 228, No. 2, (Jun. 2002), pp. 319-341, ISSN 0010-8545.

Bogé, G. & Roche, H. (1996). Cytotoxicity of phenolic compounds on Dicentrarchus labrax erythrocytes. *Bull Environ Contam Toxicol.,* Vol. 57, No. 2, (Mar. 1996), pp. 171-178, ISSN 0007-4861

Bondy, S. C. (2010). The neurotoxicity of environmental aluminum is still an issue. *NeuroToxicology,* Vol.31, No.5, (Sep. 2010), pp. 575-581, ISSN 0161-813X.

Bornhorst, J., Ebert, F., Hartwig, A., Michalke, B. & Schwerdtle T. Manganese inhibits poly(ADP-ribosyl)ation in human cells: a possible mechanism behind manganese-induced toxicity? *J. Environ. Monit.,* Vol. 12, No. 11, (Nov. 2010), pp. 2062-9, ISSN 1464-0325.

Botchway, S.W., Stevens, D.L., Hill, M.A., Jenner, T.J. & O'Neill, P. (1997). Induction and rejoining of DNA double-strand breaks in Chinese hamster V79-4 cells irradiated with characteristic aluminum K and copper L ultrasoft X rays. *Radiation Research*, Vol. 148, No. 4, (Oct. 1997), pp. 317–324, ISSN 0033-7587.

Brega, S.M., Vassilieff, I., Almeida, A., Mercadante, A., Bissacot, D., Cury, P.R. & Freire-Maia, D.V. (1998). Clinical, cytogenetic and toxicological studies in rural workers exposed to pesticides in Botucatu, São Paulo, Brazil. *Reports in Public Health*, Vol. 14, Suppl. 3, (1998), pp. 109–115, ISSN 0102-311X.

Busser, J., Geldmacher, D.S., Herrup, K. (1998). Ectopic cell cycle proteins predict the sites of neuronal cell death in Alzheimer's disease brain. *The Journal of neuroscience : the official journal of the Society for Neuroscience*, Vol. 18, No 8, (Apr. 1998), pp. 2801-2807, ISSN 0270-6474.

Bush, A.I. (2003). The metallobiology of Alzheimer's disease. *Trends Neuroscience*, Vol. 26, No. 4, (Apr. 2003), pp. 207-214, ISSN 0166-2236.

Butterworth, R. F. (2010). Metal Toxicity, Liver Disease and Neurodegeneration. *Neurotoxicity Research*, Vol. 18 , No. 1, (Apr. 2010), pp. 100-105, ISSN 1029-8428.

Campbell, A., Bondy, S.C. (2000). Aluminum induced oxidative events and its relation to inflammation: a role for the metal in Alzheimer's disease. *Cellular and Molecular Biology*, Vol. 46, No. 4, (Jun. 2000), pp. 721-730, ISSN 1098-5549.

Chen, J., Cohen, M.L., Lerner, A.J., Yang, Y. & Herrup, K. (2010). DNA damage and cell cycle events implicate cerebellar dentate nucleus neurons as targets of Alzheimer's disease. *Molecular Neurodegeneration*, Vol. 5, No. 60, (Dec. 2010), pp.1-11, ISSN 1750-1326.

Cherny, R. A., Legg, J. T., McLean, C. A., Farlie, D.P., Huang, X., Atwood, C.S., Beyreuther, K., Tanzi, R.E., Masters, C.L. & Bush, A.L. (1999). Aqueous dissolution of Alzheimer's disease Aβ amyloid deposits by biometal depletion. *Journal of Biological Chemistry*, Vol. 274 , No. 33 , (Aug. 1999), pp. 23223-23228, ISSN 1083-351X.

Connor, J. R., Benkovic, S. A. (1992). Iron regulation in the brain: histochemical, biochemical, and molecular consider- ations. *Annals of Neurology*, Vol. 32 , No. Suppl (1992), pp. S51-S61, ISSN 0364-5134.

Corain, B., Bombi, G.G., Tapparo, A., Perazzolo, M., Zatta, P. (1996). Aluminium toxicity and metal speciation: established data and open questions. *Coordination Chemistry Reviews*, Vol. 149, (May 1996), pp.11-22, ISSN 0010-8545.

Cox, P.A., (1995). *The elements on earth: inorganic chemistry in the environment*. Oxford University Press, ISBN 0198562411, Oxford, New York.

Crapper, D.R., Krishnan, S.S., Quittkat, S. (1976). Aluminium, neurofibrillary degeneration and Alzheimer's disease. *Brain: a Journal of Neurology*, Vol. 99, No.1, (Mar. 1976), pp. 67-80, ISSN 0006-8950.

De Meo, M., Laget, M., Castegnaro, M. & Dumenil, G. (1991). Genotoxic activity of potassium permanganate in acidic solutions. *Mutation Research*, Vol. 260, No. 3, (Jul. 1991), pp. 295–306, ISSN 0027-5107.

Demougeot, C., Methy, D., Prigent-Tessier, A., Garnier, P., Bertrand, N., Guilland, J.C., Beley, A. & Marie C. (2003). Effects of a direct injection of liposoluble iron into rat striatum. Importance of the rate of iron delivery to cells. *Free Radical Research*, Vol. 37, No.1, (Jan. 2003), pp. 59-67, ISSN 1071-5762.

Dennis, J., Selkoe, M.D. (2000). The Origins of Alzheimer Disease. *Journal of American Medical Association*. Vol. 283, No.12 (2000), pp.1615–1617, ISSN 1538-3598.

Deskin R., Bursian S.J. & Edens F.W. (1980). Neurochemical alterations induced by manganese chloride in neonatal rats. *Neurotoxicology*, Vol. 2, No. 1, (Jan. 1980), pp. 65–73, ISSN 0161-813X.

Donaldson, J., McGregor, D., LaBella, F. (1982). Manganese neurotoxicity: A model of free radical mediated neurodegeneration? *Canadian Journal of Physiology and Pharmacology*, Vol. 60, No. 11, (1982), pp. 1398-1405, ISSN 0008-4212.

Dong, J., Atwood, C.S., Anderson, V.E., Siedlak, S.L., Smith, M.A., Perry, G. & Carrey, P.R. (2003). Metal binding and oxidation of amyloid-beta within isolated senile plaque cores: Raman microscopic evidence. *Biochemistry*, Vol. 42, No. 10, (Mar 2003), pp. 2768-2773, ISSN 0264-6021.

Double K.L., Gerlach M., Youdim M.B., Riederer P. (2000). Impaired iron homeostasis in Parkinson's disease. *Journal of Neural Transmission Supplementum*, 60, 37-58. Vol. 60, No.1, (2000), pp. 37-58, ISSN 0303-6995.

Dovgaliuk, A.I., Kaliniak, T.B. & Blium, I.B. (2001b). Cytogenetic effects of toxic metal salts on apical meristem cells of Allium cepa L. seed roots. *TSitologiia i Genetika*, Vol. 35, No. 2, (Mar./Apr. 2001), pp. 3–10, ISSN 0564-3783.

Dovgaliuk, A.I., Kaliniak, T.B., Blium, I.B. (2001a). Assessment of phytoand cytotoxic effects of heavy metals and aluminum compounds using onion apical root meristem. *TSitologiia i Genetika*, Vol. 35, No. 1, (Jan./Feb. 2001), pp. 3–9, ISSN 0564-3783.

Drago, D., Bettella, M., Bolognin, S., Cendron, L., Scancar, J., Milacic, R., Richelli, R., Casini, A., Messori, L., Tagnon, G. & Zatta, P. (2008). Potential pathogenic role of beta-amyloid(1-42)-aluminum complex in Alzheimer's disease. The International Journal of Biochemistry & Cell Biology, Vol. 40, No. 4, (Oct. 2008), pp. 731-746, ISSN 1357-2725.

Dunkel, V.C., San, R.H., Seifried, H.E. & Whittaker, P. (1999). Genotoxicity of iron compounds in Salmonella typhimurium and L5178Y mouse lymphoma cells. *Environmental and Molecular Mutagenesis*, Vol. 33, No. 1 (Feb. 1999), pp. 28-41, ISSN 0893-6692.

Durante, M., Gialanella, G., Grossi, G., Pugliese, M., Scampoli, P.,Kawata, T., Yasuda, N. & Furusawa, Y. (2002). Influence of the shielding on the induction of chromosomal aberrations in human lymphocytes exposed to high-energy iron ions. *Radiation Research*, Vol. 43, Suppl. S, (Dec. 2002), pp. 107–111, ISSN 0449-3060.

Dutta, D., Devi, S.S., Krishnamurthi, K. & Chakrabarti, T. (2006). Anticlastogenic effect of redistilled cow's urine distillate in human peripheral lymphocytes challenged with manganese dioxide and hexavalent chromium. *Biomedical and Environmental Sciences*, Vol. 19, No. 6, (Dec. 2006), pp. 487-494, ISSN 0895-3988.

Eidelberg, D., Sotrel, A., Joachim, C., Selkoe, D., Forman, A., Pendlebury, W.W. & Perl, D.P. (1987). Adult onset Hallervorden-Spatz disease with neurofibrillary pathology. *Brain*, Vol. 110, No. 4, (Aug. 1987), pp. 993-1013, ISSN 1460-2156.

Elmore, A.R. (2003). Final report on the safety assessment of aluminum silicate, calcium silicate, magnesium aluminum silicate, magnesium silicate, magnesium trisilicate, sodium magnesium silicate, zirconium silicate, attapulgite, bentonite, Fuller's earth, hectorite, kaolin, lithium magnesium silicate, lithium magnesium sodium silicate, montmorillonite, pyrophyllite and zeolite. *International Journal of Toxicology*, Vol. 22, Suppl. 1, (2003), pp. 37–102, ISSN 1091-5818.

Erbe, M.C., Ramsdorf, W.A., Vicari, T. & Cestari, M.M. (2011). Toxicity evaluation of water samples collected near a hospital waste landfill through bioassays of genotoxicity piscine micronucleus test and comet assay in fish Astyanax and ecotoxicity Vibrio fischeri and Daphnia magna. *Ecotoxicology*, Vol. 20, No. 2, (Mar. 2011), pp. 320-328, ISSN 0963-9292.

Eriksson, H., Lenngren, S. & Heilbronn, E. (1987). Effect of long-term administration of manganese on biogenic amine levels in discrete striatal regions of rat brain. *Archives of Toxicology*, Vol. 59, No. 6, (Apr. 1987), pp. 426–431, ISSN 0340-5761.

Evans, H.H., Horng, M.F., Ricanati, M., Diaz-Insua, M., Jordan, R. & Schwartz, J.L. (2001). Diverse delayed effects in human lymphoblastoid cells surviving exposure to high-LET (56)Fe particles or low-LET (137)Cs gamma radiation. *Radiation Research*, Vol. 156, No. 3, (Sep. 2001), pp. 259–271, ISSN 0449-3060.

Evans, H.H., Horng, M.F., Ricanati, M., Diaz-Insua, M., Jordan, R. & Schwartz, J.L. (2003). Induction of genomic instability in TK6 human lymphoblasts exposed to 137Cs gamma radiation: comparison to the induction by exposure to accelerated 56Fe particles. *Radiation Research*, Vol. 159, No. 6, (Jun. 2003), pp. 737–747, ISSN 0449-3060.

Ferrer, A. (2003). Metal poisoning. *Anales del Sistema Sanitario de Navarra*, Vol. 26, pp. 141–153., ISSN 1137-6627.

Florence, T.M., Stauber, J.L. (1989). Manganese catalysis of dopamine oxidation. *The Science of the Total Environment*, Vol. 78, No. 1, (Jan. 1989), pp. 233-240, ISSN 0048-9697.

Franke, S.I.R., Prá, D., Giulian, R., Dias, J.F., Yoneama, M.L., Silva, J., Erdtmann, B. & Henriques, J.A.P. (2006). Influence of orange juice in the levels and in the genotoxicity of iron and copper. *Food and Chemical Toxicology* , Vol. 44, No. 3, (Mar. 2006), pp. 425–435, ISSN 0278-6915.

García-Medina, S., Razo-Estrada, C., Galar-Martinez, M., Cortéz-Barberena, E., Gómez-Oliván, L.M., Alvarez-González, I. & Madrigal-Bujaidar, E. (2011). Genotoxic and cytotoxic effects induced by aluminum in the lymphocytes of the common carp (Cyprinus carpio). *Comp. Biochem. Physiol. C. Toxicol. Pharmacol.* Vol. 153, No. 1, (Jan 2011), pp. 113-118, ISSN 1532-0456.

Garruto, R.M., Shankar, S.K., Yanagihara, R., Salazar, A.M., Amyx, H.L., Gajdusek, D.C. (1989). Low- calcium, high-aluminum diet-induced motor neuron pathology in cynomolgus monkeys. *Acta Neuropathologica (Berl)*, Vol. 78, No. 2, (1989), pp. 210-219, ISSN: 0001-6322.

Garry, S., Nesslany, F., Aliouat, E., Haguenoer, J.M. & Marzin, D. (2003). Hematite (Fe(2)O(3)) enhances benzo[a]pyrene genotoxicity in endo-tracheally treated rat, as determined by Comet Assay. *Mutation Research*, Vol. 538, No. 1-2, (Jul. 2003), pp.19–29, ISSN 13835742.

George, K.A., Hada, M., Jackson, L.J., Elliott, T., Kawata, T., Pluth, J.M. & Cucinotta, F.A. (2009). Dose response of gamma rays and iron nuclei for induction of chromosomal aberrations in normal and repair-deficient cell lines. *Radiation Research*, Vol. 171, No. 6, (Jun. 2009), pp. 752-63, ISSN 0033-7587.

Gerber, G.B., Leonard, A. & Hantson, P. (2002). Carcinogenicity, mutagenicity and teratogenicity of manganese compounds. *Critical Reviews in Oncology/Hematology*, Vol. 42, No. 1, (Apr. 2002), pp. 25–34 ISSN 1040-8428.

Gerlach, M., Double, K.L., Youdim, M.B., Riederer, P. (2006). Potential sources of increased iron in the substantia nigra of parkinsonian patients. *The Journal of* Neural Transmission Supplementa, Vol. 70, No. 1, (2006), pp. 133-142, ISSN: 0303-6995.

Ghetti, B., Musicco, M., Morton, J., Bugiani, O. (1985). Nerve cell loss in the progressive encephalopathy induced by aluminum powder: A morphologic and semiquantitative study of the Purkinje cells. *Neuropathology and Applied Neurobiology*, Vol. 11, No. 1, (Jan. - Feb. 1985), pp. 31-53, ISSN: 0305-1846.

Glei, M., Latunde-Dada, G.O., Klinder, A., Becker, T.W., Hermann, U., Voigt, K. & Pool-Zobel, B.l. (2002). Iron-overload induces oxidative DNA damage in the human colon carcinoma cell line HT29 clone 19A. *Mutation Research*, Vol. 519, No. 1-2, (Aug. 2002), pp. 151–161, ISSN 0027-5107.

Good, P.F., Olanow, C.W., Perl, D.P. (1992). Neuromelanin- containing neurons of the substantia nigra accumulate iron and aluminum in Parkinson's disease: a LAMMA study. *Brain Research*, Vol. 593, No. 2, (Oct. 1992), pp. 343-346, ISSN 0006-8993.

Griffiths, P.D., Dobson, B.R., Jones, G.R. & Clarke, D.T. (1999). Iron in the basal ganglia in Parkinson's disease. An in vitro study using extended X-ray absorption fine structure and cryo-electron microscopy. *Brain*, Vol. 122, No. 4, (Nov. 1999), pp. 667-673, ISSN 1460-2156.

Guilarte T. R. (2010.) "APLP1, Alzheimer's-like pathology and neu- rodegeneration in the frontal cortex of manganese-exposed non-human primates". *NeuroToxicology*, Vol.31, No.5, (Sep. 2010), pp. 572-574, ISSN:0161-813X.

Gupta, V.B., Anitha, S., Hegde, M.L., Zecca, L., Garruto, R.M., Ravid, R., Shankar, S.K., Stein, R., Shanmugavelu, P., Jagannatha Rao, K.S. (2005). Aluminium in Alzheimer's disease: are we still at a crossroad? *Cellular and Molecular Life Sciences*, Vol. 62, No.2, (Jan. 2005), pp. 143-158, ISSN 1420-682X.

Guy, S.P., Jones, D., Mann, D.A.M, Itzhaki, R.F. (1991). Human neuroblastoma cells treated with aluminium express an epitope associated with Alzheimer's disease neurofibrillary tangles. *Neuroscience Letters*, Vol. 121, No. 1-2, (Jan. 1991), pp. 166-168, ISSN 0304-3940.

Hardy, J., Selkoe., D.J. (2002). The amyloid hypothesis of Alzheimer's disease: Progress and problems on the road to therapeutics. Science, Vol. 297 , No. 5580 (Jul. 2002), pp. 353-356, ISSN: 1095-9203.

Hasan, M.R., Morishima, D., Tomita, K., Katsuki, M. & Kotani, S. (2005). Identification of a 250 kDa putative microtubule-associated protein as bovine ferritin. Evidence for a ferritin–microtubule interaction. *The FEBS Journal*, Vol. 272, No. 3, (Dec. 2005), pp. 822–831, ISSN 0014-2956.

Hegde, M. L., Hegde, P. M., Holthauzen, L.M.F., Hazra, T. K., Rao, K. S.J., Mitra, S. (2010). Specific inhibition of NEIL-initiated repair of oxidized base damage in human genome by copper and iron: potential etiological linkage to neurodegenerative diseases. *The Journal of Biological Chemistry*, Vol. 285, No. 37, (Jul. 2010), pp. 28812-28825, ISSN 0021–9258.

Heidelberger, C., Freeman, A.E., Pienta, R.J., Sivak, A., Bertram, J.S., Casto, B.C., Dunkel, V.C., Francis, M.W., Kakunaga, T., Little, J.B. & Schechtman, L.M. (1983). Cell transformation by chemical agents - a review and analysis of the literature. A report of the US Environmental Protection Agency Gene-Tox Program. *Mutation Research*, Vol. 114, No. 3, (Apr. 1983), pp. 283–385, ISSN 0027-5107.

Hollenberg P.F. (2010). Introduction: Mechanisms of Metal Toxicity. *Chemical Research in Toxicology*, Vol. 23, No. 15, pp. 292–293, ISSN 0893-228X.

House, E., Collingwod, J., Khan, A., Korchazkina, O., Berthon, G., Exley, C. (2004). Aluminium, iron, zinc and copper influence the *in vitro* formation of amyloid fibrils of Abeta42 in a manner which may have consequences for metal chelation therapy in Alzheimer's disease. *Journal Alzheimer's Disease*, 6: 291-301 Vol. 6, No. 3, (Jun. 2004), pp. 291-301, ISSN 1387-2877.

Hurley, L.S., Keen, C.L. (1987). Manganese. In: *Trace elements in human and animal nutrition*, W. Mertz, (Ed.), Vol. 1. pp. 185–223, Academic Press, New York, NY.

International Labour Organization (ILO), (1997). Encyclopaedia of occupational health and safety. Metals: chemical properties and toxicity. 4th ed. Geneve, 6368 pp, ISBN 978-92-2-109816-4.

Iwami, O., Watanabe, T., Moon, C.S., Nakatsuka, H. & Ikeda, M. (1994). Motor neuron disease on the Kii Peninsula of Japan: excess manganese intake from food coupled with low magnesium in drinking water as a risk factor. *The Science of the Total Environment*, 149(1-2), 121-35. Vol.149, No.1-2, (Jun. 1994), pp. 121-135, ISSN 0048-9697.

Kawahara, M., Muramoto, K., Kobayashi, K., Mori, H. & Kuroda Y., (1994). Aluminum promotes the aggregation of Alzheimer's amyloid beta- protein *in vitro. Biochemical and Biophysical Research* Communication, Vol. 198, No. 2, (Jan. 1994), pp. 531-535, ISSN 0006-291X.

Kawahara, M., Kato, M., Kuroda, Y. (2001). Effects of aluminium on the neurotoxicity of primary cultured neurons and on the aggregation of beta-amyloid protein. *Brain Research Bulletin*, Vol. 55, No. 2, (May 2001), pp. 211-217, ISSN 0361-9230.

Kell, D. B., Towards a unifying, systems biology understand- ing of large-scale cellular death and destruction caused by poorly liganded iron: Parkinson's, Huntington's, Alzheimer's, prions, bactericides, chemical toxicology and others as examples. *Archives of Toxicology*, Vol. 84, No. 11, (Nov. 2010), pp. 825-889, ISSN 1432-0738.

Kontush, A., Berndt, C., Weber, W., Akopyan, V., Arlt, S., Schippling, S. & Beisiegel, U. (2001). Amyloid-beta is an antioxidant for lipoproteins in cerebrospi- nal fluid and plasma. *Free Radical Biology & Medicine*, Vol. 30, No.1, (Dec. 2001), pp. 119-128, ISSN 0891-5849.

Kostoryz, E.L. & Yourtee, D.M. (2001). Oxidative mutagenesis of doxorubicin–Fe(III) complex. *Mutation Research*, Vol. 490, No. 2, (Feb. 2001), pp. 131–139, ISSN 0027-5107.

Kruman, I.I., Wersto, R.P., Cardozo-Pelaez, F., Smilenov, L., Chan, S.L., Chrest, F.J., Emokpae, R., Gorospe, M., Mattson, M.P. (2004). Cell cycle activation linked to neuronal cell death initiated by DNA damage. *Neuron*, Vol. 41, No 4, (Feb. 2004), pp. 549-561, ISSN 1097-4199.

Kumar, V., Gill, K.D. (2009). Aluminium neurotoxicity: neurobehavioural and oxidative aspects. *Archives of Toxicology*, Vol. 83, No. 11, (Nov. 2009), pp. 730-735. ISSN 0340-5761.

LaFerla, F. M., Green, K. N. Oddo, S. (2007). Intracellular amyloid-β in Alzheimer's Disease. *Nature Reviews Neuroscience*, Vol. 7 No. 8 (Jul. 2007), pp. 499- 509, ISSN 1471-003X.

Lai, J.C., Leung T.K. & Lim L. (1984). Differences in the neurotoxic effects of manganese during development and aging: Some observations on brain regional neurotransmitter and non- neurotransmitter metabolism in a developmental rat model of chronic manganese encephalopathy. *NeuroToxicology*, Vol. 5, No. 1, (spring 1984), pp. 37–47, ISSN 0161-813X.

Lan, J., Jiang, D.H. (1997). Excessive iron accumulation in the brain: a possible potential risk of neurodegeneration in Parkinson´s disease. *Journal of Neural Transmission*, Vol. 104, No. 6-7, (1997), pp. 649-660, ISSN 0300-9564.

Lankoff, A., Banasik, A., Duma, A., Ochniak, E., Lisowska, H., Kuszewski, T., Góźdz, S. & Wojcik A. (2006). A comet assay study reveals that aluminium induces DNA damage and inhibits the repair of radiation-induced lesions in human peripheral blood lymphocytes. *Toxicology Letters*, Vol. 161, No. 1, (Feb. 2006), pp. 27–36, ISSN 0378-4274.

Lapresle, J., Duckett, S., Galle, P., Cartier, L. (1975). Clinical, anatomical and biophysical data on a case of encephalopathy with aluminum deposition. *Comptes rendus des séances de la Société de biologie et de ses filiales*, Vol. 169, No. 2, (1975), pp. 282-285, ISSN 0037-9026.

Lee, D.W. Andersen, J.K. (2010). Iron elevations in the aging Parkinsonian brain: a consequence of impared iron homeostasis? *Journal of Neurochemistry*, Vol. 112, No. 2, (Jan. 2010), pp. 332-339. ISSN 0022-3042.

Léonard A. (1988). Mechanisms in metal genotoxicity: the significance of in vitro approaches. *Mutation Research*, Vol. 198, No. 2, (Apr. 1988), pp. 321–6, ISSN 1383-5742.

Li, H., Campbell, A., Ali, S.F., Cong, P., Bondy, S.C. (2008). Chronic exposure to low levels of aluminum alters cerebral cell signaling in response to acute MPTP treatment. Toxicology and Industrial Health, Vol. 23, No. 2, (Jan. 2008), pp. 515-524, ISSN 0748-2377.

Liu G., Huang W., Moir R. D., Vanderburg, C.R,, Lai, B., Peng, Z., Tanzi, R.E., Rogers, J.T. & Huang, X. (2006). Metal exposure and Alzheimer's pathogenesis. *Journal of Structura Biology*, Vol. 155, No. 1, (Jul. 2006), pp. 45-51, ISSN 1047-8477.

Lima, P.D., Leite, D.S., Vasconcellos, M.C., Cavalcanti, B.C., Santos, R.A., Costa-Lotufo, L.V., Pessoa, C., Moraes, M.O. & Burbano, R.R. (2007). Genotoxic effects of aluminum chloride in cultured human lymphocytes treated in different phases of cell cycle. *Food and Chemical Toxicology*, Vol. 45, No. 7, (Jul. 2007), pp. 1154–1159, ISSN 0278-6915.

Lima, P.D., Vasconcellos, M.C., Bahia, M.O., Montenegro, R.C., Pessoa, C.O., Costa-Lotufo, L.V., Moraes, M.O. & Burbano, R.R. (2008). Genotoxic and cytotoxic effects of manganese chloride in cultured human lymphocytes treated in different phases of cell cycle. *Toxicology In Vitro*, Vol. 22, No. 4, (Jun. 2008), pp. 1032-1037, ISSN 0887-2333.

Lima, P.D., Vasconcellos, M.C., Montenegro, R.A., Sombra, C.M., Bahia, M.O., Costa-Lotufo, L.V., Pessoa, C.O., Moraes, M.O. & Burbano, R.R. (2008). Genotoxic and cytotoxic effects of iron sulfate in cultured human lymphocytes treated in different phases of cell cycle. *Toxicology In Vitro*, Vol. 22, No. 3, (Apr. 2008) pp. 723-729, ISSN 0887-2333.

Lovell, M.A., Ehmann, W.D., Markesbery, W.R. (1993). Laser mi- croprobe analysis of brain aluminum in Alzheimer's disease. *Annals of Neurology*, Vol. 33, No. 1, (Jan. 1993), pp. 36-42, ISSN 0364-5134.

Lovell, M.A., Robertson, J.D., Teesdale, W.J., Campbell, J.L. & Markesbery, W.R. (1998). Copper, iron and zinc in Alzheimer's disease senile plaques. *Journal of the Neurological Science*, Vol. 158, No. 1, (Jun. 1998), pp. 47-52, ISSN 0022-510X.

Lu, T., Pan, Y., Kao, S.Y., Li, C., Kohane, I., Chan, J., Yankner, B.A. (2004) Gene regulation and DNA damage in the ageing human brain. *Nature*, Vol. 429, No. 6994, (Jun. 2004), pp. 883-891, ISSN 0028-0836.

Lukiw W.J. & Pogue A.I. (2007). Induction of specific micro RNA (miRNA) species by ROS-generating metal sulfates in primary human brain cells. Journal of Inorganic *Biochemistry*, Vol. 101, No. 9, (Sep. 2007), pp. 1265-1269, ISSN 0162-0134.

Lukiw W.J. (2007). Micro-RNA speciation in fetal, adult and Alzheimer'sdisease hippocampus. *Neuroreport*. Vol. 18, No. 3, (Feb. 2007), pp. 297-300, ISSN 0959-4965.

Lukiw W.J. In: Aluminum and Alzheimer's Disease, the Science that Describes the Link. Exley C, (Ed.), pp. 147–168, Elsevier Publishers, London.

Lukiw, W.J. (2001). Aluminum and Gene Transcription in the Mammalian Central Nervous System—Implications for Alzheimer's Disease, In: *Aluminum and Alzheimer's Disease: the Science that Describes the Link,* Exley, C., pp. 147–68, Elsevier Publishers, ISBN, 978-0-444-50811-9, London.

Maynard, C.J., Bush, A.I., Masters, C.L., Cappai, R. & Li, Q.X. (2005). Metals and amyloid beta in Alzheimer's disease. International Journal of Experimental Pathology, Vol. 86, No. 3, (Jun. 2005), pp. 147-159, ISSN 1365- 2613.

Maenosono, S., Suzuki, T. & Saita, S. (2007). Mutagenicity of water-soluble FePt nanoparticles in Ames test. *The Journal of Toxicological Sciences*, Vol. 32, No. 5, (Dec. 2007), pp. 575-579, ISSN 0388-1350.

Mark, R.J., Lovell, M.A., Markesbery, W.R. Uchida, K., Mattson, M.P. (1997). A role for 4-hydroxynonenal, an aldehydic product of lipid peroxidation, in disruption of ion homeostasis and neuronal death induced by amyloid beta-peptide. *Journal of Neurochemistry*, Vol. 66, No. 1, (Jan. 1997), pp. 255-264. ISSN 0022-3042.

Mark, R.J., Pang, Z., Geddes, J.W., Uchida, K. & Mattson, M.P. (1997). Amyloid beta-peptide impairs glucose transport in hippocampal and cortical neurons: involvement of membrane lipid peroxidation. *The Journal of Neuroscience*, Vol. 17, No. 3, (Feb. 1997), pp. 1046-1054, ISSN 0270-6474.

Martin, W.R.W., Wiler, M. (2008). Midbrain iron content in early Parkinson disease. A potential biomarker of disease status. *Neurology*, Vol. 70, No. 16 pt 2, (Apr. 2008), pp. 1411-1417, ISSN 1473-6551.

McLachlan, D.R.C., Bergeron, C., Smith, J.E., Boomer, D. & Rifat, S.L. (1996). Risk for neuropathologically confirmed Alzheimer's disease and residual aluminum in municipal drinking water employing weighted residential histories. *Neurology*, Vol. 46, No. 2, (Apr. 1996), pp. 401-405, ISSN 1473-6551.

Mills, E., Dong, X. P., Wang, F., Xu, H. (2010). Mechanisms of brain iron transport: insight into neurodegeneration and CNS disorders. *Future Medicinal Chemistry*, Vol. 2, No. 1, (2010), pp. 51-64, ISSN 1756-8919.

Miu, A.C., Benga, O. (2006). Aluminum and Alzheimer's disease: a new look. Journal of Alzheimer's disease, Vol. 10, No. 2-3, (Nov. 2006), pp. 179-201, ISSN 1387-2877.

Montgomery, E.B.J. (1995). Heavy metals and the etiology of Parkinson's disease and other movement disorders. *Toxicology,* Vol. 97, No. 1-3, (Mar. 1995), pp. 3-9, ISSN 0300-483X.

Moreno, E.A., Rojas, G.F., Frenk, F.H., De La Huerta, A.O., Belmares, R.Q. & Vargas, A.R.O. (1997). In vitro induction of abnormal anaphases by contaminating atmospheric dust from the City of Mexicali, Baja California, Mexico. *Archives of Medical Research,* Vol. 28, No. 4, (Dec. 1997), pp. 549–53, ISSN 0188-4409.

Morgan, D.M., Dong, J., Jacob, J., Lu, K., Apkarian, R.P., Thiyagarajan, P. & Lynn, D.G. (2002). Metal switch for amyloid formation: insight into the structure of the nucleus. Journal of the American Chemical Society, Vol. 124, No. 43, (Oct. 2002), pp. 12644-12645, ISSN 0002-7863.

Myung, N.H., Zhu, X., Castellani, R.J., Petersen, R.B., Siedlak, S.L., Perry, G., Smith, M.A., Lee, H.G. (2008). Evidence of DNA damage in Alzheimer disease: phosphorylation of histone H2AX in astrocytes. *Age (Dordrecht, Netherlands),* Vol. 30, No 4, (Apr. 2008), pp. 209-215, ISSN 1574-4647.

Nachtman, J.P., Tubben R.E. & Commissaris, R.L. (1986). Behavioral effects of chronic manganese administration in rats: Locomotor activity studies. *Neurobehavioral Toxicology and Teratology,* Vol. 8, No. 6, (Nov. - Dec. 1986), pp. 711–715, ISSN 0275-1380.

Nakano, M. (1993). A possible mechanism of iron neurotoxicity. *European Neurology,* Vol. 33, No. 1, (1993), pp. 44-51, ISSN 0014- 3022.

Nayak, P. (2002). Aluminum: Impacts and Disease. Environmental Research, Vol. 89, No. 2, (Jun. 2002), pp. 101-115. ISSN 0013-9351.

Nayak, P., Chatterjee, A.K. (1999). Biochemical view of aluminum-induced neurohazards. *Journal of environmental biology,* Vol. 20, No. (1999), pp. 77-84, ISSN 0254-8704.

Newland, M.C., Ceckler, T.L., Kordower, J.H., Weiss, B. (1989). Visualizing manganese in the primate basal ganglia with magnetic resonance imaging. *Expiremental Neurology,* Vol. 106, No. 3, (Dec. 1989), pp. 251-258. ISSN 0014-4886.

Ogawa, H.I., Shibahara, T., Iwata, H., Okada, T., Tsuruta, S., Kakimoto, K., Sakata, K., Kato, Y., Ryo, H. & Itoh, T. (1994). Genotoxic activities in vivo of cobaltous chloride and other metal chlorides as assayed in the Drosophila wing spot test. *Mutation Research,* Vol. 320, No. 1-2, (Jan. 1994), pp. 133–140, ISSN 0027-5107.

Olanow, C.W., Good, P.F., Shinotoh, H., Hewitt, K.A., Vingerhoets, F., Snow, B.J., Beal, M.F., Calne, D.B. & Perl, D.P. (1996). Manganese intoxication in the rhesus monkey: a clinical, imaging, pathologic, and biochemical study. *Neurology,* Vol. 46, No. 2, (Feb. 1996), pp. 492–8 ISSN 0028-3878.

O´Neil, P., (1994). Major elements in the earth´s crust - Iron. In: *Environmental chemistry 2nd ed.,* Chapman and Hall (Eds.), pp. 151-168, ISBN 0045510865, New York,

Ong, W. Y., Farooqui, A. A. (2005). Iron, neuroinflammation, and Alzheimer's disease. *Journal of Alzheimer's Disease,* Vol. 8, No. 2, (Nov. 2005), pp. 183-200, ISSN 1387-2877.

Orgel A. & Orgel L.E. (1965). Induction of mutations in bacteriophage T4 with divalent manganese. *Journal of Molecular Biology,* Vol. 14, No. 2, (Dec. 1965), pp. 453–457, ISSN 0022-2836.

Park, J.H. & Park, E. (2011). Influence of iron-overload on DNA damage and its repair in human leukocytes in vitro. *Mutat. Res.*, Vol. 718, No. 1-2, (Jan. 2011), pp. 56-61, ISSN 1383-5742.

Park, D.S., Morris, E.J., Padmanabhan, J., Shelanski, M.L., Geller, H.M., Greene, L.A. (1998). Cyclin-dependent kinases participate in death of neurons evoked by DNA-damaging agents. *The Journal of cell biology*, Vol. 143, No. 2, (1998), pp. 457-467, ISSN 540-8140.

Petrik, M.S., Wong, M.C., Tabata, R.C., Garry, R.F., Shaw, C.A. (2007). Aluminum adjuvant linked to Gulf War illness induces motor neuron death in mice. *NeuroMolecular Medicine*, Vol. 9, No. 1, (2007), pp. 89-100, ISSN 1559-1174.

Prá, D., Franke, S.I., Giulian, R., Yoneama, M.L., Dias, J.F., Erdtmann, B. & Henriques, J.A. (2008). Genotoxicity and mutagenicity of iron and copper in mice. *Biometals*, Vol. 21, No. 3, (Jun. 2008), pp. 289-297, ISSN 0966-0844.

Pratico, D., Uryu, K., Sung, S., Tang, S., Trojanowski, J.Q., Lee, V.M. (2002). Aluminum modulates brain amyloidosis through oxidative stress in APP transgenic mice. *The FASEB Journal*, Vol. 16, No. 9, (Jul. 2002), pp. 1138-1140, ISSN 0892-6638.

Prikhojan, A., Brannan, T., Yahr, M.D. (2002). Intrastriatal iron perfusion releases dopamine: an in-vivo microdialysis study. *Journal of Neural Transmission*, Vol. 109, No. 5-6, (May 2002), pp. 645-649, ISSN 1435-1463.

Qiu, W.O., Folstein. M. (2006). Insulin, insulin-degrading enzyme and amyloid-β peptide in Alzheimer's disease: review and hypothesis. *Neurobiology of Aging*, Vol. 27 No. 2 (Feb. 2006), pp. 190–198, ISSN 0197-4580.

Rass, U., Ahel, I., West, S.C. (2007). Defective DNA repair and neurodegenerative disease. *Cell*, Vol. 130, No 6, (Sep. 2007), pp. 130:991-1004, ISSN 0092-8674.

Rauk A. (2009). The chemistry of Alzheimer's disease (AD). Chemical Society Reviews, Vol. 38, No. 9, (Aug. 2008), pp. 2698-2715, ISSN 0306-0012.

Ribes, D., Colomina, M.T., Vicens, P., Domingo, J.L. (2010). Impaired spatial learning and unaltered neurogenesis in a transgenic model of Alzheimer's disease after oral aluminum exposure. *Current Alzheimer Research* , Vol. 7, No. 5, (Aug. 2010), pp. 401-408, ISSN 1567-2050.

Ricchelli F, Drago D, Filippi B, Tognon G, Zatta P. (2005). Aluminum- triggered structural modifications and aggregation of beta- amyloids. Cellular and Molecular Life Sciences, Vol. 62, No. 15, (Aug. 2005), pp. 1724-1733, ISSN 1420-9071.

Riederer, P., Sofic, E., Raush, W.D. (1989). Transition metals, ferritin, glutathione, and ascorbic acid in parkinsonian brain. *Journal of Neurochemistry*, 52, 515-520. Vol. 52, No. 2, (Feb. 1989), pp. 515-520. ISSN 0022-3042.

Rondeau, V., Commenges, D., Jacqmin-Gadda, H., Dartigues, J.F. (2001). Relation between aluminum concentrations in drinking water and Alzheimer's disease: an 8-year follow- up study. *American Journal of Epidemiology*, Vol. 154, No. 3, (Aug. 2001), pp. 159- 166, ISSN 1476-6256.

Rossman T.G. & Molina M., 1986. The genetic toxicology of metal compounds: II. Enhancement of ultraviolet light-induced mutagenesis in Escherichia coli WP2. *Environmental Mutagenesis*, Vol. 8, No. 2, (1986), pp. 263–71, ISSN 0192-2521.

Rossman T.G. & Molina M., Meyer L.W. (1984). The genetic toxicology of metal compounds: I. Induction of lambda prophage in E coli WP2s(lambda). *Environmental Mutagenesis*, Vol. 6, No. 1, (1984), pp. 59–69, ISSN 0192-2521.

Rouault, T. A. (2001). Systemic iron metabolism: a review and implications for brain iron metabolism. *Pediatric Neurology, Journal of Neurochemistry,* Vol. 25, No. 2, (Aug. 2001), pp. 130-137, ISSN 1304-2580.

Roy, A.K., Sharma A. & Talukder, G. (1991). Effects of aluminium salts on bone marrow chromosomes in rats in vivo. *Cytobios,* Vol. 66, No. 265 (1991), pp. 105–11, ISSN 0011-4529.

Santiago, M., Matarredona, E.R., Granero, L., Cano, J., Machado, A. (2000). Neurotoxic relationship between dopamine and iron in the striatal dopaminergic nerve terminals. *Brain Research,* Vol. 858, No. 1, (Mar. 2000), pp. 26-32, ISSN 0006-8993.

Sakae, Y., Shigeo, K., Akihiro, O., Akira, I. (2009). Demonstration of aluminum in amyloid fibers in the cores of senile plaques in the brains of patients with Alzheimer's disease. *Journal of Inorganic Biochemistry,* Vol. 103, No. 11, (Nov. 2009), pp. 1579-1584 ISSN 0162-0134.

Salvador, G.A., Uranga, R.M., Giusto, N.M. (2010). Iron and Mechanisms of Neurotoxicity. *International Journal of Alzheimer's Disease,* Vol. 2011, No. 1, (Dec. 2010), pp. 1-9, ISSN 2090-0252.

Santamaria, A.B., Sulsky, S.I. (2010). Risk assessment of an essential element: manganese. *Journal of Toxicology and Environmental Healt A,* Vol. 73, No. 2, (2010), pp. 128-155, ISSN 1087-2620.

Savory, J., Jagannatha Rao K.S., Huang, Y., Letada, P.R. & Herman, M.M. (1999). Age-related hippocampal changes in Bcl-2:Bax ratio, oxidative stress, redox-active iron and apoptosis associated with aluminium- induced neurodegeneration: increased susceptibility with aging. *NeuroToxicology,* Vol. 20, No. 5, (Oct. 2008), pp. 805-818, ISSN 0161-813X.

Sarkander H.I., Balb, G., Schlosser, H., Stoltenburg, G. & Lux, R.M. (1983). In: *Brain Aging: Neuropathology and Neuropharmacology,* Cervos-Navarro, J. & Sarkander, H.I., pp. 259–274, Raven Press, New York

Sayre, L. M., Zagorski, M. G., Surewicz, W. K., Krafft, G. A. & Perry, G. (1997). Mechanism of neurotoxicity associated with amyloid β deposition and the role of free radicals in the pathogenesis of Alzheimer's disease: a critical appraisal. *Chemical Research in Toxicology,* Vol. 10, No. 5 (May 1997), pp.518–526, ISSN 0893-228X.

Sayre, L. M., Zelasko, D.A., Harris, P.L.R., Perry, G., Salomon, R.G. & Smith, M.A. (1997). 4-Hydroxynonenal-derived advanced lipid peroxidation end products are increased in Alzheimer's disease. *Journal of Neurochemistry,* Vol. 68, No. 5, (May 1997), pp. 730-735. ISSN 0022-3042.

Sayre, L.M., Moreira, P.I., Smith, M.A., Perry, G. (2005). Metal ions and oxida- tive protein modification in neurological disease. Annali dell'Istituto Superiore di Sanità, Vol. 41, No. 2, (2005), pp. 143-164, ISSN 0021-2571.

Scalon, M.C., Rechenmacher, C., Siebel, A.M., Kayser, M.L., Rodrigues, M.T., Maluf, S.W., Rodrigues, M.A. & Silva, L.B. (2010). Evaluation of Sinos River water genotoxicity using the comet assay in fish. *Braz. J. Biol.,* Vol. 70, No. 4 (Suppl), (2010), pp. 1217-22, ISSN 1519-6984.

Schneider, J. S., Decamp, E., Clark, K., Bouquio, C., Syversen, T. & Guilarte, T. R. (2009). Effects of chronic manganese exposure on working memory in non-human primates. *Brain Research,* Vol. 1258, No. 3, (Dec. 2009), pp. 86-95, ISSN 0006-8993.

Sethi, P., Jyoti, A., Singh, R., Hussain, E., Sharma, D. (2008). Aluminium-induced electrophysiological, biochemical and cognitive modifications in the hippocampus of aging rats. *NeuroToxicology*, Vol. 29, No.2, (Nov. 2008), pp. 1069-1079, ISSN 0161-813X.

Sienko, M.J., Plane, R.A., (1977). Elementos de transição II. In: *Química 5 ed*, Sienko, M.J., Plane, R.A. (Eds.), pp. 436-454. São Paulo.

Smith, M. A., Tabaton, M., Perry, G. (1996). Early contribution of oxidative glycation in Alzheimer disease. *Neuroscience Letters*, Vol. 217, No. 2-3, (Oct. 1996), pp. 210-211, ISSN 0304-3940.

Smith, M. A., Harris, P. L. R., Sayre, L. M., Perry, G. (1997) Iron accumulation in Alzheimer disease is a source of redox- generated free radicals. *Proceedings of the National Academy of Sciences of the United States of America*, Vol. 94, No. 18, (Sep. 1997), pp. 9866-9868, ISSN 0027-8424.

Sriram, K., Lin G.X., Jefferson, A.M., Roberts, J.R., Chapman, R.S., Chen, B.T., Soukup, J.M., Ghio, A.J. & Antonini, J.M. (2010). Dopaminergic neurotoxicity following pulmonary exposure to manganese-containing welding fumes. *Archives of Toxicology*, Vol. 84, No. 7, (Jul. 2010), pp. 521-540, ISSN 0340-5761.

Stankiewicz, J.M., Brass, S.D. (2009). Role of iron in neurotoxicity: a cause for concern in the elderly? *Current Opinion in Clinical Nutrition and Metabolic Care*, Vol. 12, No. 1, (Jan. 2009), pp. 22-29, ISSN 1363-1950.

Su, B., Wang, X., Nunomura, A., Moreira, P.I., Lee, H.-gon, Perry, G., Smith, M.A. & Zhu., X. (2008). Oxidative Stress Signaling in Alzheimer's Disease. *Current Alzheimer Research*, Vol. 5, No. 6, (Dec. 2008), pp.525-532, ISSN 1567-2050.

Subhash, M.N. & Padmashree, T.S. (1990). Regional distribution of dopamine β-hydroxylase and monoamine oxidase in the brains of rats exposed to manganese. *Food Chemistry and Toxicology*, Vol. 28, No. 8, (Aug. 1990), pp. 567–570, ISSN 0278-6915.

Suh, S.W., Jensen, K.B., Jensen, M.S., Silva, D.S., Kesslak, P.J., Danscher, G. & Frederickson, C.J. (2000). Histochemically-reactive zinc in amyloid plaques, an- giopathy,and degenerating neurons of Alzheimer's diseased brains. *Brain Research*, Vol. 852, No. 2, (Jan. 2000), pp. 274-278, ISSN 0006-8993.

Sullivan, E. V., Adalsteinsson, E., Rohlfing, T., Pfeffer-baum A. (2009). Relevance of iron deposition in deep gray matter brain structures to cognitive and motor on performance in healthy elderly men and women: exploratory findings. *Brain Imaging and Behavior, Journal of Neurochemistry*, Vol. 3, No. 2, (Jun. 2009), pp. 167-175, ISSN 1931-7565.

Suwalsky, M., Ungerer, B., Villena, F., Norris, B., Cardenas, H., Zatta, P., (2001). Effects of AlCl3 on toad skin, human erythrocytes, and model cell membranes. *Brain research bulletin*, Vol. 55, No 2, (May 2001), pp. 205-210, ISSN . 0361-9230.

Terry, R.D., Pena, C. (1965). Experimental production of neurofibrillary degeneration (2) Electron microscopic, phosphatase histochemistry and electron probe analysis. *Journal of Neuropathology and Experimental Neurology*, Vol. 24, No.1, (Apr. 1965), pp. 200-210, ISSN 0022-3069.

Timchenko, O.I., Paran´Ko, N.M., Shantyr, E.E. & Kuz´Menko, S.D. (1991). The cytogenetic effects of separate and combined exposures to a manganese dioxide aerosol and wide-band noise. *Gigiena i Sanitariia*, No. 11, (Nov. 1991), pp. 70–72 , ISSN 0016-9900.

Trippi, F., Botto, N., Scarpato, R., Petrozzi, L., Bonuccelli, U., Latorraca, S., Sorbi, S. & Migliore, L. (2001). Spontaneous and induced chromosome damage in somatic cells of sporadic and familial Alzheimer's disease patients. *Mutagenesis*, Vol. 16, No. 4, (Jul. 2001), pp. 323–327, ISSN 0267-8357.

Troncoso, J.C., Price, D.L., Griffin, J.W. & Perhad, I.M. (1982). Neurofibrillary axonal pathology in aluminum intoxication. *Annals of Neurology*, Vol. 12, No. 3, (Sep. 1982), pp. 278-283, ISSN 0364-5134.

Tucker, J.D., Auletta, A., Cimino, M.C., Dearfield, K.L., Jacobson-Kram, D., Tice, R.R. & Carrano, A.V. (1993). Sister-chromatid exchange: second report of the Gene-Tox Program. *Mutation Research*, Vol. 297, No. 2, (Sep. 1993), pp. 101–180, ISSN 0027-5107.

Van de Sande, J.H., McIntosh, I.P. & Jovin, T.N. (1982). Mn^{2+} and other transition metals at low concentrations at low concentration induce the right-to-left helical transformation of poly d(G–C). *The EMBO Journal*, Vol. 1, No. 7, (1982), pp. 777–782, ISSN 0261-4189.

Varadarajan. S., Yatin, S., Aksenova, M. Butterfield, D.A. (2000). Review: Alzheimer's amyloid beta-peptide-associated free radical oxidative stress and neurotoxicity. *Journal of Structural Biology*, Vol. 130, No. 2-3, (Jun. 2000), pp. 184-208, ISSN 1095-8657.

Varner, J.A., Jensen, K.F., Hovarth, W., Issacson, R.L., (1998). Chronic administration of aluminium fluoride or sodium fluoride to rats in drinking water: Alterations in neuronal and cerebrovascular integrity. *Brain Research*, Vol. 784, No. 16, (Feb. 1998), pp. 284-298, ISSN 0006-8993.

Varella, S.D., Pozetti, G.L., Vilegas, W. & Varanda, E.A. (2004). Mutagenic activity in waste from an aluminum products factory in Salmonella/microsome assay. *Toxicology In Vitro*, Vol. 18, No. 8, (Dec. 2004), pp. 895–900, ISSN 0887-2333.

Veldman, B.A., Widn, A.M., Knoers, N., Pramstra, P., Horstink, M.W., (1998). Genetic and environmental risk factors in Parkinson's disease. *Clinical neurology and neurosurgery*, Vol. 100, No. 1, (Mar. 1998), pp. 295-301, ISSN 0303-8467.

Vidal, L., Alfonso, M., Campos, F., Faro, L.R., Cervantes, R.C. & Duran, R. (2005). Effects of manganese on extracellular levels of dopamine in rat striatum: an analysis in vivo by brain microdialysis. *Neurochemical Research*, Vol. 30, No. 9, (Sep. 2005), pp. 147-1154, ISSN 1573-6903.

Weiss, B. (2010). Lead, Manganese, and Methylmercury as risk factors for neurobehavioral impairment in advanced age. *International Journal of Alzheimer's Disease*, Vol. 2011, No. 27, (Dec. 2010), pp. 1-11 ,ISSN 2090-0252.

Wen-zhen, Z., Wei-de, Z., Wei, W., Chuan-jia, Z., Cheng-yuan, W., Jian-pin, Q., Jian-zhi, W. & Ting, L. (2009). Quantitative MR phase-corrected imaging to investigate increased brain iron deposition of patients with Alzheimer disease. *Radiology*, Vol. 253, No. 2, (Nov. 2009), pp. 497-504, ISSN 1527- 1315.

Willmore, L.J., Rubin, J.J. (1984). The effect of tocopherol and dimethyl sulfoxide on focal edema and lipid peroxidation induced by isocortical injection of ferrous chloride. *Brain Research*, Vol. 296, No. 2, (Apr. 1984), pp. 389-392, ISSN 0006-8993.

Winder, B.S., Salmon, A.G., Marty, M.A. (2010). Inhalation of an essential metal: development of reference exposure levels for manganese. *Regulatory Toxicology and Pharmacology*, Vol. 57, No. 2-3, (Jul. - Aug. 2010), pp. 195-199, ISSN 0273-2300.

Wright, J.A., Brown, D.R. (2008). Alpha-synuclein and its role in metal binding: relevance to Parkinson's disease. *The Journal of Neuroscience Research,* Vol. 86, No. 3, (Feb. 2008), pp. 496-503, ISSN 0360-4012.

World Health Organization (WHO), (1996). Guidelines for drinking - water quality recommendations. 2nd ed. Geneva.

World Health Organization (WHO). (1997). Aluminium. Environmental Health Criteria, N° 194, Geneva.

World Health Organization (WHO). (1998). Trace elements in human nutrition and health.

World Health Organization (WHO), (1999). Manganese and its compounds. Concise International Chemical Assessment Document 12. WHO, Geneva.

Wu, Z., Du, Y., Xue, H., Wu, Y. & Zhou, B. (2010). Aluminum induces neurodegeneration and its toxicity arises from increased iron accumulation and reactive oxygen species (ROS) production. *Neurobiol of Aging.* Jul 29. [Epub ahead of print], ISSN 0197-4580.

Xu J, Chen S, Ahmed SH, Chen H, Ku G, Goldberg MP, Hsu, C.Y. (2001). Amyloid-beta peptides are cytotoxic to oligodendrocytes. *The Journal of Neuroscience,* Vol. 21, No. 1, (Jan. 2001), pp. 1-6, ISSN 0270-6474.

Yang, Y., Mufson, E.J., Herrup, K. (2003). Neuronal cell death is preceded by cell cycle events at all stages of Alzheimer's disease. *The Journal of neuroscience : the official journal of the Society for Neuroscience,* Vol. 23, No. 7, (Apr. 2003), pp. 2557-2563, ISSN 0270-6474.

Yasui, M., Kihira, T., Ota, K. (1992). Calcium, magnesium and aluminum concentrations in Parkinson´s disease. *NeuroToxicology,* Vol. 13, No. 3, (1992), pp. 593-600, ISSN 0161-813X.

Yi, M., Yi, H., Li, H. & Wu, L. (2010). Aluminum induces chromosome aberrations, micronuclei, and cell cycle dysfunction in root cells of Vicia faba. *Environmental Toxicology,* Vol. 25, No. 2, (Apr. 2010), pp. 124-9, ISSN 1520-4081.

Yumei, W., Jinfeng, J., Xiaohong, Z. & Baoshan, Y. (1998). Genotoxicity of the dust organic extract and its fractions derived from an aluminium electrolytic plant. *Toxicology Letters,* Vol. 98, No. 3, (Sep. 1998), pp. 147–153, ISSN 0378-4274.

Yokel, R.A. (1994). Aluminum exposure produces learning and memory deficits, a model of Alzheimer's disease. In: *Toxin-Induced Models of Neurological Disorders,* Woodruff, M.L. and Nonneman, A.J., pp. 301-318, Plenum, ISBN 03064-46146, New York.

Youdim, M. B. H., Fridkin, M., Zheng, H. (2005). Bifunctional drug derivatives of MAO-B inhibitor rasagiline and iron chelator VK-28 as a more effective approach to treatment of brain ageing and ageing neurodegenerative. diseases.*Mechanisms of Ageing and Development,* Vol. 126, No. 2, (Feb. 2005), pp. 317-326, ISSN 0047-6374.

Yumoto, S., Nagai, H., Matsuzaki, H., Matsumura, H., Tada, W., Nagatsma, E., Kobayashi, K. (2001). Aluminium incorporation into the brain of rat fetuses and sucklings. *Brain Research Bulletin,* Vol.55, No. 2, (May 2001), pp. 229-234, ISSN 0361-9230.

Zatta, P.F., Nicolini, M., Corain B. (1991). Aluminum (III) toxicity and blood-brain barrier permeability. In: *Aluminum in Chemistry, Biology and Medicine,* Nicolini, M., Zatta, P.F., Corain, B., pp. 97-12, Cortina International, ISBN 3642105580, Verona.

Zecca, L., Gallorini, M., Schunemann, V., Trautwein, A. X., Gerlach, M., Riederer, P., Vezzoni, P., Tampellini, D. (2001). Iron, neuro- melanin and ferritin content in the substantia nigra of normal subjects at different ages: consequences for iron storage and neurodegenerative processes. *Journal of Neurochemistry*, Vol. 76, No. 6, (Mar. 2001), pp. 1766-1773, ISSN 0022-3042.

Zheng, W., Ren, S., Graziano, J.H., (1998). Manganese inhibits mitochondrial aconitase: a mechanism of manganese neurotoxicity. *Brain Research,* Vol. 799, No. 2, (Jul. 1998), pp. 334-342, ISSN 0006-8993.

5

Impact of Oxidative-Nitrosative Stress on Cholinergic Presynaptic Function

Stefanie A.G. Black and R. Jane Rylett
Molecular Brain Research Group, Robarts Research Institute, Schulich School of Medicine & Dentistry, University of Western Ontario, London, ON Canada

1. Introduction

Cholinergic neurotransmission plays an essential role in a variety of physiological processes in both the central and peripheral nervous systems. Cholinergic neurons use the classical neurotransmitter acetylcholine (ACh) to communicate with their target cells. In the periphery, ACh is the neurotransmitter used at the skeletal neuromuscular junction, at all pre- and postganglionic parasympathetic synapses and at preganglionic sympathetic synapses. In the central nervous system, the actions of ACh are widespread with cholinergic neurotransmission involved in attention, learning and memory, cognition, sleep, wakefulness, and modulation of sensory information (Hasselmo, 2006; Sarter & Parihk, 2005; Woolf & Butcher, 2010). Dysfunction of cholinergic neurotransmission in the central nervous system is apparent in a number of neurological disorders, such as Alzheimer's, Parkinson's, and Huntington's diseases, schizophrenia and amyotrophic lateral sclerosis (Bohnen & Albin, 2010; Mesulam, 2004; Oda, 1999).

Cholinergic neurons innervate almost all areas of the brain, where this can be mediated by either intrinsic interneurons or by extrinsic projection neurons. Cholinergic interneurons localized in the striatum are involved in motor function, cognition, and behavior (Woolf & Butcher, 2010). The basal forebrain, which is comprised of the nucleus basalis of Meynert, medial septum, diagonal band of Broca, the magnocellular preoptic nucleus, and substantia innominata, contains the cell bodies of cholinergic neurons that project to the hippocampus, amygdala, olfactory bulb, and all areas of the cerebral cortex (Woolf & Butcher, 2010). Collectively, basal forebrain cholinergic neuron activity plays a role in attention, learning, memory, perception, and consciousness (Sarter et al., 2003; Woolf, 1998; Woolf & Butcher, 2010). Cholinergic neurons in the mesopontine region (the pedunculopontine and laterodorsal nuclei) project to the thalamus, hypothalamus, basal forebrain, medial frontal cortex, brainstem and spinal cord (Woolf & Butcher, 2010). Descending cholinergic projections from the mesopontine area decrease muscle tone during rapid eye movement sleep while ascending cholinergic projections are involved in cognitive functions and consciousness (Woolf & Butcher, 2010). Cholinergic projections to the interpeduncular nucleus originate from neurons with cell bodies in the medial habenula; these neurons regulate electroencephalogram patterns and rapid eye movement sleep (Woolf & Butcher, 2010).

The cycle of ACh synthesis, storage, release and degradation has been well-characterized at the cellular and molecular levels and is depicted in Figure 1. ACh is synthesized in the cytoplasm of cholinergic neurons from the precursors choline and acetylCoenzyme-A by the enzyme choline acetyltransferase (ChAT), and it is then taken up into synaptic vesicles for storage by the vesicular acetylcholine transporter (VAChT) (Prado et al., 2002). Depolarization of the nerve terminal causes exocytotic fusion of synaptic vesicles with the presynaptic membrane at specialized release sites called active zones (Garner et al., 2000); this is a calcium-dependent process that involves the coordinated actions of many presynaptic proteins such as SNARE and Rab proteins (Sudhof, 2008). When vesicles fuse with the presynaptic membrane, ACh diffuses into the synaptic cleft where it can bind to nicotinic and muscarinic receptors located on both pre- and postsynaptic cells (Gotti et al., 2009; Nathanson, 2008). ACh signalling is terminated by its diffusion away from the synaptic cleft and by its rapid hydrolysis into choline and acetate by acetylcholinesterase (AChE) (Lane et al., 2006). After fusion, synaptic vesicles recycle (S.M. Smith et al., 2008) and are re-filled with neurotransmitter in preparation for another round of depolarization-induced release. The choline derived from ACh hydrolysis is recycled into the presynaptic terminal by the sodium-dependent, high-affinity choline transporter CHT for re-synthesis of ACh (Birks & MacIntosh, 1961; Collier & MacIntosh, 1969; Collier & Katz, 1974; Haga, 1971; Okuda et al., 2000; Yamamura & Snyder, 1972). Mechanistic details of the molecular regulation of these processes in both health and disease are lacking.

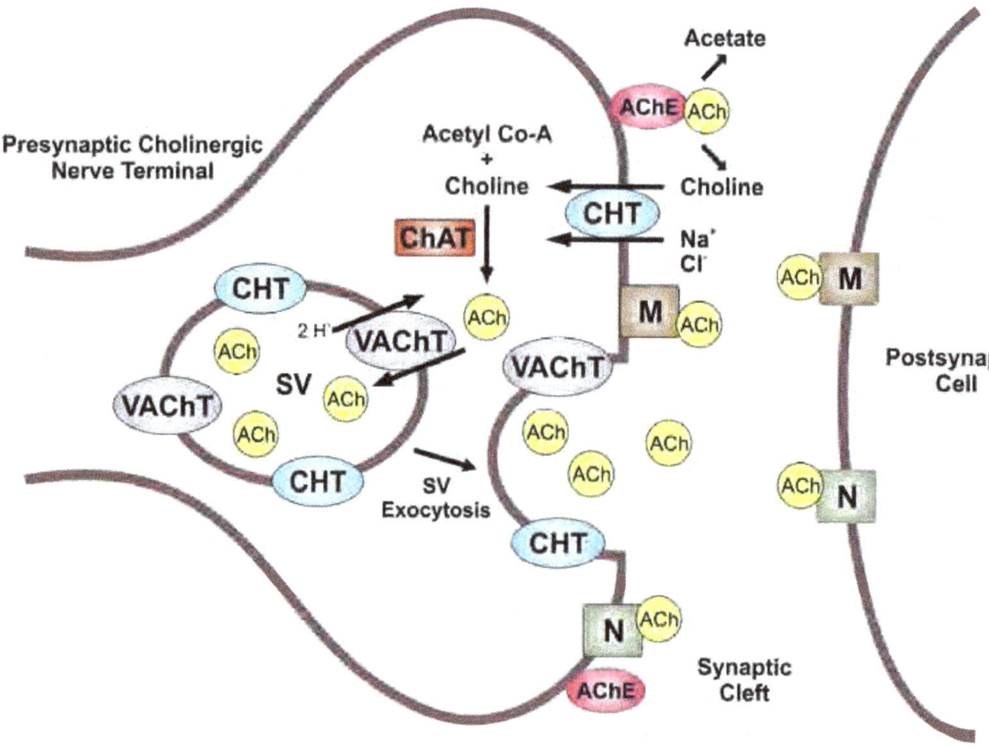

Fig. 1. Mechanisms involved in the synthesis, storage, release and degradation of ACh at the cholinergic synapse. Abbreviations: Acetyl Co-A, acetylCoenzyme-A; ACh, acetylcholine; AChE, acetylcholinesterase; ChAT, choline acetyltransferase; CHT, sodium-dependent, high-affinity choline transporter; M, muscarinic receptor; N, nicotinic receptor; SV, synaptic vesicle; VAChT, vesicular ACh transporter.

Age-related changes in brain that lead to neuronal and vascular pathology frequently compromise synaptic transmission. Many reports associate neurological and cardiovascular diseases with cholinergic neuron dysfunction, and draw parallels between the reduction in cholinergic neurotransmission and cognitive deficits. However, little is known about the actual mechanisms by which these changes impact cholinergic neuron function or the extent to which this can be prevented or reversed. Some of these changes are initiated by oxidative and nitrosative stress which then increases as the pathology progresses. There is also a relationship with altered amyloid precursor protein (APP) metabolism and β-amyloid peptide (Aβ) production that is likely due to changes in the expression or activity of enzymes directing APP into an amyloidogenic pathway. Modified APP/Aβ metabolism is a hallmark of Alzheimer's disease, but is also a result of cardiovascular disease including ischemia (Bennett et al., 2000; Lee et al., 2006; Nihashi et al., 2001; Shi et al., 2000), stroke (Petcu et al., 2008) and hypertension (Gentile et al., 2009; Skoog et al., 1996; Skoog et al., 2006). Age-related increases in soluble oligomeric Aβ acutely modulate synaptic communication at concentrations far below those causing neurodegeneration, and play a central role in Alzheimer's-related synaptic changes (Marcello et al., 2008). The tissue stress response and the generation of reactive oxygen (ROS) and nitrogen species (RNS) in aging brain and early stages of vascular and neuronal disease are attributed partly to increasing Aβ (De Felice et al., 2007). Increased ROS-RNS can initiate changes that result in both reversible and irreversible alterations in protein structure and function. This Chapter focuses on studies of ChAT and CHT structure and function in conditions with altered exposure to ROS-RNS, and the consequences for cholinergic neuron communication related to Alzheimer's disease pathology and potential outcomes related to neuroprotection.

2. Cholinergic neuron function in aging brain

A large literature addresses the role of cholinergic neurons in cognition and attentional processes, and their involvement in Alzheimer's disease (Sarter & Bruno, 1997; Sarter & Bruno, 2004; Schliebs & Arendt, 2006). The current opinion is that while dysfunction of cholinergic neurons is not the cause of this disease, loss of their function is central to changes that occur in brain with normal aging and in a spectrum of disorders that includes mild cognitive impairment (MCI) (Mesulam, 2004). Studies in aging humans and animal models show that some cholinergic pathways have diminished function compared to younger groups. Cognitive decline correlates with elevated oxidative stress in a cohort of normal aging human subjects (Foster, 2006). Also, in aging rats, spatial learning deficits are associated with elevated markers of oxidative stress (Nicolle et al., 2001). However, the small loss of forebrain cholinergic neurons does not relate strongly to cognitive status (McKinney & Jacksonville, 2005) providing compelling evidence that other dynamic cholinergic processes must be affected that are not detected simply by counting the number of neurons.

A comparison of two cholinergic pathways in aged rat brain suggests that neurons in different brain areas can respond differentially to age-related stressors. Basal forebrain cholinergic neurons lose the activity or expression of essential proteins that maintain chemical transmission and their numbers are reduced, whereas brainstem cholinergic neurons in the pontine nuclei are preserved (Baskerville et al., 2006). This is reinforced by the observation that cultured pontine neurons are resistant to ROS-RNS whereas basal forebrain cholinergic neurons are vulnerable (Fass et al., 2000; McKinney et al., 2004). The reasons for this are not known, but age-related oxidative stress in the cortex (Nicolle et al.,

2001) may elevate basal forebrain neuron metabolism. Oxidatively-stressed aged cortex is less responsive to ACh and may compensate for this by requiring enhanced input from basal forebrain neurons thereby causing increased neuron firing rates and/or changes such as increased expression of genes that are involved in energy production (Baskerville et al., 2008; Ongwijitwat et al., 2006; Yang et al., 2006). Alternatively, up-regulation of expression of metabolic genes may be normal and an "adaptive" consequence of aging in basal forebrain neurons that precedes their degeneration (Baskerville et al., 2008). Elevated metabolic activity may also precede increased ROS-RNS levels and, along with pathology such as increased Aβ levels, may mediate their selective vulnerability. It is important to note that basal forebrain cholinergic neurons project to regions with Aβ deposits, whereas pontine cholinergic neurons do not.

A shift in thinking about the timing and nature of changes in cholinergic neuron function in aging and disease came about with reports that ChAT activity is unchanged or even increased in the hippocampus and cortex of subjects with MCI (DeKosky et al., 2002; Ikonomovic et al., 2003; Mufson et al., 2003). This is in sharp contrast to reports of large decreases in cholinergic neuron markers and numbers in Alzheimer's disease (Davies, 1979; Francis et al., 1985; Perry et al., 1977; Rylett et al., 1982; Sims et al., 1983). Mechanisms underlying this apparent increase in cholinergic neuron function are unknown, but it was suggested that basal forebrain cholinergic neurons undergo sprouting in an attempt to maintain neurotransmission or to repair entorhinal cortex damage (Ikonomovic et al., 2003). This has stimulated studies on the functional status of cholinergic neurons in MCI and early Alzheimer's disease; a pivotal study used pharmacological-functional magnetic resonance imaging (fMRI) to document that cholinergic neurotransmission is compromised (Goekoop et al., 2006). It is important to note that most of the studies reported to date have monitored postsynaptic events for insight into the status of cholinergic neurotransmission and to reveal alterations that would result in decreased cholinergic synaptic function and neuron responsiveness in MCI and Alzheimer's disease (Grön et al., 2006). There is a large gap in knowledge about the effects that perturbations such as ROS-RNS, Aβ or altered antioxidant defense mechanisms have on cholinergic presynaptic functions, and the role that this has in compromised neurotransmission. Moreover, most studies have assayed static measures such as neuron numbers or enzyme levels that do not accurately reflect the more dynamic aspects of neurotransmission (Mesulam, 2004), and this may give an incorrect assessment as they do not reveal changes in the capacity for neurotransmitter synthesis and release.

3. Cholinergic neurons have a role in regulation of APP metabolism

A critical link has emerged between cholinergic neurons and APP processing. These neurons are particularly susceptible to the adverse effects of Aβ, and this may partially underlie their vulnerability in amyloidogenic diseases (Auld et al., 1998; Tran el al., 2002). Of note however, cholinergic neurons are also integral in the development of amyloid-based pathology (Auld et al., 1998; Francis et al., 1999; Tran et al., 2002) as they can regulate APP processing and, in turn, Aβ can decrease ACh synthesis and release (Heinitz et al., 2006; Hoshi et al., 1996, 1997; Kar et al., 1996, 1998; Pederson et al., 1996; Pederson & Blusztajn, 1997; Satoh et al., 2001). The stimulation of either nicotinic or muscarinic ACh receptors on cholinoreceptive neurons can promote non-amyloidogenic APP cleavage, thereby potentially decreasing the production of toxic Aβ (Isacson et al., 2002; Seo et al., 2001; Tran et al., 2002; Unger et al., 2005; Verhoeff, 2005). Thus, the activation of either α7- or α4β2-nicotinic receptors (Lahiri et al., 2002; Shimohama & Kihara, 2001; Zamani & Allen, 2001) can decrease Aβ toxicity by protecting neurons through activation of PI3-kinase and increasing levels of Bcl-2 and Bcl-x50. Taken together, the loss of cholinergic neuron innervation may promote Aβ-based pathology, and therapies that would enable cholinergic neurotransmission may indirectly decrease neurodegeneration by reducing Aβ production.

Aβ can assume various physical conformations that may differ in their biological actions. These various Aβ peptides are produced both intracellularly and extracellularly and appear in brain tissue as soluble oligomers and diffusible ligands (Gong et al., 2003; Klein, 2002; Klein et al., 2004) that can aggregate to form insoluble plaques (Kuo et al., 1996; Lue et al., 1999; Walsh et al., 2002a, 2002b; J. Wang et al., 1999). The increased levels of soluble Aβ correlate with synaptic loss and cognitive impairment, and it is now known that synaptic neurotransmission is impacted directly by soluble Aβ with this leading to decreased memory (Klein, 2002). Aβ can bind to a number of different cell surface receptors, modulate synaptic events, lead to generation of ROS-RNS or the release of inflammatory mediators, and disrupt cellular calcium homeostasis (W.W. Smith et al., 2006; Tran et al., 2002). In animal models having chronic delivery of Aβ into rat brain there is increased iNOS expression and disruption of hippocampal cholinergic transmission and memory impairment (Tran et al., 2001).

4. Aβ promotes oxidative stress that can affect neuron function

The inside of cells is normally a reducing environment that maintains proteins in their native reduced states. However, even under these "reducing" conditions some proteins do exist in their *S*-glutathionylated forms (Klatt & Lamas, 2000). Moreover, if ROS-RNS generation exceeds the antioxidant capacity of the cell, then oxidative-nitrosative stress can occur with modification of cellular constituents causing loss of their function. Aβ, particularly the toxic Aβ(1-42), can be involved both directly (Butterfield & Bush, 2004) and indirectly (Lahiri & Greig, 2004) in the generation of ROS-RNS in the brain, thus causing oxidation of lipids and proteins (Qi et al., 2005) and nitration of tyrosine residues in proteins. As it is critical that the oxidative balance inside of the cell is tightly regulated, compensatory mechanisms become upregulated in normal cells that have been exposed to oxidant stress. These adaptive processes are found in the brain, but they can become dysregulated during aging (Mattson & Magnus, 2006) and in pathological states (Mattson, 2004; Zhu et al., 2004). Mitochondria are a source of hydrogen peroxide (H_2O_2), and Aβ in the presence of redox-active ions such as iron and copper can lead to the generation of excess H_2O_2 (Pedersen & Blusztajn, 1997). This ROS may induce cellular damage, particularly by the generation of highly-reactive superoxide radical anion (•O2-) or hydroxyl radical (•OH), the latter being formed in the Fenton reaction in the presence of redox-active iron. However, under some conditions protective mechanisms such as the activation of stress-activated protein kinase (SAPK) pathways are engaged with the induction of downstream antioxidant enzymes (Tamagno et al., 2003). Thus, Aβ alone or in combination with other constituents can lead to the generation of ROS-RNS that can damage macromolecules and result in the modulation of neurotransmission and cause neurotoxicity.

Cholinergic presynaptic function is affected by low levels of Aβ (pM-nM), with the result being decreased pyruvate dehydrogenase activity (Hoshi et al., 1996, 1997), ACh synthesis (Hoshi et al., 1996, 1997; Pederson et al., 1996; Pederson & Blusztajn, 1997) and release (Heinitz et al., 2006; Kar et al., 1996, 1998; Satoh et al., 2001). However, there are conflicting reports on the effects of Aβ on the functions of both ChAT and CHT proteins. Hippocampal ChAT activity is decreased after several days of Aβ administration into rat brain (Nitta et al., 1994, 1997), but this may be due to the loss of neurons rather than to a direct effect on the enzyme. The acute addition of Aβ to neural cells can either reduce ChAT activity (McMillian et al., 1995; Pederson et al., 1996) or have no effect (Hoshi et al., 1996, 1997; Kar et al., 1998); it is difficult to interpret these studies as the Aβ conformation was not determined and it is increasingly clear that the oligomeric, fibrillar or other forms of Aβ have quite different cellular effects. Experiments that involve the use of a variety of model systems indicate that the high-affinity choline uptake activity of CHT can be modulated by Aβ, but the results are also variable. Some reports show that Aβ can actually increase high-affinity choline uptake activity (Bales et al., 2006; Kristofikova et al., 2006), whereas others suggest that Aβ impairs choline uptake (Apelt et al., 2002; Kar et al., 1998; Klingner et al., 2003; Kristofikova et al., 2001, 2008; Opazo et al., 2006; Payette et al., 2007) or that Aβ has no effect on high-affinity uptake of choline (Forgon et al., 1998; Hartmann et al., 2004; Melo et al., 2002). It is known that cholinergic neurochemical function is affected directly by Aβ in a manner that is not related to neuron degeneration, but it is not known to what extent these effects are due to the oxidant stress engaged by increasing Aβ. Unfortunately, for the most part these results are descriptive in nature rather than being mechanistic and do not offer insight into the potential reversibility of the functional changes or information that would be useful for the development of approaches to support cholinergic neuron function.

5. ROS – RNS cause reversible and irreversible modification of proteins

Reactive cysteine (Cys) thiol groups are ionized at physiological pH, and proteins having reactive Cys thiols are found in cells in multiple forms as they are modified by ROS and RNS or form homo- and hetero-protein complexes. Figure 2 shows common modifications that reactive Cys thiols can undergo using ChAT as the model because it is an outstanding example of a protein that has an unusually high number of Cys residues. The modification of reactive Cys thiols during oxidative or nitrosative stress is a key regulator of protein activity (Klatt & Lamas, 2000), and can result in either loss- or gain-of-function (Barrett et al., 1999; Borges et al., 2002; Fukuda et al., 2005; Humphries et al., 2002; Ishii et al., 2005; Jaffrey et al., 2001; Lind et al., 2002; J. Wang et al., 2001). There are cellular mechanisms that protect proteins from irreversible inactivation by oxidation that involve the reversible addition of antioxidant peptides, particularly reduced glutathione (GSH) (Townsend, 2007). The formation of protein-GSH mixed disulphide conjugates can protect vulnerable thiol groups in proteins from further damage during transient oxidative stress (Borges et al., 2002; Jaffreyet al., 2001). A critical point is that protein-GSH mixed disulphide formation is reversible, with the native protein being regenerated as the interior of the cell returns to a more reduced state. However, the more highly oxidized forms of proteins, sulphinic (Pr-SO_2H) and sulphonic (Pr-SO_3H) acids, are not reduced in cells with this leading to irreversible loss-of-function of the target protein. Brain and other tissues can take a double hit during aging by increased ROS–RNS levels and decreased antioxidant mechanisms, with this characterized by a decreased ratio of reduced to oxidized GSH [GSH:GSSG]. This is illustrated in necropsy brain fractions from subjects that were neurologically normal or that had MCI or Alzheimer's disease. The effects of oxidative stress were localized mostly to synaptic regions, with the largest changes seen in presynaptic [synaptosome] fractions as significant decreases in antioxidant levels and increases in markers of oxidative damage (Ansari & Scheff, 2010). These changes occurred early in the disease and the free radical burden increased as an active persistent process in aging and disease (Ansari & Scheff, 2010). Similar findings are seen in aging rodents (Gilmer et al., 2010).

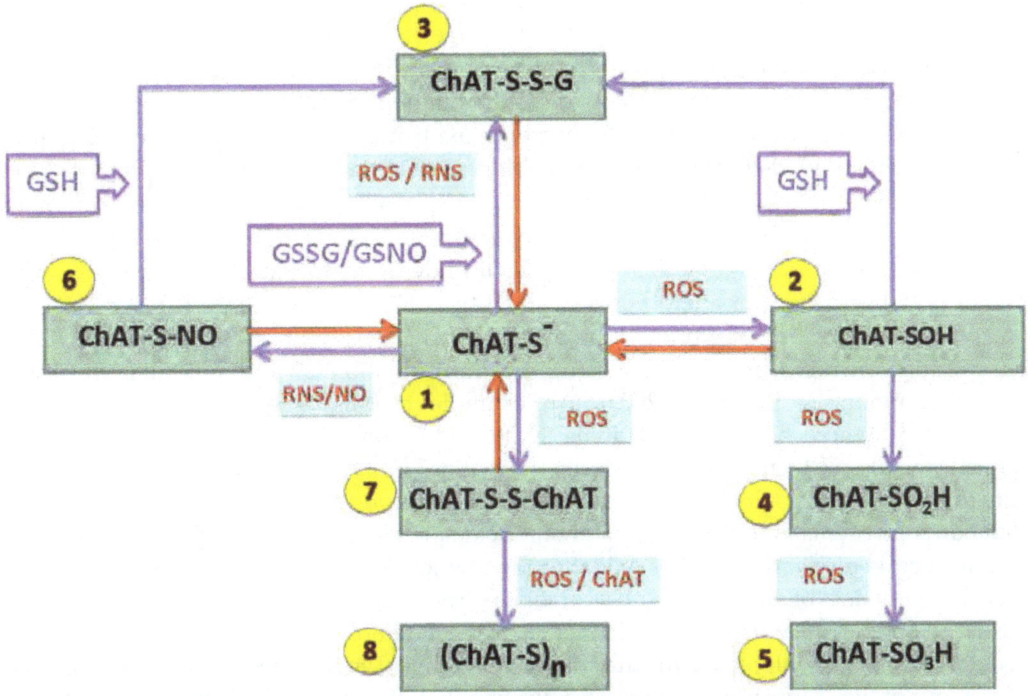

Fig. 2. ROS–RNS can cause reversible and irreversible modification of proteins at reactive cysteine thiol residues. The common modifications that reactive Cys thiols can undergo are shown using ChAT as an example to illustrate that the protein can be found in cells in multiple forms that are modified by ROS and RNS with the potential formation of homo- and hetero-protein complexes. Unmodified ChAT-S^- (1) is oxidized by low levels of H_2O_2 to its sulphenic acid, ChAT-S-OH (2); ChAT-S-OH reacts non-enzymatically with glutathione (GSH) to form ChAT-GSH mixed disulphide, ChAT-S-S-G (3) that protects Cys from further oxidation. ChAT-S-OH (2) is further oxidized by excess ROS to inactive sulphinic ChAT-SO_2H (4) and sulphonic ChAT-SO_3H (5) acids when GSH is depleted. Also, ChAT-S^- (1) can react with NO to form *S*-nitrosylated ChAT, ChAT-S-NO (6) by reaction at reactive Cys thiols. ChAT-S-NO (6) can also react with GSH to give ChAT-S-S-G (3). Alternatively, ChAT-S^- (1) can be converted to ChAT-S-S-G (3) by reaction with *S*-nitrosoglutathione (GSNO). In the absence of GSH, ChAT-S^- (1) can be converted by ROS to intermolecular dimers ChAT-S-S-ChAT (7) or higher-order oligomers (8) that may precipitate from the cytoplasm. [*Adapted from Giustarini et al., 2004*].

6. Effects of oxidative and nitrosative stress alter ChAT activity

It is striking that ChAT contains twenty Cys residues, which is a substantially greater proportion of Cys (3.2%) than is normally found in intracellular proteins (~ 1%). This could make ChAT particularly vulnerable to oxidative-nitrosative stress. Indeed, ChAT activity is decreased by acute exposure of either the purified protein (Guermonprez et al., 2001; Kim et al., 2006; Morris, 1967; Roskoski, 1973) or brain fractions or cells (Liu et al., 1999) to ROS-RNS agents, with some protection being given by the addition of thioreductants (Liu et al., 1999; Morris, 1967). We found that the activity of purified human ChAT is rapidly lost in the absence of reducing agents and that its activity is partially recovered by the addition of fresh reducing agents (Kim et al., 2005). Nitric oxide (NO) donors can also inactivate ChAT with this effect being partially reversed by GSH (Liu et al., 1999). A common site for post-translational modification and redox regulation of proteins is at reactive Cys thiols with this leading to protein *S*-glutathionylation or *S*-nitrosylation. Reactive Cys thiols (Cys-S^-) are ionized at physiological pH and are more easily oxidized than are fully-reduced Cys (Cys-SH). ROS-RNS could also cause both reversible and irreversible changes to ChAT resulting in it having altered structure and function. The functional consequences of the oxidation of reactive Cys thiols in ChAT could include regulation or inactivation of catalysis, homo- or hetero-dimerization or oligomerization by disulphide bond formation, altered binding to cellular protein partners, or altered protein stability.

Structural reorganization of a protein can also serve to protect vulnerable reversibly-oxidized Cys residues during acute oxidative stress by the formation of intramolecular disulphide bonds (Cumming & Schubert, 2005). An example of this is seen in protein tyrosine phosphatases where a reactive catalytic Cys residue undergoes reversible oxidation to sulphenic acid, and then participates in the formation of an intramolecular disulphide bond with one of two "backdoor" Cys residues in the catalytic site to protect it from further oxidation to irreversible sulphinic or sulphonic acid species (Chen et al., 2009). The disulphide bond formed is resistant to further oxidation by low levels of ROS and can be re-reduced by GSH. Re-reduction of the catalytic Cys thiolate drives oxidation of the two backdoor Cys causing them to form a disulphide and facilitates regeneration of the active phosphatase. This model is significant with regard to ChAT as there are five Cys residues in its catalytic site, and at least four of these are arranged in a configuration that disulphide bonds may be able to form with only minor changes in side chain torsion angles (Kim et al., 2006).

7. Subcellular trafficking of CHT proteins, an important mode of regulation of high-affinity choline uptake, is altered by nitrosative stress

In many experimental paradigms, high-affinity choline uptake by CHT proteins is the rate-limiting step in the production of ACh, and it is modulated by neuronal activity and dependent upon the sodium electrochemical gradient (Birks & MacIntosh, 1961; Guyenet et al., 1973; Haga, 1971; Simon & Kuhar, 1975; Yamamura & Snyder, 1972). With molecular tools becoming available since the cloning of the CHT gene in the year 2000 (Okuda et al., 2000), the importance of the subcellular trafficking of CHT proteins as a regulatory mechanism for choline uptake, and thus for ACh production, has emerged. CHT proteins are distributed between the plasma membrane and subcellular compartments such as endosomes and synaptic vesicles (Ferguson et al., 2003; Nakata et al., 2004; Ribeiro et al., 2003). It was discovered that CHT proteins are internalized from the plasma membrane to endocytic vesicles via clathrin-mediated endocytosis (Ribeiro et al., 2003), a process that is dependent on a dileucine-like internalization motif located in the cytosolic carboxyl-terminal tail of CHT (Ribeiro et al., 2005); dileucine internalization motifs interact with the adaptor protein 2 complex of the clathrin-mediated endocytosis machinery (Traub, 2009). A subsequent study showed that internalized CHT undergoes constitutive recycling to the plasma membrane; importantly, potassium-mediated depolarization increases the rate of CHT recycling in neural cells, but not in non-neural cells (Ribeiro et al., 2007b). In addition, a recent report indicates that preventing CHT entry into the endosomal compartment using a selective endosomal ablation strategy decreases both CHT levels at the cell surface and choline uptake activity in a time-dependent manner (Ivy et al., 2010).

Since subcellular trafficking of CHT proteins is such a crucial mode of regulation of high-affinity choline uptake, it is important to address the question of how oxidative/nitrosative stress affects the proteins involved in vesicle trafficking. It has been demonstrated by a number of groups that oxidative stress perturbs the dynamic endocytosis of cell surface proteins such as receptors and transporters, with this having key roles in regulating their trafficking and activity. This may involve either the modification of specific amino acids in cargo proteins or be related to changes in the interaction of these receptors or transporters with other cellular proteins involved in their trafficking. For example, the dopamine transporter is inactivated by the RNS peroxynitrite by an action on a Cys residue in its third intracellular loop, with this resulting in toxicity to dopamine neurons (Park et al., 2002). This is prevented, but not reversed, by GSH and some reducing agents. Other studies reveal that the effects of ROS-RNS agents on cell surface proteins can be mediated indirectly by an action on components of the protein trafficking machinery, and this can likely involve changes in both clathrin-mediated and clathrin-independent pathways (Ozawa et al., 2008). Interestingly, this does not always involve inhibition of function of the protein; NO can regulate endocytosis by *S*-nitrosylation of dynamin which then affects endocytic vesicle budding thus facilitating internalization of some membrane proteins (G. Wang et al., 2006). This gain-of-function example illustrates the physiological role for low levels of NO. It has also been demonstrated that peroxynitrite stimulates synaptic vesicle exocytosis and induces the nitration of tyrosine residues in SNARE complex proteins (Di Stasi et al., 2002). However, another recent report showed that the fusion of synaptic vesicles with the presynaptic plasma membrane is impaired by oxidative stress (Arai et al., 2011).

Guermonprez and coworkers (2001) determined that peroxynitrite decreases CHT activity in synaptosomes from *Torpedo marmorata*. We have undertaken studies to identify the mechanisms by which oxidative-nitrosative stress alter choline uptake activity thereby interfering with cholinergic neurotransmission. Thus, we found that peroxynitrite causes a rapid, dose-dependent inhibition of CHT activity that is attenuated specifically by scavengers of peroxynitrite (Pinthong et al., 2008). Other oxidants such as H_2O_2 have no effect on CHT activity (Guermonprez et al., 2001; Pinthong et al., 2008). Importantly, doses of SIN-1, a peroxynitrite-generating molecule, that significantly decrease CHT activity do not compromise membrane integrity or alter cellular membrane potential (Pinthong et al., 2008). The SIN-1-induced decreases in choline uptake activity correlate with decreased CHT cell surface levels that result from accelerated endocytosis of CHT proteins by a clathrin-dependent mechanism (Pinthong et al., 2008).

Based on the important role that neuronal activity has in regulating the levels of CHT that are available at the plasma membrane to take up choline as substrate for ACh synthesis, it is predicted that the reduction in synaptic efficacy that is associated with elevated oligomeric

Aβ levels (Selkoe, 2002) would decrease the movement of CHT to the cell surface as constituents of synaptic vesicles. Thus, under conditions of oxidative-nitrosative stress, this effect of reduced synaptic efficacy associated with increasing oligomeric Aβ could further negatively impact CHT protein levels at the plasma membrane. This in turn would lead to diminished cholinergic signalling, a process found to be crucial in maintaining the cholinergic phenotype and regulating APP metabolism (Isacson et al., 2002; Seo et al., 2001; Tran et al., 2002; Unger et al., 2005; Verhoeff, 2005).

8. ROS-RNS may affect post-translational modifications and protein-protein interactions that regulate CHT and ChAT activities

Post-translational modifications can greatly influence both the function and subcellular localization of proteins. Phosphorylation, the reversible addition of a phosphate group to serine, threonine or tyrosine residues, is an important signalling event that has been shown to regulate both ChAT and CHT proteins. The activities of both ChAT and CHT are altered by treatments that modulate protein kinases or change the levels of protein phosphorylation in the cell (Black et al., 2010; Breer & Knipper, 1990; Cancela et al., 1995; Cooke & Rylett, 1997; Dobransky & Rylett, 2005; Ford et al., 1999; Gates et al., 2004; Guermonprez et al., 2002; Issa et al., 1996; Ivy et al., 2001; Knipper et al., 1992; Vogelsberg et al., 1997). Both ChAT and CHT proteins are phosphorylated in neural cells (Bruce & Hersh 1989; Dobransky et al., 2000; Gates et al., 2004; Habert et al. 1992; Schmidt & Rylett 1993). ChAT is a substrate for protein kinase C (PKC), casein kinase 2 and calcium/calmodulin-dependent kinase II (Dobransky et al., 2000), and CHT activity is modulated by activation of PKC (Black et al., 2010; Gates et al., 2004). Thus, pathological changes in protein kinase levels or functions could affect the functions of ChAT and/or CHT. For example, diminished PKC protein levels and signalling are seen in Alzheimer's disease (Alkon et al., 2007). However, ROS can lead to enhanced PKC activity (Zhao et al., 2011). Since PKC plays an important role in regulation of both ChAT and CHT function, it will be interesting to determine how oxidative stress alters phosphorylation-dependent regulation of ChAT, CHT and ACh synthesis, and the role that this plays in the failure of cholinergic neurotransmission in Alzheimer's disease and related disorders.

Protein-protein interactions are another molecular mode of regulation of protein function and/or subcellular localization, and some protein binding partners for ChAT and CHT have now been identified (Bales et al., 2006; Dobransky et al. 2003; Ribeiro et al., 2007a; B. Wang et al., 2007; Xie & Guo, 2004). In general, the interaction of CHT with other cellular proteins regulates it subcellular distribution. Notably, it has been determined that CHT interacts with the carboxyl-terminus of amyloid precursor protein (APP) family members (B. Wang et al., 2007) and with Aβ peptide (Bales et al., 2006). Mice lacking both APP and APP-like protein 2 have reduced levels of CHT protein at nerve terminals and this is seen as decreased high-affinity choline uptake activity; APP appears to be a modulator of both presynaptic localization and endocytosis of CHT proteins (B. Wang et al., 2007). Recent data indicate that modulation of APP metabolism or processing is an early cellular response to oxidative stress (Recuero et al., 2010). Based on the intimate relationship between oxidative/nitrosative stress and Aβ production, ROS-RNS generation could impact CHT activity by altering the interactions of this transporter with APP or Aβ. However, the mechanisms by which oxidative/nitrosative stress directly affects the interactions of ChAT and CHT with their protein binding partners have not been investigated.

9. Conclusion

The regulation of cellular proteins related to their reactions with ROS and RNS are described by the nitroso- and disulphide proteomes, and this has emerged as a critical modulator of protein function in both physiological and pathological situations (Ghezzi & Benetto, 2003; Lopez-Sanchez et al., 2009; Torta et al., 2008; Yano et al., 2002). A crucial point is that cellular mechanisms of limited capacity are normally in place, such as the formation of protein mixed-disulphides with glutathione (GSH), that transiently protect proteins from detrimental effects of ROS-RNS until redox balance is restored in the cell. S-glutathionylation at critical reactive Cys residues may even result in a gain-of-function for some proteins. However, during aging and disease, GSH levels are decreased and this can lead to irreversible oxidation and loss-of-function of vulnerable proteins. Investigations that are combining a range of proteomic, cell biology and *in vivo* experimental approaches have begun to characterize the dynamic responses of cholinergic neurons to the changes in brain that are induced by oxidative-nitrosative stress. A critical outcome of these studies is the identification of conditions that determine if the structural and functional modifications to ChAT and CHT that occur with tissue stress have the potential to be reversible or whether they are persistent. Future studies should focus on defining changes that are consistent with healthy and successful brain aging compared to changes that are associated with the onset of age-related disorders such as Alzheimer's disease. This will give insight into changes that are potentially reversible and that are amenable to intervention, and assist with the identification of therapeutic targets for protection of these proteins in normal aging and in diseases that may involve Aβ-induced / oxidative stress-induced changes.

10. Acknowledgment

Research grants from the Canadian Institutes of Health Research (CIHR) and Alzheimer's Association, USA were awarded to RJR. SAGB is the recipient of a CIHR Doctoral Research Award.

11. References

Alkon, D.L.; Sun, M.K. & Nelson, T.J. (2007). PKC signalling deficits: a mechanistic hypothesis for the origins of Alzheimer's disease. *Trends in Pharmacological Sciences*, Vol. 28, No. 2, (February 2007), pp. 51-60, ISSN 1873-3735

Ansari, M.A. & Scheff, S.W. (2010). Oxidative stress in the progression of Alzheimer disease in the frontal cortex. *Journal of Neuropathology and Experimental Neurology*, Vol. 69, No. 2, (February 2010), pp. 155-167, ISSN 0022-3069

Apelt, J.; Kumar, A. & Schliebs, R. (2002). Impairment of cholinergic neurotransmission in adult and aged transgenic Tg2576 mouse brain expressing the Swedish mutation of human beta-amyloid precursor protein. *Brain Research*, Vol. 953, No. 1-2, (October 2002), pp. 17-30, ISSN 1872-6240

Arai, M.; Saito, M.; Takatsu, H.; Fukui, K. & Urano, S. (2011). Dysfunction of the Fusion of Pre-Synaptic Plasma Membranes and Synaptic Vesicles Caused by Oxidative Stress, and its Prevention by Vitamin E. *Journal of Alzheimer's Disease*, (Feb 2011) [Epub ahead of print], ISSN 1387-2877

Auld, D.S.; Kar, S. & Quirion, R. (1998). Beta-amyloid peptides as direct cholinergic neuromodulators: a missing link? *Trends in Neurosciences,* Vol. 21, No. 1, (January 1998), pp. 43-49, ISSN 1878-108X

Bales, K.R.; Tzavara, E.T.; Wu, S.; Wade, M.R.; Bymaster, F.P.; Paul, S.M. & Nomikos, G.G. (2006). Cholinergic dysfunction in a mouse model of Alzheimer disease is reversed by an anti-A beta antibody. *Journal of Clinical Investigation,* Vol. 116, No. 3, (March 2006), pp. 825-832, ISSN 1558-8238

Barrett, W.C.; DeGnore, J.P.; Konig, S.; Fales, H.M.; Keng, Y.F.; Zhang, Z.Y.; Yim, M.B. & Chock, P.B. (1999). Regulation of PTP1B via glutathionylation of the active site cysteine 215. *Biochemistry,* Vol. 38, No. 20, (May 1999), pp. 6699-6705, ISSN 1520-4995

Baskerville, K.A.; Kent, C.; Nicolle, M.; Gallagher, M. & McKinney, M. (2006). Aging causes partial loss of basal forebrain but no loss of pontine reticular cholinergic neurons. *NeuroReport,* Vol. 17, No. 17, (November 2006), pp. 1819-1823, ISSN 1473-558X

Baskerville, K.A.; Kent, C.; Personett, D.; Lai, W.R.; Park, P.J.; Coleman, P. & McKinney, M. (2008). Aging elevates metabolic gene expression in brain cholinergic neurons. *Neurobiology of Aging,* Vol. 29, No. 12, (December 2008), pp. 1874-1893, ISSN 1558-1497

Bennett, S.A.; Pappas, B.A.; Stevens, W.D.; Davidson, C.M.; Fortin, T. & Chen, J. (2000). Cleavage of amyloid precursor protein elicited by chronic cerebral hypoperfusion. *Neurobiology of Aging,* Vol. 21, No. 2, (March-April 2000), pp 207-214, ISSN 1558-1497

Birks, R. & MacIntosh, F.C. (1961). Acetylcholine metabolism of a sympathetic ganglion. *Canadian Journal of Biochemistry and Physiology,* Vol. 39, pp. 787-827, ISSN 0576-5544

Black, S.A.; Ribeiro, F.M.; Ferguson, S.S. & Rylett, R.J. (2010). Rapid, transient effects of the protein kinase C activator phorbol 12-myristate 13-acetate on activity and trafficking of the rat high-affinity choline transporter. *Neuroscience,* Vol. 167, No. 3, (May 2010), pp. 765-773, ISSN 1873-7544

Bohnen, N.I. & Albin, R.L. (2010). The cholinergic system and Parkinson disease. *Behavioural Brain Research,* (January 2010), doi:10.1016/j.bbr.2009.12.048, ISSN 1872-7549

Borges, C.R.; Geddes, T.; Watson, J.T. & Kuhn, D.M. (2002). Dopamine biosynthesis is regulated by S-glutathionylation. Potential mechanism of tyrosine hydroxylase inhibition during oxidative stress. *Journal of Biological Chemistry,* Vol. 277, No. 50, (December 2002), pp. 48295-48302, ISSN 1083-351X

Breer, H. & Knipper, M. (1990). Regulation of high affinity choline uptake. *Journal of Neurobiology,* Vol. 21, No. 2, (March 1990), pp. 269-275, ISSN 1097-4695

Bruce, G. & Hersh, L.B. (1989). The phosphorylation of choline acetyltransferase. *Neurochemical Research,* Vol. 14, No. 7, (July 1989), pp. 613–620, ISSN 1573-6903

Butterfield, D.A. & Bush, A.I. (2004). Alzheimer's amyloid beta-peptide (1-42): involvement of methionine residue 35 in the oxidative stress and neurotoxicity properties of this peptide. *Neurobiology of Aging,* Vol. 25, No. 5, (May-June 2004), pp. 563-568, ISSN 1558-1497

Cancela, J.M.; Bertrand, N. & Beley, A. (1995). Involvement of cAMP in the regulation of high affinity choline uptake by rat brain synaptosomes. *Biochemical and Biophysical Research Communications,* Vol. 213, No. 3, (August 1995), pp. 944-949, ISSN 1090-2104

Chen, C.Y.; Willard, D. & Rudolph, J. (2009). Redox regulation of SH2-domain-containing protein tyrosine phosphatases by two backdoor cysteines. *Biochemistry,* Vol. 48, No. 6, (February 2009), pp. 1399-1409, ISSN 1520-4995

Collier, B. & MacIntosh, F.C. (1969). The source of choline for acetylcholine synthesis in a sympathetic ganglion. *Canadian Journal of Biochemistry and Physiology,* Vol. 47, pp. 127-135, ISSN 0576-5544

Collier, B. & Katz, H.S. (1974). Acetylcholine synthesis from recaptured choline by a sympathetic ganglion. *Journal of Physiology,* Vol. 238, No. 3, (May 1974), pp. 639-655, ISSN 1469-7793

Cooke, L.J. & Rylett, R.J. (1997). Inhibitors of serine/threonine phosphatases increase membrane-bound choline acetyltransferase activity and enhance acetylcholine synthesis. *Brain Research,* Vol. 751, No. 2, (March 1997), pp. 232-238, ISSN 1872-6240

Cumming, R.C. & Schubert, D. (2005). Amyloid-beta induces disulfide bonding and aggregation of GAPDH in Alzheimer's disease. *FASEB Journal,* Vol. 19, No. 14, (December 2005), pp. 2060-2062, ISSN 1530-6860

Davies, P. (1979). Biochemical changes in Alzheimer's disease-senile dementia: neurotransmitters in senile dementia of the Alzheimer's type. *Research Publications – Association for Research in Nervous and Mental Disease,* Vol. 57, pp. 153-66, ISSN 0091-7443

De Felice, F.G.; Velasco, P.T.; Lambert, M.P.; Viola, K.; Fernandez, S.J.; Ferreira, S.T. & Klein, W.L. (2007). Abeta oligomers induce neuronal oxidative stress through an N-methyl-D-aspartate receptor-dependent mechanism that is blocked by the Alzheimer drug memantine. *Journal of Biological Chemistry,* Vol. 282, No. 15, (April 2007), pp. 11590-11601, ISSN 1083-351X

DeKosky, S.T.; Ikonomovic, M.D.; Styren, S.D.; Beckett, L.; Wisniewski, S.; Bennett, D.A.; Cochran, E.J.; Kordower, J.H. & Mufson, E.J. (2002). Upregulation of choline acetyltransferase activity in hippocampus and frontal cortex of elderly subjects with mild cognitive impairment. *Annals of Neurology,* Vol. 51, No. 2, (February 2002), pp. 145-155, ISSN 1531-8249

Di Stasi, A.M.; Mallozzi, C.; Macchia, G.; Maura, G.; Petrucci, T.C. & Minetti, M. (2002). Peroxynitrite affects exocytosis and SNARE complex formation and induces tyrosine nitration of synaptic proteins. *Journal of Neurochemistry,* Vol. 82, No. 2, (July 2002), pp. 420-429, ISSN 1471-4159

Dobransky, T.; Davis, W.L.; Xiao, G.H. & Rylett, R.J. (2000). Expression, purification and characterization of recombinant human choline acetyltransferase: phosphorylation of the enzyme regulates catalytic activity. *Biochemical Journal,* Vol. 349, No. 1, (July 2000), pp. 141-151, ISSN 1470-8728

Dobransky, T.; Brewer, D.; Lajoie, G. & Rylett, R.J. (2003). Phosphorylation of 69-kDa choline acetyltransferase at threonine 456 in response to amyloid-beta peptide 1–42. *Journal of Biological Chemistry,* Vol. 278, No. 8, (February 2003), pp. 5883–5893, ISSN 1083-351X

Dobransky, T. & Rylett, R.J. (2005). A model for dynamic regulation of choline acetyltransferase by phosphorylation. *Journal of Neurochemistry,* Vol. 95, No. 2, (October 2005), pp. 305-13, ISSN 1471-4159

Fass, U.; Panickar, K.; Personett, D.; Bryan, D.; Williams, K.; Gonzales, J.; Sugaya, K. & McKinney, M. (2000). Differential vulnerability of primary cultured cholinergic neurons to nitric oxide excess. *NeuroReport,* Vol. 11, No. 5, (April 2000), pp. 931-936, ISSN 1473-558X

Ferguson, S.M.; Savchenko, V.; Apparsundaram, S.; Zwick, M.; Wright, J.; Heilman, C.J.; Yi, H.; Levey, A.I. & Blakely, R.D. (2003). Vesicular localization and activity-dependent trafficking of presynaptic choline transporters. *Journal of Neuroscience,* Vol. 23, No. 30, (October 2003), pp. 9697-9709, ISSN 1529-2401

Ford, B.D.; Ivy, M.T.; Mtshali, C.P. & Townsel, J.G. (1999). The involvement of protein kinase C in the regulation of choline cotransport in *Limulus. Comparative Biochemistry and Physiology. Part A, Molecular and Integrative Physiology,* Vol. 123, No. 3, (July 1999), pp. 255-261, ISSN 1095-6433

Forgon, M.; Farkas, Z.; Gulya, K.; Pakaski, M.; Penke, B. & Kasa, P. (1998). Amyloid beta-peptide and its fragments induce acetylcholine release in in vitro basal forebrain tissue slices of rat brain, but do not affect the choline uptake. *Neurobiology (Budapest, Hungary),* Vol. 6, No. 3, pp. 359-361, ISSN 1216-8068

Foster, T.C. (2006). Biological markers of age-related memory deficits: treatment of senescent physiology. *CNS Drugs,* Vol. 20, No. 2, pp. 153-156, ISSN 1172-7047

Francis, P.T.; Palmer, A.M.; Sims, N.R.; Bowen, D.M.; Davison, A.M.; Esiri, M.M.; Neary, D.; Snowden, J.S. & Wilcock, G.K. (1985). Neurochemical studies of early-onset Alzheimer's disease. Possible influence on treatment. *New England Journal of Medicine,* Vol. 313, No. 1, (July 1985), pp. 7-11, ISSN 1533-4406

Francis, P.T.; Palmer, A.M.; Snape, M. & Wilcock, G.K. (1999). The cholinergic hypothesis of Alzheimer's disease: a review of progress. *Journal of Neurology, Neurosurgery, and Psychiatry,* Vol. 66, No. 2, (February 1999), pp. 137-147, ISSN 1468-330X

Fukuda, K.; Davies, S.S.; Nakajima, T.; Ong, B.H.; Kupershmidt, S.; Fessel, J.; Amarnath, V.; Anderson, M.E.; Boyden, P.A.; Viswanathan, P.C.; Roberts, L.J. 2nd & Balser, J.R. (2005). Oxidative mediated lipid peroxidation recapitulates proarrhythmic effects on cardiac sodium channels. *Circulation Research,* Vol. 97, No. 12, (December 2005), pp. 1262-1269, ISSN 0009-7300

Garner, C.C.; Kindler, S. & Gundelfinger, E.D. (2000). Molecular determinants of presynaptic active zones. *Current Opinion in Neurobiology,* Vol. 10, No. 3, (June 2000), pp. 321-327, ISSN 0959-4388

Gates, J. jr.; Ferguson, S.M. & Blakely, R.D. (2004). Regulation of choline transporter surface expression and phosphorylation by protein kinase C and protein phosphatase 1/2. *Journal of Pharmacology and Experimental Therapeutics,* Vol. 310, No. 2, (August 2004), pp. 536-545, ISSN 1521-0103

Gentile, M.T.; Poulet, R.; Di Pardo, A.; Cifelli, G.; Maffei, A.; Vecchione, C.; Passarelli, F.; Landolfi, A.; Carullo, P. & Lembo, G. (2009). Beta-amyloid deposition in brain is enhanced in mouse models of arterial hypertension. *Neurobiology of Aging,* Vol. 30, No. 2, (February 2009), pp. 222-228, ISSN 1558-1497

Ghezzi, P. & Benetto, V. (2003). Redox proteomics: identification of oxidatively modified proteins. *Proteomics,* Vol. 3, No. 7, (July 2003), pp. 1145-1153, ISSN 1615-9861

Gilmer, L.K.; Ansari, M.A.; Roberts, K.N. & Scheff, S.W. (2010). Age-related changes in mitochondrial respiration and oxidative damage in the cerebral cortex of the Fischer 344 rat. *Mechanisms of Ageing and Development,* Vol. 131, No. 2, (February 2010), pp. 133-143, ISSN 0047-6374

Giustarini, D.; Rossi, R.; Milzani, A.; Colombo, R. & Dalle-Donne, I. (2004). S-glutathionylation: from redox regulation of protein functions to human diseases. Journal of Cellular and Molecular Medicine, Vol. 8, No. 2, (April-June 2004), pp. 201-212, ISSN 1582-4934

Goekoop, R.; Scheltens, P.; Barkhof, F. & Rombouts, S.A. (2006). Cholinergic challenge in Alzheimer patients and mild cognitive impairment differentially affects hippocampal activation--a pharmacological fMRI study. *Brain,* Vol. 129, No. 1, (January 2006), pp. 141-157, ISSN 1460-2156

Gong, Y.; Chang, L.; Viola, K.L.; Lacor, P.N.; Lambert, M.P.; Finch, C.E.; Krafft, G.A. & Klein, W.L. (2003). Alzheimer's disease-affected brain: presence of oligomeric A beta ligands (ADDLs) suggests a molecular basis for reversible memory loss. *Proceedings of the National Academy of Sciences of the United States of America,* Vol. 100, No. 18, (September 2003), pp. 10417-10422, ISSN 1091-6490

Gotti, C.; Clementi, F.; Fornari, A.; Gaimarri, A.; Guiducci, S.; Manfredi, I.; Moretti, M.; Pedrazzi, P.; Pucci, L. & Zoli, M. (2009). Structural and functional diversity of native brain neuronal nicotinic receptors. *Biochemical Pharmacology,* Vol. 78, No. 7, (October 2009), pp. 703-711, ISSN 1873-2968

Grön, G.; Brandenburg, I.; Wunderlich, A.P. & Riepe, M.W. (2006). Inhibition of hippocampal function in mild cognitive impairment: targeting the cholinergic hypothesis. *Neurobiology of Aging,* Vol. 27, No. 1, (January 2006), pp. 78-87, ISSN 1558-1497

Guermonprez, L.; Ducrocq, C. & Gaudry-Talarmain, Y.M. (2001). Inhibition of acetylcholine synthesis and tyrosine nitration induced by peroxynitrite are differentially prevented by antioxidants. *Molecular Pharmacology,* Vol. 60, No. 4, (October 2001), pp. 838-846, ISSN 1521-0111

Guermonprez, L.; O'Regan, S.; Meunier, F.M. & Morot-Gaudry-Talarmain, Y. (2002). The neuronal choline transporter CHT1 is regulated by immunosuppressor-sensitive pathways. *Journal of Neurochemistry,* Vol. 82, No. 4, (August 2002), pp. 874-884, ISSN 1471-4159

Guyenet, P.; Lefresne, P.; Rossier, J.; Beaujouan, J.C. & Glowinski, J. (1973). Inhibition by hemicholinium-3 and antiparkinson drugs on (14C)acetylcholine synthesis and (3H)choline uptake in rat striatal synaptosomes. *Brain Research,* Vol. 62, No. 2, (November 1973), pp. 523-529, ISSN 1872-6240

Habert, E.; Birman, S. & Mallet, J. (1992). High-level synthesis and fate of acetylcholine in baculovirus-infected cells: characterization and purification of recombinant rat choline acetyltransferase. *Journal of Neurochemistry,* Vol. 58, No. 4, (April 1992), pp. 1447-1453, ISSN 1471-4159

Haga, T. (1971). Synthesis and release of (14C)acetylcholine in synaptosomes. *Journal of Neurochemistry,* Vol. 18, No. 6, (June 1971), pp. 781-798, ISSN 1471-4159

Hartmann, J.; Erb, C.; Ebert, U.; Baumann, K.H.; Popp, A.; König, G. & Klein, J. (2004). Central cholinergic functions in human amyloid precursor protein knock-in/presenilin-1 transgenic mice. *Neuroscience,* Vol. 125, No. 4, pp. 1009-1017, ISSN 1873-7544

Hasselmo, M.E. (2006). The role of acetylcholine in learning and memory. *Current Opinion in Neurobiology,* Vol. 16, No. 6, (December 2006), pp. 710-715, ISSN 0959-4388

Heinitz, K.; Beck, M.; Schliebs, R. & Perez-Polo, J.R. (2006). Toxicity mediated by soluble oligomers of beta-amyloid(1-42) on cholinergic SN56.B5.G4 cells. *Journal of Neurochemistry,* Vol. 98, No. 6, (September 2006), pp. 1930-1945, ISSN 1471-4159

Hoshi, M.; Takashima, A.; Noguchi, K.; Marayama, M.; Sato, M.; Kondo, S.; Saitoh, Y.; Ishiguro, K.; Hoshino, T. & Imahori, K. (1996). Regulation of mitochondrial pyruvate dehydrogenase activity by tau protein kinase I/glycogen synthase kinase 3beta in brain. *Proceedings of the National Academy of Sciences of the United States of America,* Vol. 93, No. 7, (April 1996), pp. 2719-2723, ISSN 1091-6490

Hoshi, M.; Takashima, A.; Murayama, M.; Yasutake, K.; Yoshida, N.; Ishiguro, K.; Hoshino, T. & Imahori, K. (1997). Nontoxic amyloid beta peptide 1-42 suppresses acetylcholine synthesis. Possible role in cholinergic dysfunction in Alzheimer's disease. *Journal of Biological Chemistry,* Vol. 272, No. 4, (January 1997), pp. 2038-2041, ISSN 1083-351X

Humphries, K.M.; Juliano, C. & Taylor, S.S. (2002). Regulation of cAMP-dependent protein kinase activity by glutathionylation. *Journal of Biological Chemistry,* Vol. 277, No. 45, (November 2002), pp. 43505-43511, ISSN 1083-351X

Ikonomovic, M.D.; Mufson, E.J.; Wuu, J.; Cochran, E.J.; Bennet, D.A. & DeKosky, S.T. (2003). Cholinergic plasticity in hippocampus of individuals with mild cognitive impairment: correlation with Alzheimer's neuropathology. *Journal of Alzheimer's Disease,* Vol. 5, No. 1, (February 2003), pp. 39-48, ISSN 1387-2877

Isacson, O.; Seo, H.; Lin, L.; Albeck, D. & Granholm, A.C. (2002). Alzheimer's disease and Down's syndrome: roles of APP, trophic factors and ACh. *Trends in Neurosciences,* Vol. 25, No. 2, (February 2002), pp. 79-84, ISSN 1878-108X

Ishii, T.; Sakurai, T.; Usami, H. & Uchida, K. (2005). *Biochemistry,* Vol. 44, No. 42, (October 2005), pp. 13893-13901, ISSN 1520-4995

Issa, A.M.; Gauthier, S. & Collier, B. (1996). Effects of the phosphatase inhibitors calyculin A and okadaic acid on acetylcholine synthesis and content of rat hippocampal formation. *Journal of Neurochemistry,* Vol. 66, No. 5, (May 1996), pp. 1924-1932, ISSN 1471-4159

Ivy, M.T.; Newkirk, R.F.; Karim, M.R.; Mtshali, C.M. & Townsel J.G. (2001). Hemicholinium-3 mustard reveals two populations of cycling choline cotransporters in *Limulus. Neuroscience,* Vol. 102, No. 4, pp. 969-978, ISSN 1873-7544

Ivy, M.T.; Newkirk, R.F.; Wang, Y. & Townsel, J.G. (2010). A novel choline cotransporter sequestration compartment in cholinergic neurons revealed by selective endosomal ablation. *Journal of Neurochemistry,* Vol. 112, No. 5, (March 2010), pp. 1295-1304, ISSN 1471-4159

Jaffrey, S.R.; Erdjument-Bromage, H.; Ferris, C.D.; Tempst, P. & Snyder, S.H. (2001). Protein S-nitrosylation: a physiological signal for neuronal nitric oxide. *Nature Cell Biology,* Vol. 3, No. 2, (February 2001), pp. 193-197, ISSN 1476-4679

Kar, S.; Seto, D.; Gaudreau, P. & Quirion, R. (1996). Beta-amyloid-related peptides inhibit potassium-evoked acetylcholine release from rat hippocampal slices. *Journal of Neuroscience,* Vol. 16, No. 3, (February 1996), pp. 1034-1040, ISSN 1529-2401

Kar, S.; Issa, A.M.; Seto, D.; Auld, D.S.; Collier, B. & Quirion, R. (1998). Amyloid beta-peptide inhibits high-affinity choline uptake and acetylcholine release in rat hippocampal slices. *Journal of Neurochemistry,* Vol. 70, No. 5, (May 1998), pp. 2179-2187, ISSN 1471-4159

Kim, A.R.; Doherty-Kirby, A.; Lajoie, G.; Rylett, R.J. & Shilton, B.H. (2005). Two methods for large-scale purification of recombinant human choline acetyltransferase. *Protein Expression and Purification,* Vol. 40, No. 1, (March 2005), pp. 107-117, ISSN 1096-0279

Kim, A.R.; Rylett, R.J. & Shilton, B.H. (2006). Substrate binding and catalytic mechanism of human choline acetyltransferase. *Biochemistry,* Vol. 45, No. 49, (December 2006), pp. 14621-14631, ISSN 1520-4995

Klatt, P. & Lamas, S. (2000). Regulation of protein function by S-glutathiolation in response to oxidative and nitrosative stress. *European Journal of Biochemistry,* Vol. 267, No. 16, (August 2000), pp. 4928-4944, ISSN 1432-1033

Klein, W.L. (2002). Abeta toxicity in Alzheimer's disease: globular oligomers (ADDLs) as new vaccine and drug targets. *Neurochemistry International,* Vol. 41, No. 5, (November 2002), pp. 345-352, ISSN 1872-9754

Klein, W.L.; Stine, W.B. Jr. & Teplow, D.B. (2004). Small assemblies of unmodified amyloid beta-protein are the proximate neurotoxin in Alzheimer's disease. *Neurobiology of Aging,* Vol. 25, No. 5, (May-June 2004), pp. 569-580, ISSN 1558-1497

Klingner, M.; Apelt, J.; Kumar, A.; Sorger, D.; Sabri, O.; Steinbach, J.; Scheunemann, M. & Schliebs, R. (2003). Alterations in cholinergic and non-cholinergic neurotransmitter receptor densities in transgenic Tg2576 mouse brain with beta-amyloid plaque pathology. *International Journal of Developmental Neuroscience,* Vol. 21, No. 7, (November 2003), pp. 357-369, ISSN 1873-474X

Knipper, M.; Kahle, M. & Breer, H. (1992). Regulation of hemicholinium binding sites in isolated nerve terminals. *Journal of Neurobiology,* Vol. 23, No. 2, (March 1992), pp. 163-172, ISSN 1097-4695

Krishnaswamy, A. & Cooper, E. (2009). An activity-dependent retrograde signal induces the expression of the high-affinity choline transporter in cholinergic neurons. *Neuron,* Vol. 61, No. 2, (January 2009), pp. 272-286, ISSN 1097-4199

Kristofiková, Z.; Tejkalová, H. & Klaschka, J. (2001). Amyloid beta peptide 1-40 and the function of rat hippocampal hemicholinium-3 sensitive choline carriers: effects of a proteolytic degradation in vitro. *Neurochemical Research,* Vol. 26, No. 3, (March 2001), pp. 203-212, ISSN 1573-6903

Kristofiková, Z.; Rícný, J.; Kozmiková, I.; Rípová, D.; Zach, P. & Klaschka, J. (2006). Sex-dependent actions of amyloid beta peptides on hippocampal choline carriers of postnatal rats. *Neurochemical Research,* Vol. 31, No. 3, (March 2006), pp. 351-360, ISSN 1573-6903

Kristofiková, Z.; Kopecký, V. Jr.; Hofbauerová, K.; Hovorková, P. & Rípová, D. (2008). Complex of amyloid beta peptides with 24-hydroxycholesterol and its effect on hemicholinium-3 sensitive carriers. *Neurochemical Research,* Vol. 33, No. 3, (March 2008), pp. 412-421, ISSN 1573-6903

Kuo, Y.M.; Emmerling, M.R.; Viog-Pelfrey, C.; Kasunic, T.C.; Kirkpatrick, J.B.; Murdoch, G.H.; Ball, M.J. & Roher, A.E. (1996). Water-soluble Abeta (N-40, N-42) oligomers in normal and Alzheimer disease brains. *Journal of Biological Chemistry,* Vol. 271, No. 8, (February 1996), pp. 4077-4081, ISSN 1083-351X

Lahiri, D.K.; Utsuki, T.; Chen, D.; Farlow, M.R.; Shoaib, M.; Ingram, D.K. & Greig, N.H. (2002). Nicotine reduces the secretion of Alzheimer's beta-amyloid precursor protein containing beta-amyloid peptide in the rat without altering synaptic proteins. *Annals of the New York Academy of Sciences,* Vol. 965, (June 2002), pp. 364-372, ISSN 1749-6632

Lahiri, D.K. & Greig, N.H. (2004). Lethal weapon: amyloid beta-peptide, role in the oxidative stress and neurodegeneration of Alzheimer's disease. *Neurobiology of Aging,* Vol. 25, No. 5, (May-June 2004), pp. 581-587, ISSN 1558-1497

Lane, R.M.; Potkin, S.G. & Enz, A. (2006). Targeting acetylcholinesterase and butyrylcholinesterase in dementia. *International Journal of Neuropsychopharmacology,* Vol. 9, No. 1, (February 2006), pp. 101-124, ISSN 1469-5111

Lee, P.H.; Hwang, E.M.; Hong, H.S.; Boo, J.H.; Mook-Jung, I. & Huh, K. (2006). Effect of ischemic neuronal insults on amyloid precursor protein processing. *Neurochemical Research,* Vol. 31, No. 6, (June 2006), pp. 821-827, ISSN 1573-6903

Lind, C.; Gerdes, R.; Hamnell, Y.; Schuppe-Koistinen, I.; von Lowenhielm, H.B.; Holmgren, A. & Cotgreave, I.A. (2002). Identification of S-glutathionylated cellular proteins during oxidative stress and constitutive metabolism by affinity purification and proteomic analysis. *Archives of Biochemistry and Biophysics,* Vol. 406, No. 2, (October 2002), pp. 229-240, ISSN 1096-0384

Liu, M.; Huang, Y.; Wu, J.; Wang, E. & Wang, Y. (1999). Effect of cysteine residues on the activity of arginyl-tRNA synthetase from *Escherichia coli. Biochemistry,* Vol. 38, No. 34, (August 1999), pp. 11006-11011, ISSN 1520-4995

Lopez-Sanchez, L.M.; Muntane, J.; de la Mata, M. & Rodriguez-Ariza, A. (2009). Unraveling the S-nitrosoproteome: tools and strategies. *Proteomics,* Vol. 9, No. 4, (February 2009), pp. 808-818, ISSN 1615-9861

Lue, L.F., Kuo, Y.M.; Roher, A.E.; Brachova, L.; Shen, Y.; Sue, L.; Beach, T.; Kurth, J.H.; Rydel, R.E. & Rogers, J. (1999). Soluble amyloid beta peptide concentration as a predictor of synaptic change in Alzheimer's disease. *American Journal of Pathology,* Vol. 155, No. 3, (September 1999), pp. 853-862, ISSN 1525-2191

Marcello, E.; Epis, R. & Di Luca, M. (2008). Amyloid flirting with synaptic failure: towards a comprehensive view of Alzheimer's disease pathogenesis. *European Journal of Pharmacology,* Vol. 585, No. 1, (May 2008), pp. 109-118, ISSN 1879-0712

Mattson, M.P. (2004). Pathways towards and away from Alzheimer's disease. *Nature,* Vol. 430, No. 7000, (August 2004), pp. 631-639, ISSN 1476-4687

Mattson, M.P. & Magnus, T. (2006). Ageing and neuronal vulnerability. *Nature Reviews. Neuroscience,* Vol. 7, No. 4, (April 2006), pp. 278-294, ISSN 1471-0048

McKinney, M.; Williams, K.; Personett, D.; Kent, C.; Bryan, D.; Gonzalez, J. & Baskerville, K. (2004). Pontine cholinergic neurons depend on three neuroprotection systems to resist nitrosative stress. *Brain Research,* Vol. 1002, No. 1-2, (March 2004), pp. 100-109, ISSN 1872-6240

McKinney, M. & Jacksonville, M.C. (2005). Brain cholinergic vulnerability: relevance to behavior and disease. *Biochemical Pharmacology,* Vol. 70, No. 8, (October 2005), pp. 1115-1124, ISSN 1873-2968

McMillian, M.; Kong, L.Y; Sawin, S.M.; Wilson, B.; Das, K.; Hudson, P.; Hong, J.S. & Bing, G. (1995). Selective killing of cholinergic neurons by microglial activation in basal forebrain mixed neuronal/glial cultures. *Biochemical and Biophysical Research Communications,* Vol. 215, No. 2, (October 1995), pp. 572-577, ISSN 1090-2104

Melo, J.B.; Agostinho, P. & Oliveira, C.R. (2002). Amyloid beta-peptide 25-35 reduces [3H]acetylcholine release in retinal neurons. Involvement of metabolic dysfunction. *Amyloid*, Vol. 9, No. 4, (December 2002), pp. 221-228, ISSN 1744-2818

Mesulam, M. (2004). The cholinergic lesion of Alzheimer's disease: pivotal factor or side show? *Learning and Memory,* Vol. 11, No. 1, (January-February 2004), pp. 43-49, ISSN 1549-5485

Morris, D. (1967). The effect of sulphydryl and other disulphide reducing agents on choline acetyltransferase activity estimated with synthetic acetyl-CoA. *Journal of Neurochemistry,* Vol. 14, No. 1, (January 1967), pp. 19-27, ISSN 1471-4159

Mufson, E.J.; Ginsberg, S.D.; Ikonomovic, M.D. & DeKosky, S.T. (2003). Human cholinergic basal forebrain: chemoanatomy and neurologic dysfunction. *Journal of Chemical Neuroanatomy,* Vol. 26, No. 4, (December 2003), pp. 233-242, ISSN 1873-6300

Nakata, K.; Okuda, T. & Misawa, H. (2004). Ultrastructural localization of high-affinity choline transporter in the rat neuromuscular junction: enrichment on synaptic vesicles. *Synapse,* Vol. 53, No. 1, (July 2004), pp. 53-56, ISSN 1098-2396

Nathanson, N.M. (2008). Synthesis, trafficking, and localization of muscarinic acetylcholine receptors. *Pharmacology and Therapeutics,* Vol. 119, No. 1, (July 2008), pp. 33-43, ISSN 0163-7258

Nicolle, M.M.; Gonzalez, J.; Sugaya, K.; Baskerville, K.A.; Bryan, D.; Lund, K.; Gallagher, M. & McKinney, M. (2001). Signatures of hippocampal oxidative stress in aged spatial learning-impaired rodents. *Neuroscience,* Vol. 107, No. 3, pp. 415-431, ISSN 1873-7544

Nihashi, T.; Inao, S.; Kajita, Y.; Kawai, T.; Sugimoto, T.; Niwa, M.; Kabeya, R.; Hata, N.; Hayashi, S. & Toshida, J. (2001). Expression and distribution of beta amyloid precursor protein and beta amyloid peptide in reactive astrocytes after transient middle cerebral artery occlusion. *Acta Neurochirurgica (Wien),* Vol. 143, No. 3, pp. 287-295, ISSN 0942-0940

Nitta, A.; Itoh, A.; Hasegawa, T. & Nabeshima, T. (1994). beta-Amyloid protein-induced Alzheimer's disease animal model. *Neuroscience Letters,* Vol. 170, No. 1, (March 1994), pp. 63-66, ISSN 1872-7972

Nitta, A.; Fukuta, T.; Hasegawa, T. & Nabeshima, T. (1997). Continuous infusion of beta-amyloid protein into the rat cerebral ventricle induces learning impairment and neuronal and morphological degeneration. *Japanese Journal of Pharmacology,* Vol. 73, No. 1, (January 1997), pp. 51-57, ISSN 1347-3506

Oda, Y. (1999). Choline acetyltransferase: the structure, distribution and pathologic changes in the central nervous system. *Pathology International,* Vol. 49, No. 11, (November 1999), pp. 921-937, ISSN 1440-1827

Okuda, T.; Haga, T.; Kanai, Y.; Endou, H.; Ishihara, T. & Katsura, I. (2000). Identification and characterization of the high-affinity choline transporter. *Nature Neuroscience,* Vol. 3, No. 2, (February 2000), pp. 120-125, ISSN 1546-1726

Ongwijitwat, S.; Liang, H.L.; Graboyes, E.M. & Wong-Riley, M.T. (2006). Nuclear respiratory factor 2 senses changing cellular energy demands and its silencing down-regulates cytochrome oxidase and other target gene mRNAs. *Gene,* Vol. 374, (June 2006), pp. 39-49, ISSN 1879-0038

Opazo, P.; Saud, K.; de Saint Pierre, M.; Cárdenas, A.M.; Allen, D.D.; Segura-Aguilar, J.; Caviedes, R. & Caviedes, P. (2006). Knockdown of amyloid precursor protein normalizes cholinergic function in a cell line derived from the cerebral cortex of a trisomy 16 mouse: An animal model of down syndrome. *Journal of Neuroscience Research,* Vol. 84, No. 6, (November 2006), pp. 1303-1310, ISSN 1872-8111

Ozawa, K.; Whalen, E.J.; Nelson, C.D.; Mu, Y.; Hess, D.T.; Lefkowitz, R.J. & Stamler, J.S. (2008). S-nitrosylation of beta-arrestin regulates beta-adrenergic receptor trafficking. *Molecular Cell,* Vol. 31, No. 3, (August 2008), pp. 395-405, ISSN 1097-4164

Park, S.U.; Ferrer, J.V.; Javitch, J.A. & Kuhn, D.M. (2002). Peroxynitrite inactivates the human dopamine transporter by modification of cysteine 342: potential mechanism of neurotoxicity in dopamine neurons. *Journal of Neuroscience,* Vol. 22, No. 11, (June 2002), pp. 4399-4405, ISSN 1529-2401

Payette, D.J.; Xie, J. & Guo, Q. (2007). Reduction in CHT1-mediated choline uptake in primary neurons from presenilin-1 M146V mutant knock-in mice. *Brain Research,* Vol. 1135, No. 1, (March 2007), pp. 12-21, ISSN 1872-6240

Pedersen, W.A.; Kloczewiak, M.A. & Blusztajn, J.K. (1996). Amyloid beta-protein reduces acetylcholine synthesis in a cell line derived from cholinergic neurons of the basal forebrain. *Proceedings of the National Academy of Sciences of the United States of America,* Vol. 93, No. 15, (July 1996), pp. 8068-8071, ISSN 1091-6490

Pedersen, W.A. & Blusztajn, J.K. (1997). Characterization of the acetylcholine-reducing effect of the amyloid-beta peptide in mouse SN56 cells. *Neuroscience Letters,* Vol. 239, No. 2-3, (December 1997), pp. 77-80, ISSN 1872-7972

Perry, E.K.; Perry, R.H.; Blessed, G. & Tomlinson, B.E. (1977). Necropsy evidence of central cholinergic deficits in senile dementia. *Lancet,* Vol. 1, No. 8004, (January 1977), p. 189, ISSN 1474-547X

Petcu, E.B.; Sfedel, V.; Platt, D.; Herndon, J.G.; Kessler, C. & Popa-Wagner, A. (2008). Cellular and molecular events underlying the dysregulated response of the aged brain to stroke: a mini-review. *Gerontology,* Vol. 54, No. 1, pp. 6-17, ISSN 1423-0003

Pinthong, M.; Black, S.A.; Ribeiro, F.M.; Pholpramool, C.; Ferguson, S.S. & Rylett, R.J. (2008). Activity and subcellular trafficking of the sodium-coupled choline transporter CHT is regulated acutely by peroxynitrite. *Molecular Pharmacology,* Vol. 73, No. 3, (March 2008), pp. 801-812, ISSN 1521-0111

Prado, M.A.; Reis, R.A.; Prado, V.F.; de Mello, M.C.; Gomez, M.V. & de Mello, F.G. (2002). Regulation of acetylcholine synthesis and storage. *Neurochemistry International,* Vol. 41, No. 5, (November 2002), pp. 291-299, ISSN 1872-9754

Qi, X.L.; Xiu, J.; Shan, K.R.; Xiao, Y.; Gu, R.; Liu, R.Y. & Guan, Z.Z. (2005). Oxidative stress induced by beta-amyloid peptide(1-42) is involved in the altered composition of cellular membrane lipids and the decreased expression of nicotinic receptors in human SH-SY5Y neuroblastoma cells. *Neurochemistry International,* Vol. 46, No. 8, (June 2005), pp. 613-621,ISSN 1872-9754

Ribeiro, F.M.; Alves-Silva, J.; Volknandt, W.; Martins-Silva, C.; Mahmud, H.; Wilhelm, A.; Gomez, M.V.; Rylett, R.J.; Ferguson, S.S.; Prado, V.F. & Prado, M.A. (2003). The hemicholinium-3 sensitive high affinity choline transporter is internalized by clathrin-mediated endocytosis and is present in endosomes and synaptic vesicles. *Journal of Neurochemistry,* Vol. 87, No. 1, (October 2003), pp. 136-146, ISSN 1471-4159

Ribeiro, F.M.; Black, S.A.; Cregan, S.P.; Prado, V.F.; Prado, M.A.; Rylett, R.J. & Ferguson, S.S. (2005). Constitutive high-affinity choline transporter endocytosis is determined by a carboxyl-terminal tail dileucine motif. *Journal of Neurochemistry*, Vol. 94, No. 1, (July 2005), pp. 86-96, ISSN 1471-4159

Ribeiro F.M.; Ferreira, L.T.; Marion, S.; Fontes, S.; Gomez, M.; Ferguson, S.S.; Prado, M.A. & Prado, V.F. (2007a). SEC14-like protein 1 interacts with cholinergic transporters. *Neurochemistry International*, Vol. 50, No. 2, (January 2007), pp. 356-364, ISSN 1872-9754

Ribeiro, F.M.; Pinthong, M.; Black, S.A.; Gordon, A.C.; Prado, V.F.; Prado, M.A.; Rylett, R.J. & Ferguson, S.S. (2007b). Regulated recycling and plasma membrane recruitment of the high-affinity choline transporter. *European Journal of Neuroscience*, Vol. 26, No. 12, (December 2007), pp. 3437-3448, ISSN 1460-9568

Recuero M, Muñoz T, Aldudo J, Subías M, Bullido MJ, Valdivieso F. (2010). A free radical-generating system regulates APP metabolism/processing. *FEBS Letters*, Vol. 584, No. 22, (November 2010), pp. 4611-4618, ISSN 1873-3468

Roskoski, R. (1973). Choline acetyltransferase. Evidence for an acetyl-enzyme reaction intermediate. *Biochemistry*, Vol. 12, No. 19, (September 1973), pp. 3709-3714, ISSN 1520-4995

Ruan, C.J.; Zhang, L.; Chen, D.H.; Li, Z.; Du, G.H. & Sun, L. (2010). Effects of trans-2,4-dimethoxystibene against the neurotoxicity induced by Abeta(25-35) both in vitro and in vivo. *Neuroscience Research*, Vol. 67, No. 3 (July 2010), pp. 209-214, ISSN 1872-8111

Rylett, R.J.; Ball, M.J. & Colhoun, E.H. (1982). Evidence for high affinity choline transport in synaptosomes prepared from hippocampus and neocortex of patients with Alzheimer's disease. *Brain Research*, Vol. 289, No. 1-2, (December 1982), pp. 169-175, ISSN 1872-6240

Sarter, M. & Bruno, J.P. (1997). Cognitive functions of cortical acetylcholine: toward a unifying hypothesis. *Brain Research Reviews*, Vol. 23, No. 1-2, pp. 28-46, ISSN 1872-6321

Sarter, M.; Bruno, J.P. & Givens, B. (2003). Attentional functions of cortical cholinergic inputs: what does it mean for learning and memory? *Neurobiology of Learning and Memory*, Vol. 80, No. 3, (November 2003), pp. 245-56, ISSN 1095-9564

Sarter, M. & Bruno, J.P. (2004). Developmental origins of the age-related decline in cortical cholinergic function and associated cognitive abilities. *Neurobiology of Aging*, Vol. 25, No. 9, (October 2004), pp. 1127-1139, ISSN 1558-1497

Sarter, M. & Parikh, V. (2005). Choline transporters, cholinergic transmission and cognition. *Nature Reviews. Neuroscience*, Vol. 6, No. 1, (January 2005), pp. 48-56, ISSN 1471-0048

Satoh, Y.; Hirakura, Y.; Shibayama, S.; Hirashima, N.; Suzuki, T. & Kirino, Y. (2001). Beta-amyloid peptides inhibit acetylcholine release from cholinergic presynaptic nerve endings isolated from an electric ray. *Neuroscience Letters*, Vol. 302, No. 2-3, (April 2001), pp. 97-100, ISSN 1872-7972

Schliebs, R. & Arendt, T. (2006). The significance of the cholinergic system in the brain during aging and in Alzheimer's disease. *Journal of Neural Transmission*, Vol. 113, No. 11, (November 2006), pp. 1625-1644, ISSN 1435-1463

Schmidt, B.M. & Rylett, R.J. (1993). Phosphorylation of rat brain choline acetyltransferase and its relationship to enzyme activity. *Journal of Neurochemistry*, Vol. 61, No. 5, (November 1993), pp. 1774-1781, ISSN 1471-4159

Selkoe, D.J. (2002). Alzheimer's disease is a synaptic failure. *Science,* Vol. 298, No. 5594, (October 2002), pp. 789-791, ISSN 1095-9203

Seo, J.H.; Kim, S.H.; Kim, H.S.; Park, C.H.; Jeong, A.J.; Lee, J.H.; Choi, K.A.; Rah, J.C.; Koo, J.; Kim, E.M. & Suh, Y.H. (2001). Effects of nicotine on APP secretion and Abeta- or CT(105)-induced toxicity. *Biological Psychiatry,* Vol. 49, No. 3, (February 2001), pp. 240-247, ISSN 1873-2402

Shi, J.; Yang, S.H.; Stubley, L.; Day, A.L. & Simpkins, J.W. (2000). Hypoperfusion induces overexpression of beta-amyloid precursor protein mRNA in a focal ischemic rodent model. *Brain Research,* Vol. 853, No. 1, (January 2000), pp. 1-4, ISSN 1872-6240

Shimohama, S. & Kihara, T. (2001). Nicotinic receptor-mediated protection against beta-amyloid neurotoxicity. *Biological Psychiatry,* Vol. 49, No. 3, (February 2001), pp. 233-239, ISSN 1873-2402

Simon, J.R. & Kuhar, M.G. (1975). Impulse-flow regulation of high affinity choline uptake in brain cholinergic nerve terminals. *Nature,* Vol. 255, No. 5504, (May 1975), pp. 162-163, ISSN 1476-4687

Sims, N.R.; Bowen, D.M.; Allen, S.J.; Smith, C.C.; Neary, D. & Davison, A.N. (1983). Presynaptic cholinergic dysfunction in patients with dementia. *Journal of Neurochemistry,* Vol. 40, No. 2, (February 1983), pp. 503-509, ISSN 1471-4159

Skoog, I.; Lernfelt, B.; Landahl, S.; Palmertz, B.; Andreasson, L.A.; Nilsson, L.; Persson, G.; Odén, A. & Svanborg, A. (1996). 15-year longitudinal study of blood pressure and dementia. *Lancet,* Vol. 347, No. 9009, (April 1996), pp. 1141-1145, ISSN 1474-547X

Skoog, I. & Gustafson, D. (2006). Update on hypertension and Alzheimer's disease. *Neurological Research,* Vol. 28, No. 6, (September 2006), pp. 605-611, ISSN 1743-1328

Smith, S.M.; Renden, R. & von Gersdorff, H. (2008). Synaptic vesicle endocytosis: fast and slow modes of membrane retrieval. *Trends in Neurosciences,* Vol. 31, No. 11, (November 2008), pp. 559-568, ISSN 1878-108X

Smith, W.W.; Gorospe, M. & Kusiak, J.W. (2006). Signaling mechanisms underlying Abeta toxicity: potential therapeutic targets for Alzheimer's disease. *CNS & Neurological Disorders Drug Targets,* Vol. 5, No. 3, (June 2006), pp. 355-361, ISSN 1996-3181

Südhof, T.C. (2008). Neurotransmitter release, In: *Handbook of Experimental Pharmacology,* Vol. 184, T.C. Südhof and K. Starke, (Eds.), pp. 1-21, Springer, ISBN: 978-3-540-74804-5, Berlin, Germany

Tamagno, E.; Parola, M.; Guglielmotto, M.; Santoro, G.; Bardini, P.; Marra, L.; Tabaton, M. & Danni, O. (2003). Multiple signaling events in amyloid beta-induced, oxidative stress-dependent neuronal apoptosis. *Free Radical Biology & Medicine,* Vol. 35, No. 1, (July 2003), pp. 45-58, ISSN 1873-4596

Torta, F.; Usuelli, V.; Malgaroli, A. & Bachi, A. (2008). Proteomic analysis of protein S-nitrosylation. *Proteomics,* Vol. 8, No. 21, (November 2008), pp. 4484-4494, ISSN 1615-9861

Townsend, D.M. (2007). S-glutathionylation: indicator of cell stress and regulator of the unfolded protein response. *Molecular Interventions,* Vol. 7, No. 6, (December 2007), pp. 313-324, ISSN 1543-2548

Tran, M.H.; Yamada, K.; Olariu, A.; Mizuno, M.; Ren, X.H. & Nabeshima, T. (2001). Amyloid beta-peptide induces nitric oxide production in rat hippocampus: association with cholinergic dysfunction and amelioration by inducible nitric oxide synthase inhibitors. *FASEB Journal,* Vol. 15, No. 8, (June 2001), pp. 1407-1409, ISSN 1530-6860

Tran, M.H.; Yamada, K. & Nabashima, T. (2002). Amyloid beta-peptide induces cholinergic dysfunction and cognitive deficits: a minireview. *Peptides*, Vol. 23, No. 7, (July 2002), pp. 1271-1283, ISSN 1873-5169

Traub, L.M. (2009). Tickets to ride: selecting cargo for clathrin-regulated internalization. *Nature Reviews. Molecular Cell Biology*, Vol. 10, No. 9, (September 2009), pp. 583-596, ISSN 1471-0080

Unger, C.; Hedberg, M.M.; Mustafiz, T.; Svedberg, M.M. & Nordberg, A. (2005). Early changes in Abeta levels in the brain of APPswe transgenic mice--implication on synaptic density, alpha7 neuronal nicotinic acetylcholine- and N-methyl-D-aspartate receptor levels. *Molecular and Cellular Neurosciences*, Vol. 30, No. 2, (October 2005), pp. 218-227, ISSN 1095-9327

Verhoeff, N.P. (2005). Acetylcholinergic neurotransmission and the beta-amyloid cascade: implications for Alzheimer's disease. *Expert Review of Neurotherapeutics*, Vol. 5, No. 2, (March 2005), pp. 277-284, ISSN 1744-8360

Vogelsberg, V.; Neff, N.H. & Hadjiconstantinou, M. (1997). Cyclic AMP-mediated enhancement of high-affinity choline transport and acetylcholine synthesis in brain. *Journal of Neurochemistry*, Vol. 68, No. 3, (March 1997), pp. 1062-1070, ISSN 1471-4159

Walsh, D.M.; Klyubin, I.; Fadeeva, J.V.; Cullen, W.K.; Anwyl, R.; Wolfe, M.S.; Rowan, M.J. & Selkoe, D.J. (2002a). Naturally secreted oligomers of amyloid beta protein potently inhibit hippocampal long-term potentiation in vivo. *Nature*, Vol. 416, No. 6880, (April 2002), pp. 535-539, ISSN 1476-4687

Walsh, D.M.; Klyubin, I.; Fadeeva, J.V.; Rowan, M.J. & Selkoe, D.J. (2002b). Amyloid-beta oligomers: their production, toxicity and therapeutic inhibition. *Biochemical Society Transactions*, Vol. 30, No. 4, (August 2002), pp. 552-557, ISSN 1470-8752

Wang, B.; Yang, L.; Wang, Z. & Zheng, H. (2007). Amyloid precursor protein mediates presynaptic localization and activity of the high-affinity choline transporter. *Proceedings of the National Academy of Sciences of the United States of America*, Vol. 104, No. 35, (August 2007), pp. 14140-14145, ISSN 1091-6490

Wang, G.; Moniri, N.H.; Ozawa, K.; Stamler, J.S. & Daaka, Y. (2006). Nitric oxide regulates endocytosis by S-nitrosylation of dynamin. *Proceedings of the National Academy of Sciences of the United States of America*, Vol. 103, No. 5, (January 2006), pp. 1295-1300, ISSN 1091-6490

Wang, J.; Dickson, D.W.; Trojanowski, J.Q. & Lee, V.M. (1999). The levels of soluble versus insoluble brain Abeta distinguish Alzheimer's disease from normal and pathologic aging. *Experimental Neurology*, Vol. 158, No. 2, (August 1999), pp. 328-337, ISSN 1090-2430

Wang, J.; Boja, E.S.; Tan, W.; Tekle, E.; Fales, H.M.; English, S.; Mieyal, J.J. & Chock, P.B. (2001). Reversible glutathionylation regulates actin polymerization in A431 cells. *Journal of Biological Chemistry*, Vol. 276, No. 51, (December 2001), pp. 47763-47766, ISSN 1083-351X

Woolf, N.J. (1998). A structural basis for memory storage in mammals. *Progress in Neurobiology*, Vol. 55, No. 1, (May 1998), pp. 59-77, ISSN 1873-5118

Woolf N.J. & Butcher L.L. (2010). Cholinergic systems mediate action from movement to higher consciousness. *Behavioural Brain Research*, (January 2010), doi:10.1016/j.bbr.2009.12.046, ISSN 1872-7549

Xie, J. & Guo, Q. (2004). Par-4 inhibits choline uptake by interacting with CHT1 and reducing its incorporation on the plasma membrane. *Journal of Biological Chemistry,* Vol. 279, No. 27, (July 2004), pp. 28266-28275, ISSN 1083-351X

Yamamura, H.I. & Snyder, S.H. (1972). Choline: high-affinity uptake by rat brain synaptosomes. *Science,* Vol. 178, No. 61, (November 1972), pp. 626-628, ISSN 1095-9203

Yang, S.J.; Liang, H.L. & Wong-Riley, M.T. (2006). Activity-dependent transcriptional regulation of nuclear respiratory factor-1 in cultured rat visual cortical neurons. *Neuroscience,* Vol. 141, No. 3, (September 2006), pp. 1181-1192, ISSN 1873-7544

Yano, H.; Kuroda, S. & Buchanan, B.B. (2002). Disulfide proteome in the analysis of protein function and structure. *Proteomics,* Vol. 2, No. 9, (September 2002), pp. 1090-1096, ISSN 1615-9861

Zamani, M.R. & Allen, Y.S. (2001). Nicotine and its interaction with beta-amyloid protein: a short review. *Biological Psychiatry,* Vol. 49, No. 3, (February 2001), pp. 221-232, ISSN 1873-2402

Zhao, F.; Ilbert, M.; Varadan, R.; Cremers, C.M.; Hoyos, B.; Acin-Perez, R.; Vinogradov, V.; Cowburn, D.; Jakob, U. & Hammerling, U. (2011). Are zinc-finger domains of protein kinase C dynamic structures that unfold by lipid or redox activation? *Antioxidants and Redox Signaling,* Vol. 14, No. 5, (March 2011), pp. 757-66, ISSN 1557-7716

Zhu, X.; Raina, A.K.; Lee, H.G.; Casadesus, G.; Smith, M.A. & Perry, G. (2004). Oxidative stress signalling in Alzheimer's disease. *Brain Research,* Vol. 1000, No. 1-2, (March 2004), pp. 32-39, ISSN 1872-6240

6

Protective Roles of the Incretin Hormones Glucagon-Like Peptide-1 and Glucose-Dependent Insolinotropic Polypeptide Hormones in Neurodegeneration

Christian Hölscher
Ulster University, Neuroscience department, School of Biomed Sci, Northern Ireland, United Kingdom

1. Introduction

Alzheimer's disease is a sporadic disease with very few risk gene links associated with it. Therefore, it is very difficult to assess what the underlying causes of this diseases are, and what the initial triggering mechanisms may be. As the disease can only be diagnosed when it has already developed, very little is known what those early phase processes are that initiate the sequence of events that evenutally lead to neurodegeneration. Another approach to investigate the contributing factors is the correlation with other conditions that increase the risk of developing AD. Several such risk factors have been identified, and interestingly, type 2 diabetes is one of these. In type 2 diabetes mellitus (T2DM), insulin is no longer able to reduce the levels of blood sugar after a meal. In fact, ensulin levels may even be increased as an attempt by the body to overcome the reduced effectiveness of insulin in the periphery, which may be caused by insulin receptor desensitisation. Due to the change of lifelstyle in the industrialised nations, an unhealthy diet in combination with lack of exercise, levels of T2DM are on the rise. This may increase the rate of AD cases in the future. A lot of research is currently conducted in developing novel treatments of T2DM (Dailey 2008, Frias & Edelman 2007, Pi-Sunyer 2008, Scheen 2008). Since insulin effectiveness is reduced in diabetes, research into other signalling pathways that support insulin actions or that reduce blood glucose independently is ongoing. One of these strategies focus on the use of the incretins, a class of peptide hormones that helps to normalise insulin signaling and also improves blood sugar levels. Incretins increase the release of insulin during high blood sugar levels, the so-called 'incretin effect'. They have little effect on normal blood sugar levels and therefore are suitable for treating non-diabetics. In addition, incretins have a range of other effects that help regulate physiological lipid and glucose levels, eg. they increase the uptake of lipids and glucose in cells that express the receptor (Baggio & Drucker 2007, Drucker & Nauck 2006, D. E. Green 2007).

T2DM has been identified as a risk factor for AD, indicating that insulin signaling impairment may be a factor in initiating or accelerating the development of AD. Epidemiological studies found a clear correlation between T2DM and the risk of developing AD or other neurodegenerative disorders at a later stage (Haan 2006, Luchsinger, Tang, Shea, & Mayeux 2004, Ristow 2004, Strachan 2005). For example, a study of patient databases of the Mayo clinic showed a clear correlation between T2DM and AD. In this study, 85% of AD patients also had T2DM or increased fasting glucose levels, compared to only 42% in the control group. T2DM was clearly identified as a risk factor that doubled the chance of developing AD (Janson et al. 2004). Reduced insulin sensitivity and efficacy is also observed in the majority of elderly people and contributes to the development of AD (Carro & Torres-Aleman 2004, Hoyer 2004). It was also shown that insulin receptors in the brain are desensitised in AD patients, which has been named 'type 3 diabetes' (Lester-Coll et al. 2006, Steen et al. 2005). A recent study reported that insulin receptor levels are downregulated in the brains of patients with AD. Insulin receptors were found to be internalised in neurons, and the second messengers IRS1 and IRS2 were reduced in total levels but had increased levels of inactivated phospho^{Ser312} (Moloney et al. 2010). This unexpected connection between T2DM and AD opened up novel research avenues to investigate what the underlying mechanisms for this may be. Insulin is a hormone that has a range of functions in the body. Its general physiological profile is that of a growth factor (see fig. 1). Insulin is crucial for cell growth and survival. Neurons also carry insulin receptors, and activating these induces dendritic sprouting, neuronal stem cell activation, and general cell growth, repair and neuroprotection (Holscher 2005, Hoyer 2004, L. Li & Hölscher 2007, Stockhorst, de Fries, Steingrueber, & Scherbaum 2004, van Dam & Aleman 2004). Furthermore, insulin has potent neuroprotective factors, and also regulates GSK3ß, the main kinase that phosphorylates Tau, which is the major component of neurofibrillary tangles found in the brains of AD (Carro & Torres 2004, L. Li & Hölscher 2007). Insulin also improves brain activity such as attention, memory formation and cognition in humans (Okereke et al. 2008, Reger, Watson, Green, Baker et al. 2008, Watson & Craft 2004, W. Q. Zhao, Chen, Quon, & Alkon 2004). Nasal application of insulin, an application route where it enters the brain more directly, had clear effects on attention and memory formation (S. Craft 2007, Reger, Watson, Green, Baker et al. 2008, Reger, Watson, Green, Wilkinson et al. 2008). A recent phase II clinical trial showed that nasal application of insulin improves memory in patients with mild cognitive impairments and early AD patients, improves the CSF amyloid1-40/1-42 ratio, showed enhancement of cortical activation in PET scans, and also showed improvement in cognitive tasks (S Craft 2010).

In animal models, a decrease in insulin receptor signalling produces cognitive impairments and a reduction in hippocampal synaptic neurotransmission and synaptic plasticity, a mechanism that may be linked to memory formation (Biessels, De Leeuw, Lindeboom, Barkhof, & Scheltens 2006, C. Hölscher 2001, Trudeau, Gagnon, & Massicotte 2004). Diabetic mice show clear imprairments in spatial learning and synaptic plasticity (LTP) in the hippocampus. Treatment with incretins effectively prevented or reversed these impairments (V. A. Gault, Porter, Flatt, & Holscher 2010, Porter, Kerr, Flatt, Holscher, & Gault 2010). People with T2DM also have cognitive impairments, and effective treatment with diabetes medication improves these impairments (Gispen & Biessels 2000, Hoyer 2004). Conversely, insulin injected into the brain can improve performance in memory tasks in animals (Stockhorst et al. 2004). Treatments of diabetic animals with insulin also rescues the impairment in synaptic plasticity (Biessels, Bravenboer, & Gispen 2004, Gispen & Biessels 2000). The basis for this neuroprotective effect is that activation of neuronal insulin receptors has been shown to induce dendritic sprouting, neuronal stem cell activation, and general cell growth, repair, and additional neurotropic effects (Holscher 2005, Hoyer 2004, L. Li & Hölscher 2007, Stockhorst et al. 2004, van Dam & Aleman 2004). Therefore it is not surprising that insulin also improves brain function such as attention, memory and cognition in humans (Okereke et al. 2008, Reger, Watson, Green, Baker et al. 2008, Watson & Craft 2004, W. Q. Zhao et al. 2004).

In conclusion, the impairment of insulin signalling in the brain appears to play a role in the development of neurodegenerative disorders, as it leaves neurons more vulnerable to cytotoxic influences (S. Craft 2005, 2007, Hallschmid & Schultes 2009, Holscher 2005, Hoyer 2004).

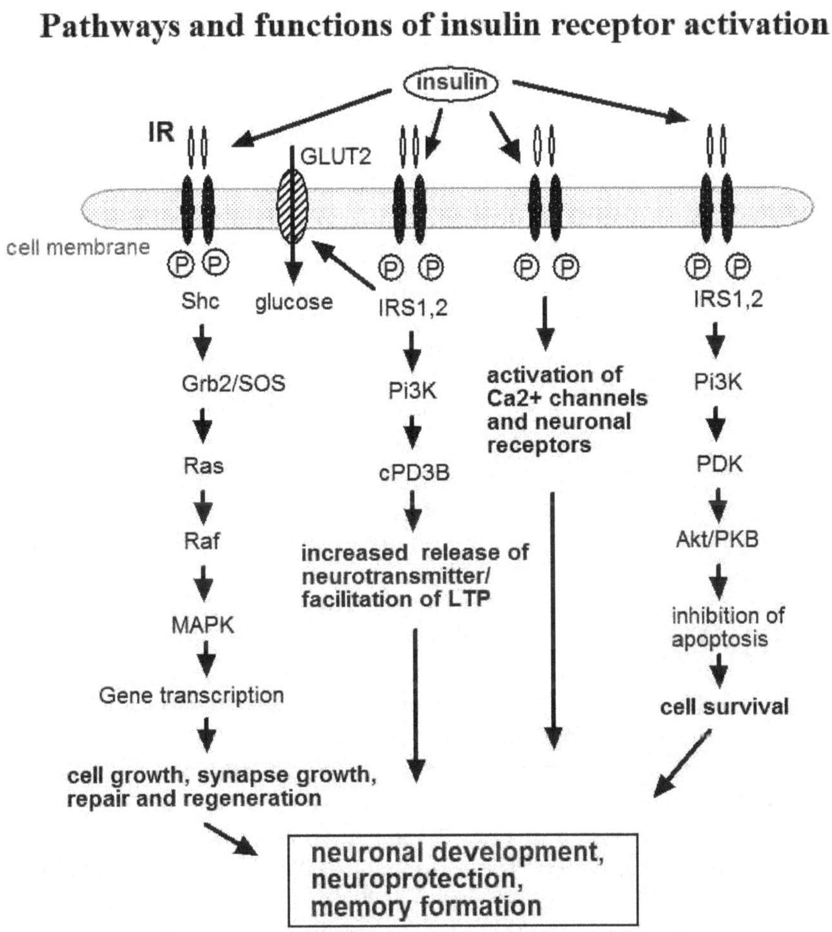

Fig. 1. An overview of some of the roles and functions of insulin receptors (IR). Traditionally, insulin is associated with its blood glucose lowering activity. This is achieved by activating a glucose uptake transporter, eg. GLUT-2. This function is only one of many of the IR. Recent research has uncovered a number of important roles in neuronal growth, synaptic development, and direct control of neurotransmitter release. During neuronal activity, insulin is released and binds to the a-subunit of the receptor. This activates the tyrosine kinase phosphorylation of the b-subunit. Then, several second messenger pathways can be activated:

1. Activation of the insulin receptor-Shc-MAP kinase pathway activates gene expression. These code for proteins that are required for cell growth, synapse growth, and for cell repair and maintenance (Biessels et al. 2006, Hoyer 1997).

2. IR activation has a direct effect on neurotransmission, and primes synapses for induction of long-term potentiation of neuronal transmission (LTP) (Biessels et al. 2004). This pathway most likely involves binding of insulin receptor substrate-1 (IRS1) and insulin receptor substrate-2 (IRS2) to phosphatidylinositol 3-kinase (PI3K). Then, the cyclic nucleotide phosphodiesterase 3B (cPD3B) is activated (A. Z. Zhao et al. 2000). This would prime the synapse for increased neurotransmitter vesicle release (de la Monte & Wands 2006). Modulation of neurotransmission will influence memory formation, information processing, and cognitive processes (C Hölscher 1999).

2. The incretins hormones: Glucagon-like Peptide-1 (GLP-1) and Glucose-dependent Insolinotropic Polypeptide (GIP)

As insulin receptors are desensitised in T2DM and in AD, and injection of insulin itself can have dangerous effects on blood sugar levels and loses its effectiveness over time, scientist in the field are investigating different strategies how to improve blood glucose level maintenance. In addition, it is not sensible to treat AD patients with insulin that do not have diabetes. However, other signalling pathways exist that also modulate blood glucose levels, eg. the incretin hormone signalling pathways - in particular GLP-1 and GIP (Frias & Edelman 2007, V. A. Gault, McClean et al. 2007).

GLP-1 is an endogenous 30-amino acid peptide hormone (fig 3a), which is released by intestinal L and K-cells after a meal. It has several physiological roles in the body to control cell metabolism (fig. 2). GLP-1 is a product of the glucagons gene which encodes the precursor peptide proglucagon. This peptide contains three glucagon-like peptides: glucagon, glucagon-like peptide 1 and glucagon-like peptide 2 (Baggio & Drucker 2007, B. D. Green et al. 2004). The GLP-1 receptor belongs to the class B family of G-protein coupled receptors. The receptors for glucagon, GLP-2 and GIP also belong to this group. Activation of the receptor activates an adenylate cyclase, increases IP3 levels, increases intracellular Ca^{2+} and affects levels of other second messengers (Baggio & Drucker 2007, Holscher 2010). GLP-1 receptor stimulation enhances beta-cell proliferation in the pancreas by activating stem cell proliferation, facilitates glucose-dependent insulin secretion and lowers blood glucose in patients with T2DM (B. D. Green et al. 2006, Lovshin & Drucker 2009).

GIP is a 42-amino acid incretin hormone which activates pancreatic islets to enhance insulin secretion and to help reduce postprandial hyperglycaemia, similar to GLP-1 (V. A. Gault, Flatt, & O'Harte 2003; Fig 3b). GIP also has been shown to promote pancreatic beta-cell growth, differentiation, proliferation and cell survival, documenting its growth-hormone properties (V. A. Gault et al. 2003). Therefore, research is ongoing to develop GIP as an therapeutic tool for T2DM treatment (Irwin et al. 2006) (see fig. 3b). GIP is a member of the vasoactive intestinal peptide seretin/glucagon family of neuroregulatory polypeptides which also include the pituitary adenylate cyclase activating peptide and the growth hormone releasing factor. It is expressed in pancreatic alpha cells, endocrine K and L cells, and also in neurons (Nyberg et al. 2005). Apart from the incretin effect of enhancing insulin release under hyperglycaemic conditions, GIPR activity in bone tissues enhances bode density, uptake of fat into adipose cells, and stem cell or neuronal progenitor cell proliferation (Baggio & Drucker 2007, Figueiredo et al. 2010). GIPR KO mice show a decrease in neuronal stem cell proliferation, and GIP analogues activate neuronal stem cells (E Faivre, McClean, & Hölscher 2010, Nyberg, Jacobsson, Anderson, & Eriksson 2007).

2.1 Incretins also play important roles in the brain

GLP-1 receptors are found on neurons in the brains of rodents and humans (Goke, Larsen, Mikkelsen, & Sheikh 1995, Perry & Greig 2005). They are predominately expressed on large size neurons, on the cell bodies and also on dendrites, indicating that they are located on the synapse (A Hamilton & Holscher 2009). Similar to insulin, GLP-1 is predominately known for its action on blood sugar levels. However, just as insulin, GLP-1 is principally a growth factor and has the main properties of all growth factors (Holscher & Li 2010). GLP-1 increases cell growth, proliferation and repair, and inhibits apoptosis (A. Hamilton, Patterson, Porter, Gault, & Holscher 2011, Perfetti, Zhou, Doyle, & Egan 2000). In the brain,

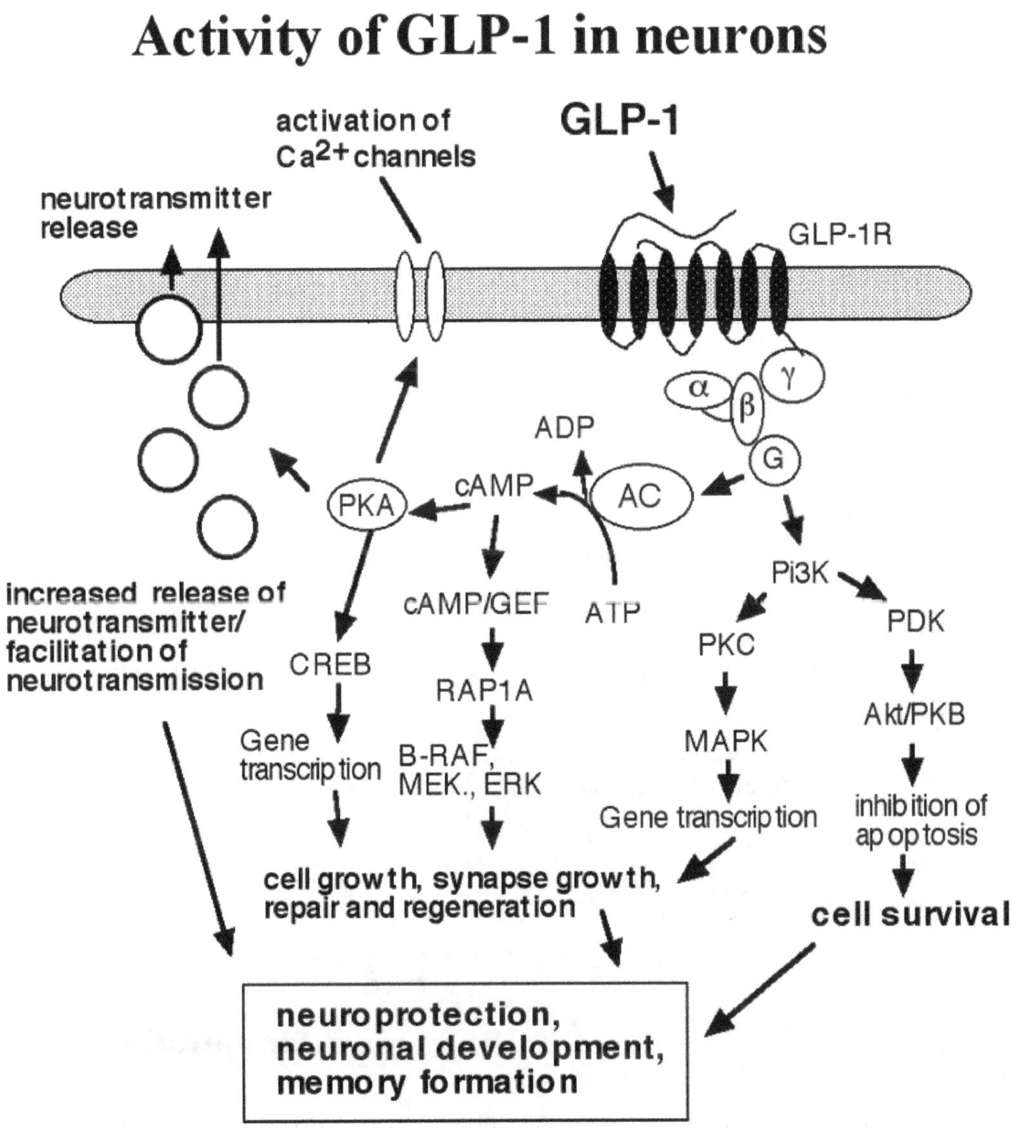

Fig. 2. Overview of the main pathways induced by GLP-1 in neurons. As compared to fig. 1, the overall mechanisms are very similar. The main physiological effects of GLP-1 on cell growth, proliferation, regeneration and inhibition of apoptosis are identical. Differences can be seen in the control of vesicle release, which is glucose-dependent in ß-cells but not in neurons. For more details see (Holscher 2010, Holscher & Li 2010).

GLP - 1 sequences

Native GLP - 1
HAEGTFTSDVSSYLEGQAAKEFIAWLVKGR

Asp(7)GLP - 1
DAEGTFTSDVSSYLEGQAAKEFIAWLVKGR

Val(8)GLP - 1
HVEGTFTSDVSSYLEGQAAKEFIAWLVKGR

Pro(9)GLP - 1
HAPGTFTSDVSSYLEGQAAKEFIAWLVKGR

Exendin - 4
HGEGTFTSDLSKQMEEEAVRLFIEWLKNGGPSSGAPPPS

Lixisenatide
HGEGTFTSDLSKQMEEEAVRLFIEWLKNGGPSSGAPPSKKKKKK - NH2

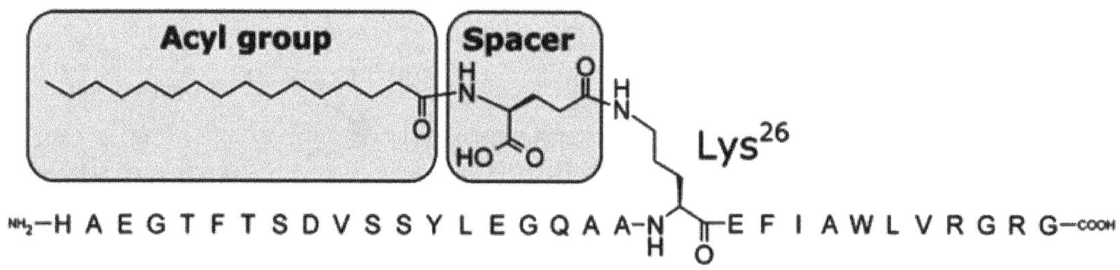

Liraglutide

Fig. 3. a. Shown are the amino acid sequences of the native GLP-1 peptide and also of some modifications of GLP-1 designed to prevent degradation by the DPP-IV protease. Shown are amino acid substitutions at position 7, 8, or 9 (Holscher 2010), and a fatty acid addition to a modified GLP-1 peptide (liraglutide). Liraglutide has the amino acid sequence of native GLP-1 with one modification, Arg34, and are derivatised at position 26 with a spacer and an acyl group (Madsen et al. 2007). The natural GLP-1 analogue exendin-4 sequence is shown. This peptide is found in the saliva of the reptile Gila monster. A derivative of this sequence is Lixisenatide, which is a long-acting GLP-1 analogue currently in clinical trials as a treatment of T2DM (Christensen, Knop, Holst, & Vilsboll 2009).

GIP sequences

Native GIP
MVATKTFALLLLSLFLAVGLGEKKEGHFSALPSLPVGSHAKV

*d*Ala(2)GIP
MAATKTFALLLLSLFLAVGLGEKKEGHFSALPSLPVGSHAKV

Pro(3)GIP
MVPTKTFALLLLSLFLAVGLGEKKEGHFSALPSLPVGSHAKV

Fig. 3. b. Shown are the amino acid sequences of the native GIP peptide and also of some of the modifications of GIP to prevent degradation by the DPP-IV protease. Shown are amino acid substitutions at position 2 and 3. The analogue D-ALA(2)GIP acts as an agonist to the receptor, while the analogue Pro(3)GIP has antagonistic properties (V. Gault et al. 2005, V. A. Gault & C. Holscher 2008, V. A. Gault, Hunter et al. 2007).

GLP-1 has been documented to induce neurite outgrowth and to protect against excitotoxic cell death and oxidative injury in cultured neuronal cells (Perry et al. 2002, Perry et al. 2003). Neurons were found to be protected against cell death induced by beta-amyloid 1-42, the peptide that aggregates in the brains of Alzheimer patients, and against oxidative stress and membrane lipid peroxidation caused by iron (Perry & Greig 2005). In addition to this, mice that overexpress GLP-1 receptors in the hippocampus showed increased neurite outgrowth and improved spatial learning. Enhanced progenitor cell proliferation in the brain was also found in this study (During et al. 2003). The novel GLP-1 analogue Liraglutide also increases the division of neuronal progenitor cells in the brain, and even increases neuronal neogenesis in the brains of a mouse model of AD (P. McClean, Parthsarathy, Faivre, & Hölscher 2011) (see fig 4). These properties are typical growth factor effects, and by activating neuronal progenitor cell proliferation and neurogenesis it may be possible to regenerate parts of the lost brain tissue and to regain some of the lost cognitive functions in patients with AD (Sugaya et al. 2007).

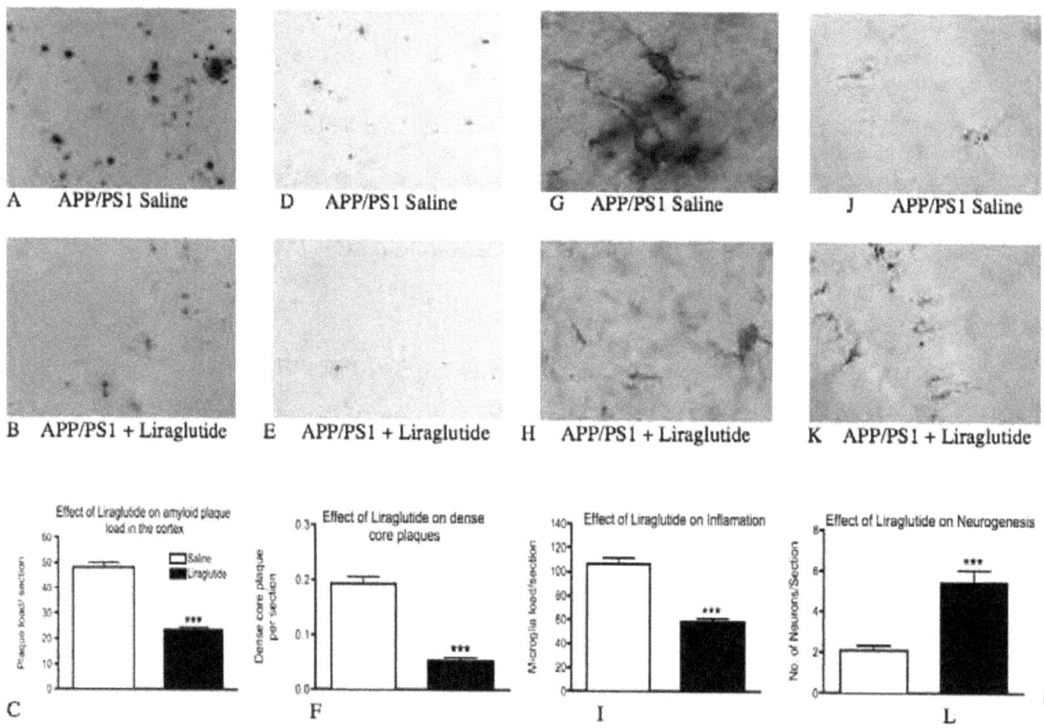

Fig. 4. Histological hallmarks of AD are improved with Liraglutide. Histological analysis of the liraglutide-injected APP/PS1 mice showed a reduction in the number of plaques in the cortex and hippocampus of Liraglutide-treated APP/PS1 mice was halved (A, B, C). The number of Congo-red positive dense core plaques was reduced to 25% (D, E, F). The inflammatory response, as shown by activated glia (IBA-1stain), was also halved (G, H, I). Mice treated with Liraglutide also had a significant increase in neurogenesis (Doublecortin positive cells) compared with saline treated animals (J, K, L). Sample micrographs show saline-treated on top, Liraglutide below, and overall quantification at bottom. ***P<0.001, (student's t-test), n=6) (P. McClean et al. 2011).

GIP is expressed in neurons and used as a neurotransmitter, and GIP receptors are also found in the brain (V. A. Gault & C. Holscher 2008, Nyberg et al. 2005, Nyberg et al. 2007). Even less is known about the roles of GIP in the brain than about the roles of GLP-1. GIP enhances neuronal progenitor proliferation in the dentate gyrus and affects learning, as discussed below (E. Faivre, Gault, Thorens, & Holscher 2011, E Faivre & Hölscher 2011).

2.2 Effects of incretins on synaptic transmission

Insulin as well as the incretins not only have growth-factor like properties in the brain, but also modulate synaptic activity. Neurons communicate via synaptic activity, and this activity can be enhanced for longer periods of time (long-term potentiation of synaptic transmission, LTP (C Hölscher 1999). One study showed that the injection of GLP-1 into the basal ganglia increased the synaptic release of the neurotransmitter glutamate (Mora, Exposito, Sanz, & Blazquez 1992). GLP-1 also increased the spontaneous firing rate of pyramidal neurons in the hippocampus (J. I. Oka, Goto, & Kameyama 1999). Interestingly, beta-amyloid fragments can directly affect synaptic transmission and impair the use-dependent upregulation of synaptic transmission (LTP). Since such a mechanism could be a used for storing information in the brain (C. Hölscher 2001), this amyloid-induced block of LTP may be in part responsible for impaired memory formation in patients with AD (Freir, Holscher, & Herron 2001, C Hölscher, Gengler, Gault, Harriott, & Mallot 2007). In addition, a recent study has shown that soluble beta-amyloid fragments directly bind to and decrease insulin receptor densities on neuronal dendrites (Xie et al. 2002, W. Q. Zhao et al. 2008). This may be a mechanism how insulin signalling in the brain becomes impaired in people with AD.

Further studies showed that direct injection of GLP-1 or long-lasting GLP-1 analogues into the brain markedly enhanced LTP in the hippocampus, a brain area that is involved in memory formation. Agonists such as Val^8-GLP-1 showed a clear upregulation of LTP, while the selective GLP-1 antagonist exendin(9-36) blocked LTP (V. Gault & C. Holscher 2008). The novel GLP-1 analogue liraglutide that has been released onto the market as a treatment for T2DM also upregulated LTP (P. L. McClean, Gault, Harriott, & Holscher 2010). Importantly, GLP-1 analogues were able to prevent the impairment of LTP that was induced by beta-amyloid fragments (V. Gault & C. Holscher 2008, Gengler, McClean, McCurtin, Gault, & Holscher 2010, P. McClean et al. 2011). These effects are most impressive and underline the fact that beta-amyloid has numerous independent effects on cell physiology; some of which may occur very early on in AD, long before amyloid aggregates appear and neuronal death is observed (Gong et al. 2003, Townsend, Shankar, Mehta, Walsh, & Selkoe 2006). Moreover, GLP-1, liraglutide and exendin-4 have been shown to reduce endogenous levels of beta-amyloid in a mouse model of AD, and to reduce levels of beta-amyloid precursor protein (APP) in neurons (P. McClean et al. 2011, Perry et al. 2003). In contrast, the elimination of the GLP-1R in a KO mouse model severely impaired learning abilities and also strongly reduced synaptic plasticity (Abbas, Faivre, & Hölscher 2009). Interestingly enough, spatial learning and synaptic plasticity is also impaired in mouse models of diabetes, and exendin-4 is able to reverse these impairments (V. A. Gault et al. 2010). These results suggest that treatment with GLP-1 or long-lasting analogues beneficially affect a number of the therapeutic targets associated with AD, such as impaired memory, impaired neuronal synaptic transmission, increased neurodegenerative processes and reduced neuronal regeneration.

Interestingly, GIP receptors are also expressed in the brain and are found on larger neurons such as the pyramidal cortical neurons (Nyberg et al. 2005), which is similar to the pattern of expression of GLP-1 receptors (A Hamilton & Holscher 2009). The peptide GIP is also expressed in neurons and serves as a neuronal transmitter (Nyberg et al. 2007). Stable analogues such as D-ala^2-GIP or N-glyc-GIP facilitate synaptic plasticity in the hippocampus, while the antagonist Pro^3-GIP impairs LTP (V. A. Gault & C. Holscher 2008). Impressively, GIP analogues can prevent the LTP impairment that beta-amyloid fragments induce on synaptic transmission in the brain (V. A. Gault & C. Holscher 2008). In a GIPR-KO mouse strain, LTP was also much reduced, and paired-pulse facilitation showed an effect on the presynapse, indicating that the release of synaptic vesicles is reduced (E. Faivre et al. 2011). The long-lasting GIP analogue D-Ala^2-GIP also had neuroprotective effects in an APP/PS1 mouse model of AD. In 12 months old mice, synaptic plasticity in area CA1 of the hippocampus and spatial memory formation was impaired in control APP/PS1 mice but was unimpaired in D-Ala^2-GIP treated APP/PS1 mice. In addition, the amyloid plaque load was much reduced, showing impressive effects in reducing the main hallmarks of AD (E Faivre & Hölscher 2011). This suggests that these analogues have neuroprotective properties in AD and protect synapses from the detrimental effects of beta-amyloid. The receptor distribution in the brain and also the effects of analogues on LTP is very similar when comparing GLP-1 analogues with GIP analogues. This would suggest that the physiological roles of these incretins may also be very similar. However, the clear results in impairing LTP (and learning) in the GLP-1R KO or GIPR KO mice show that one incretin cannot compensate the impairment or receptor loss of the another. This suggests that both incretins play distinctive roles that we currently know very little about, but also show very similar growth-factor-like effects.

2.3 Effects of incretins on memory formation

GLP-1 and longer acting analogues that can cross the BBB have beneficial effects on cognition. A behavioural study showed that the GLP-1 analogue exendin-4 can prevent the learning impairments induced by the injection of beta-amyloid fragments (J. Oka, Suzuki, & Kondo 2000). The GLP-1 analogue Val^8-GLP-1 also prevented the detrimental effect of beta-amyloid injected icv. has on learning a water maze task (Wang et al. 2010). Another study showed that GLP-1 when injected *icv.* can enhance memory formation. The study also showed that the GLP-1 analogue Ser(2)exendin(1-9) can enhance learning of a spatial task when injected *ip.*, indicting that this analogue crosses the BBB (During et al. 2003). The overexpression of the GLP-1 receptor also enhanced learning of a spatial task, while the deletion of GLP-1 receptor in KO mice impaired learning (During et al. 2003). In a different study, GLP-1 receptor KO mice were impaired in learning spatial and recognition tasks, while LTP in the hippocampus was severely impaired (Abbas et al. 2009). These results show that GLP-1 receptors do play an important role in cognitive processes in the brain, and that GLP-1 analogues can enhance learning even when injected *ip.*

Recent studies have shown that stable GIP analogues such as D-ala^2-GIP or Pro^3-GIP cross the BBB and also enhance neuronal stem cell proliferation in the brain (E Faivre et al. 2010). Furthermore, GIP analogues have clear effects on memory formation, with the GIP receptor agonist D-Ala^{2}GIP facilitating memory, and the GIP receptor antagonist Pro^3-GIP impairing memory (E Faivre et al. 2010). GIP analogues also have clear effects on synaptic plasticity in the brain. They enhance synaptic plasticity in the hippocampus, a mechanism considered by some to represent the cellular level of memory formation. Importantly, beta-amyloid impairs synaptic plasticity, and injection of GIP analogues protect synapses from the detrimental effects of beta-amyloid(25-35) (V. A. Gault & C. Holscher 2008). In another study, icv. infusion of Abeta1-40 in mice produced impairments in a water maze test, and the infusion of GIP icv. prevented the amyloid induced impairment in spatial learning (Figueiredo et al. 2010).

These properties make GIP analogues a promising target for the development of novel treatments of AD. As described earlier, spatial and non-spatial learning was greatly impaired in a GIPR- KO mouse strain, showing that the lack of GIP signalling plays an important role in memory formation, and cannot be compensated for by the still functioning insulin and GLP-1 signalling pathways (E. Faivre et al. 2011).

2.4 Novel incretin analogues have neuroprotective effects in mouse models of AD

As an important pre-clinical test, novel analogues of GLP-1 have shown neuroprotective properties in mouse models of AD. In one study, the GLP-1 analogue Val^{8}-GLP-1 had neuroprotective effects in a mouse model of AD that overexpresses the human Swedish mutated form of APP and a human mutated form of presenelin-1. The mice develop high densities of beta-amyloid plaques in the cortex and hippocampus, starting at 3 months of age (Radde et al. 2006). When injecting Val^{8}-GLP-1 chronically ip. at a dose of 25nmol/kg *ip.* once-daily for 3 weeks, synaptic plasticity in the hippocampus was protected from the effects of plaque formation and did not differ from littermate wildtype control mice. LTP was completely protected even at 18 months of age. In addition, the number of Congo red positive dense-core amyloid plaques in the brain was reduced. LTP was also improved in 18 month old *wild-type* mice when compared to controls, indicating that GLP-1 analogues also protect the brain to some degree from age-related synaptic degenerative processes (Gengler et al. 2010). Furthermore, the GLP-1 analogue exendin-4 which is currently on the market as a treatment of T2DM (Byetta®) had been tested in a triple transgenic mouse model of AD. This model also expresses the Swedish mutated form of human APP and a PS-1, and in addition expresses a mutated form of tau protein. The mice develop plaques at around 12-14 months. They also show hyperphosphorylated tau, similar to humans with AD. Exendin-4 was applied subcutaneously via osmotic pumps. To test the effects of a combination of diabetes and AD, a group of transgenic mice were made diabetic by injection of streptozotocin. The main findings were that in the diabetic mouse model of AD, beta-amyloid production had increased and plaque formation in the brain was enhanced. The treatment with exendin-4 treated the diabetes, reduced beta-amyloid production and plaque formation (Y. Li et al. 2010).

In another study, the novel GLP-1 analogue liraglutide that is also on the market as a T2DM treatment (Victoza®) enhanced memory formation and synaptic plasticity in the brains of APP/PS1 mice after ip. injection (25nmol/kg bw, once daily) for 8 weeks, at a dose that is comparable to the dose given to T2DM patients (0.9-1.8 mg subcutaneously once-daily). The learning impairments observed in untreated AD mice were reversed by liraglutide (fig. 5), and the impairment of hippocampal synaptic plasticity that develops over time in untreated mice was also prevented. More importantly, amyloid plaque formation was reduced to 50%, and the formation of Congo-red dense core plaques was reduced to 30%. In addition, the inflammation response (activated microglia) was also halved. Furthermore, increased neurogenesis was observed in the dentate gyrus of these mice, normalising the number of young neurons when compared to wild type controls (fig. 4). The level of soluble amyloid-oligomers was also greatly reduced (P. McClean et al. 2011).

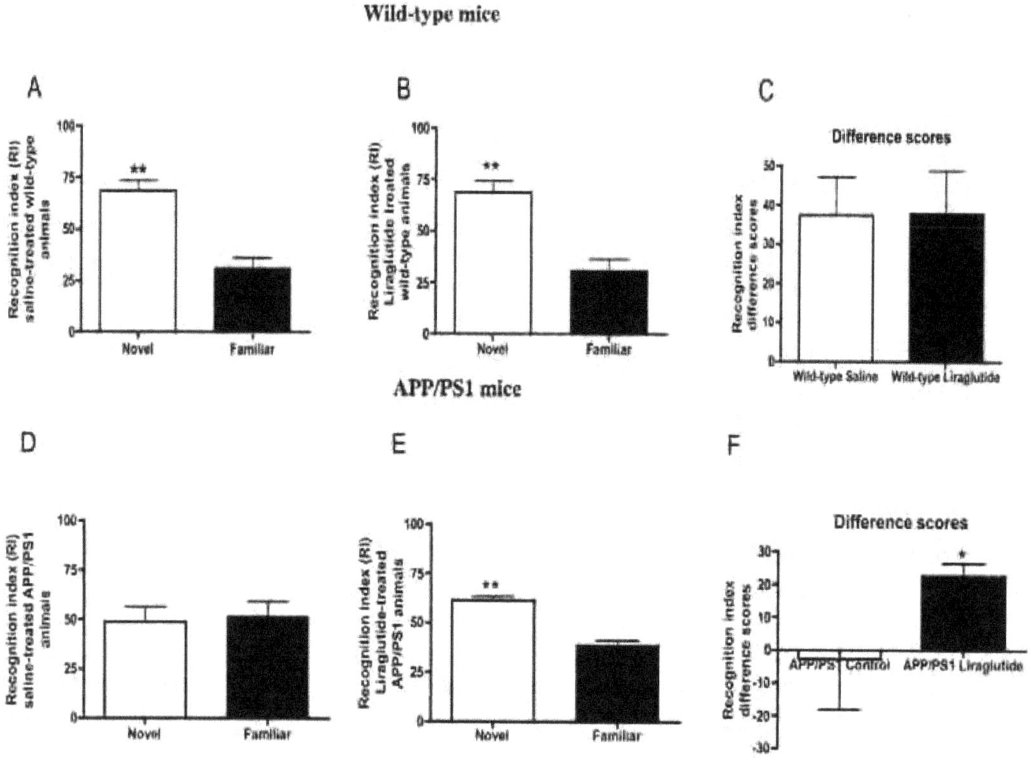

Fig. 5. Effect of the diabetes drug Liraglutide on recognition memory in APP/PS1 mice. In the object recognition task two identical objects were shown to mice for 10min, after 56 days treatment with either 0.9% Saline or Liraglutide (25nm/kg bw). After a 3h interval mice were exposed to one novel and one familiar object. Shown is the recognition index (RI) which is the % time spent exploring the novel object vs. the overall exploration time. Liraglutide treatment made no difference to the learning ability of wild-type mice (A, B), with overall difference scores comparable (C). In contrast Liraglutide rescued the recognition memory of APP/PS1 mice (E), with controls unable to discriminate between novel and familiar objects (D). Overall difference scores were significantly increased in APP/PS1 Liraglutide-treated mice. (F, student's t-test, *$p<0.05$, **$p<0.01$; all groups n=12) (P. McClean et al. 2011).

GIP analogues have shown similar effects in a APP/PS1 mouse model of AD. Injection of the GIP peptide ip. had protective effects on spatial learning in memory tasks and also reduced plaque formation and amyloid load (Figueiredo et al. 2010). In 12 months old APP/PS1 mice, spatial memory formation and object recognition memory as well as LTP was impaired in control APP/PS1 mice but was unimpaired in D-Ala^2-GIP treated APP/PS1 mice. In addition, the amyloid plaque load was much reduced, showing clear effects in reducing the main hallmarks of AD. The numer of neuronal progenitor cells in the dentate gyrus was also increased by D-Ala^2-GIP (E Faivre & Hölscher 2011).

These findings confirm that incretin analogues cross the BBB when injected peripherally and have pronounced neuroprotective effects on the main hallmarks and symptoms of AD as observed in these mouse models. This suggest that treating AD patients with novel stable

GLP-1 analogues has the potential to prevent or prolong the early phase of neurodegeneration, and potentially prevent the late phase of degeneration altogether. Since two such GLP-1 analogues are already on the market as T2DM treatment, the use of such drugs to treat neurodegenerative conditions is most promising. Importantly, clinical trials of the effects of exendin-4 in patients with Parkinson's disease (UCL, London, UK) have been started, and clinical trials in patients with MCI or early-phase AD are on their way (NIH/NIA, USA) (see an update on www.clinicaltrials.gov).

3. Acknowledgement

Dr Holscher is supported by the Alzheimer Research Trust, UK, and the Alzheimer Society, UK.

4. References

Abbas, T., Faivre, E. & Hölscher, C. (2009) Impairment of synaptic plasticity and memory formation in GLP-1 receptor KO mice: interaction between type 2 diabetes and Alzheimer's disease. *Behav Brain Res 205*: 265-271.

Baggio, L. L. & Drucker, D. J. (2007) Biology of incretins: GLP-1 and GIP. *Gastroenterology 132*(6): 2131-2157.

Biessels, G. J., Bravenboer, B. & Gispen, W. H. (2004) Glucose, insulin and the brain: modulation of cognition and synaptic plasticity in health and disease: a preface. *Eur J Pharmacol 490*(1-3): 1-4.

Biessels, G. J., De Leeuw, F. E., Lindeboom, J., Barkhof, F. & Scheltens, P. (2006) Increased cortical atrophy in patients with Alzheimer's disease and type 2 diabetes mellitus. *J Neurol Neurosurg Psychiatry 77*(3): 304-307.

Carro, E. & Torres, A. I. (2004) The role of insulin and insulin-like growth factor I in the molecular and cellular mechanisms underlying the pathology of Alzheimer's disease. *Eur J Pharmacol 490*(1-3): 127-133.

Carro, E. & Torres-Aleman, I. (2004) Insulin-like growth factor I and Alzheimer's disease: therapeutic prospects? *Expert Rev Neurother 4*(1): 79-86.

Christensen, M., Knop, F. K., Holst, J. J. & Vilsboll, T. (2009) Lixisenatide, a novel GLP-1 receptor agonist for the treatment of type 2 diabetes mellitus. *IDrugs 12*(8): 503-513.

Craft, S. (2005) Insulin resistance syndrome and Alzheimer's disease: age- and obesity-related effects on memory, amyloid, and inflammation. *Neurobiol Aging 26 Suppl 1*: 65-69.

Craft, S. (2007) Insulin resistance and Alzheimer's disease pathogenesis: potential mechanisms and implications for treatment. *Curr Alzheimer Res 4*(2): 147-152.

Craft, S. (2010). A randomized, placebo-controlled trial of intranasal insulin in amnestic MCI and early Alzheimer's, *ICAD conference* (pp. abstr. P3-455.). Hawaii, USA.

Dailey, G. (2008) Beyond insulin replacement: addressing the additional needs of the diabetes patient. *Diabetes Obes Metab 10 Suppl 2*: 83-97.

de la Monte, S. M. & Wands, J. R. (2006) Molecular indices of oxidative stress and mitochondrial dysfunction occur early and often progress with severity of Alzheimer's disease. *J Alzheimers Dis 9*(2): 167-181.

Drucker, D. J. & Nauck, M. A. (2006) The incretin system: glucagon-like peptide-1 receptor agonists and dipeptidyl peptidase-4 inhibitors in type 2 diabetes. *Lancet 368*(9548): 1696-1705.

During, M. J., Cao, L., Zuzga, D. S., Francis, J. S., Fitzsimons, H. L., Jiao, X., Bland, R. J., Klugmann, M., Banks, W. A., Drucker, D. J. & Haile, C. N. (2003) Glucagon-like peptide-1 receptor is involved in learning and neuroprotection. *Nat Med 9*(9): 1173-1179.

Faivre, E., Gault, V. A., Thorens, B. & Holscher, C. (2011) Glucose-dependent insulinotropic polypeptide receptor knockout mice are impaired in learning, synaptic plasticity, and neurogenesis. *J Neurophysiol.*

Faivre, E. & Hölscher, C. (2011). DAla2-GIP improves memory, synaptic plasticity and decreases amyloid plaques and inflammation in APP/PS1 transgenic mice, *AR-UK*. Leeds.

Faivre, E., McClean, P. & Hölscher, C. (2010). *Novel GIP analogues cross the BBB and have effects on cognitive processes and synaptic plasticity in the hippocampus.* Paper presented at the Annual conference of the Alzheimer Research Trust UK, Southampton.

Figueiredo, C. P., Pamplona, F. A., Mazzuco, T. L., Aguiar, A. S., Jr., Walz, R. & Prediger, R. D. (2010) Role of the glucose-dependent insulinotropic polypeptide and its receptor in the central nervous system: therapeutic potential in neurological diseases. *Behav Pharmacol 21*: 394-408.

Freir, D. B., Holscher, C. & Herron, C. E. (2001) Blockade of Long-Term Potentiation by beta-Amyloid Peptides in the CA1 Region of the Rat Hippocampus In Vivo. *J Neurophysiol 85*(2): 708-713.

Frias, J. P. & Edelman, S. V. (2007) Incretins and their role in the management of diabetes. *Curr Opin Endocrinol Diabetes Obes 14*(4): 269-276.

Gault, V. & Holscher, C. (2008) GLP-1 agonists facilitate hippocampal LTP and reverse the impairment of LTP induced by beta-amyloid. *Eur J Pharmacol 587*: 112-117.

Gault, V., Irwin, N., Green, B., McCluskey, J., Greer , B., Bailey, C., Harriott, P., O'Harte, F. & Flatt, P. (2005) Chemical ablation of gastric inhibitory polypeptide receptor action by daily (Pro3)GIP administration improves glucose tolerance and ameliorates insulin resistance and abnormalities of islet structure in obesity-diabetes. *Diabetes 54*: 2436-2446.

Gault, V. A., Flatt, P. R. & O'Harte, F. P. (2003) Glucose-dependent insulinotropic polypeptide analogues and their therapeutic potential for the treatment of obesity-diabetes. *Biochem Biophys Res Commun 308*(2): 207-213.

Gault, V. A. & Holscher, C. (2008) Protease-resistant glucose-dependent insulinotropic polypeptide agonists facilitate hippocampal LTP and reverse the impairment of LTP induced by beta-amyloid. *J Neurophysiol 99*(4): 1590-1595.

Gault, V. A., Hunter, K., Irwin, N., Green, B. D., Greer, B., Harriott, P., O'Harte, F. P. & Flatt, P. R. (2007) Characterisation and biological activity of Glu3 amino acid substituted GIP receptor antagonists. *Arch Biochem Biophys 461*(2): 263-274.

Gault, V. A., McClean, P. L., Irwin, N., Power, G. J., McCluskey, J. T. & Flatt, P. R. (2007) Effects of subchronic treatment with the long-acting glucose-dependent insulinotropic polypeptide receptor agonist, N-AcGIP, on glucose homeostasis in streptozotocin-induced diabetes. *Pancreas 35*(1): 73-79.

Gault, V. A., Porter, W. D., Flatt, P. R. & Holscher, C. (2010) Actions of exendin-4 therapy on cognitive function and hippocampal synaptic plasticity in mice fed a high-fat diet. *Int J Obes (Lond) 34*: 1341-1344.

Gengler, S., McClean, P., McCurtin, R., Gault, V. & Holscher, C. (2010) Val(8)GLP-1 rescues synaptic plasticity and reduces dense core plaques in APP/PS1 mice. *Neurobiol Aging DOI*: 10.1016/j.neurobiolaging.2010.1002.1014.

Gispen, W. H. & Biessels, G. J. (2000) Cognition and synaptic plasticity in diabetes mellitus. *Trends Neurosci 23*(11): 542-549.

Goke, R., Larsen, P. J., Mikkelsen, J. D. & Sheikh, S. P. (1995) Distribution of GLP-1 binding sites in the rat brain: evidence that exendin-4 is a ligand of brain GLP-1 binding sites. *Eur J Neurosci 7*(11): 2294-2300.

Gong, Y., Chang, L., Viola, K. L., Lacor, P. N., Lambert, M. P., Finch, C. E., Krafft, G. A. & Klein, W. L. (2003) Alzheimer's disease-affected brain: Presence of oligomeric A beta ligands (ADDLs) suggests a molecular basis for reversible memory loss. *Proc Natl Acad Sci U S A 100*(18): 10417-10422.

Green, B. D., Gault, V. A., Flatt, P. R., Harriott, P., Greer, B. & O'Harte, F. P. (2004) Comparative effects of GLP-1 and GIP on cAMP production, insulin secretion, and in vivo antidiabetic actions following substitution of Ala8/Ala2 with 2-aminobutyric acid. *Arch Biochem Biophys 428*(2): 136-143.

Green, B. D., Lavery, K. S., Irwin, N., O'Harte F, P., Harriott, P., Greer, B., Bailey, C. J. & Flatt, P. R. (2006) Novel GLP-1 analogue (Val8)GLP-1 results in significant improvements of glucose tolerance and pancreatic beta cell function after 3 weeks daily administration in obese diabetic (ob/ob) mice. *J Pharmacol Exp Ther 318*(2): 914-921.

Green, D. E. (2007) New therapies for diabetes. *Clin Cornerstone 8*(2): 58-63; discussion 64-55.

Haan, M. N. (2006) Therapy Insight: type 2 diabetes mellitus and the risk of late-onset Alzheimer's disease. *Nat Clin Pract Neurol 2*(3): 159-166.

Hallschmid, M. & Schultes, B. (2009) Central nervous insulin resistance: a promising target in the treatment of metabolic and cognitive disorders? *Diabetologia 52*(11): 2264-2269.

Hamilton, A. & Holscher, C. (2009) Receptors for the insulin-like peptide GLP-1 are expressed on neurons in the CNS. *Neuroreport 20*: 1161-1166.

Hamilton, A., Patterson, S., Porter, D., Gault, V. A. & Holscher, C. (2011) Novel GLP-1 mimetics developed to treat type 2 diabetes promote progenitor cell proliferation in the brain. *J Neurosci Res 89*(4): 481-489.

Holscher, C. (2005) Development of beta-amyloid-induced neurodegeneration in Alzheimer's disease and novel neuroprotective strategies. *Rev Neurosci 16*(3): 181-212.

Holscher, C. (2010) Incretin Analogues that have been Developed to Treat Type 2 Diabetes Hold Promise as a Novel Treatment Strategy for Alzheimer's Disease. *Recent Pat CNS Drug Discov 5*: 109-117.

Hölscher, C. (1999) Synaptic plasticity and learning and memory: LTP and beyond. *J Neurosci Res 58*: 62-75.

Hölscher, C. (Ed.). (2001). *Long-term potentiation induced by stimulation on the positive phase of theta rhythm: a better model for learning and memory?* Cambridge: Cambridge University Press.

Hölscher, C., Gengler, S., Gault, V., Harriott, P. & Mallot, H. (2007) Soluble beta-amyloid[25-35] reversibly impairs hippocampal synaptic plasticity and spatial learning. *Eur J Pharmacol 561*: 85-90.

Holscher, C. & Li, L. (2010) New roles for insulin-like hormones in neuronal signalling and protection: New hopes for novel treatments of Alzheimer's disease? *Neurobiol Aging 31*: 1495-1502.

Hoyer, S. (1997) Models of Alzheimer's disease: cellular and molecular aspects. *J Neural Transm 49*(11): 11-21.

Hoyer, S. (2004) Glucose metabolism and insulin receptor signal transduction in Alzheimer disease. *Eur J Pharmacol 490*(1-3): 115-125.

Irwin, N., O'Harte F, P., Gault, V. A., Green, B. D., Greer, B., Harriott, P., Bailey, C. J. & Flatt, P. R. (2006) GIP(Lys(16)PAL) and GIP(Lys(37)PAL): Novel Long-Acting Acylated Analogues of Glucose-Dependent Insulinotropic Polypeptide with Improved Antidiabetic Potential. *J Med Chem 49*(3): 1047-1054.

Janson, J., Laedtke, T., Parisi, J., O'Brien, P., Petersen, R. & Butler, P. (2004) Increased risk of type 2 diabetes in Alzheimer disease. *Diabetes 53*: 474-481.

Lester-Coll, N., Rivera, E. J., Soscia, S. J., Doiron, K., Wands, J. R. & de la Monte, S. M. (2006) Intracerebral streptozotocin model of type 3 diabetes: relevance to sporadic Alzheimer's disease. *J Alzheimers Dis 9*(1): 13-33.

Li, L. & Hölscher, C. (2007) Common pathological processes in Alzheimer Disease and Type 2 Diabetes: a review. *Brain Res Rev 56*: 384-402.

Li, Y., Duffy, K., Ottinger, M., Ray, B., Bailey, J., Holloway, H., Tweedie, D., Perry, T., Mattson, M., Kapogiannis, D., Sambamurti, K., Lahiri, D. & Greig, N. (2010) GLP-1 Receptor Stimulation Reduces Amyloid-beta Peptide Accumulation and Cytotoxicity in Cellular and Animal Models of Alzheimer's Disease. *J Alzheimers Dis 19*: 1205-1219.

Lovshin, J. A. & Drucker, D. J. (2009) Incretin-based therapies for type 2 diabetes mellitus. *Nat Rev Endocrinol 5*(5): 262-269.

Luchsinger, J. A., Tang, M. X., Shea, S. & Mayeux, R. (2004) Hyperinsulinemia and risk of Alzheimer disease. *Neurology 63*(7): 1187-1192.

Madsen, K., Knudsen, L. B., Agersoe, H., Nielsen, P. F., Thogersen, H., Wilken, M. & Johansen, N. L. (2007) Structure-activity and protraction relationship of long-acting glucagon-like peptide-1 derivatives: importance of fatty acid length, polarity, and bulkiness. *J Med Chem 50*(24): 6126-6132.

McClean, P., Parthsarathy, V., Faivre, E. & Hölscher, C. (2011) The diabetes drug Liraglutide prevents degenerative processes in a mouse model of Alzheimer's disease. *J Neurosci* 31: 6587-6594.

McClean, P. L., Gault, V. A., Harriott, P. & Holscher, C. (2010) Glucagon-like peptide-1 analogues enhance synaptic plasticity in the brain: A link between diabetes and Alzheimer's disease. *Eur J Pharmacol 630*: 158-162.

Moloney, A. M., Griffin, R. J., Timmons, S., O'Connor, R., Ravid, R. & O'Neill, C. (2010) Defects in IGF-1 receptor, insulin receptor and IRS-1/2 in Alzheimer's disease indicate possible resistance to IGF-1 and insulin signalling. *Neurobiol Aging 31*(2): 224-243.

Mora, F., Exposito, I., Sanz, B. & Blazquez, E. (1992) Selective release of glutamine and glutamic acid produced by perfusion of GLP-1 (7-36) amide in the basal ganglia of the conscious rat. *Brain Res Bull 29*(3-4): 359-361.

Nyberg, J., Anderson, M. F., Meister, B., Alborn, A. M., Strom, A. K., Brederlau, A., Illerskog, A. C., Nilsson, O., Kieffer, T. J., Hietala, M. A., Ricksten, A. & Eriksson, P. S. (2005)

Glucose-dependent insulinotropic polypeptide is expressed in adult hippocampus and induces progenitor cell proliferation. *J Neurosci 25*(7): 1816-1825.

Nyberg, J., Jacobsson, C., Anderson, M. F. & Eriksson, P. S. (2007) Immunohistochemical distribution of glucose-dependent insulinotropic polypeptide in the adult rat brain. *J Neurosci Res 85*: 2099-2119.

Oka, J., Suzuki, E. & Kondo, Y. (2000) Endogenous GLP-1 is involved in beta-amyloid protein-induced memory impairment and hippocampal neuronal death in rats. *Brain Res 878*(1-2): 194-198.

Oka, J. I., Goto, N. & Kameyama, T. (1999) Glucagon-like peptide-1 modulates neuronal activity in the rat's hippocampus. *Neuroreport 10*(8): 1643-1646.

Okereke, O. I., Selkoe, D. J., Pollak, M. N., Stampfer, M. J., Hu, F. B., Hankinson, S. E. & Grodstein, F. (2008) A profile of impaired insulin degradation in relation to late-life cognitive decline: A preliminary investigation. *Int J Geriatr Psychiatry 24*: 177-182.

Perfetti, R., Zhou, J., Doyle, M. E. & Egan, J. M. (2000) Glucagon-like peptide-1 induces cell proliferation and pancreatic-duodenum homeobox-1 expression and increases endocrine cell mass in the pancreas of old, glucose-intolerant rats. *Endocrinology 141*(12): 4600-4605.

Perry, T. & Greig, N. H. (2005) Enhancing central nervous system endogenous GLP-1 receptor pathways for intervention in Alzheimer's disease. *Curr Alzheimer Res 2*(3): 377-385.

Perry, T., Lahiri, D. K., Chen, D., Zhou, J., Shaw, K. T., Egan, J. M. & Greig, N. H. (2002) A novel neurotrophic property of glucagon-like peptide 1: a promoter of nerve growth factor-mediated differentiation in PC12 cells. *J Pharmacol Exp Ther 300*(3): 958-966.

Perry, T., Lahiri, D. K., Sambamurti, K., Chen, D., Mattson, M. P., Egan, J. M. & Greig, N. H. (2003) Glucagon-like peptide-1 decreases endogenous amyloid-beta peptide (Abeta) levels and protects hippocampal neurons from death induced by Abeta and iron. *J Neurosci Res 72*(5): 603-612.

Pi-Sunyer, F. X. (2008) The effects of pharmacologic agents for type 2 diabetes mellitus on body weight. *Postgrad Med 120*(2): 5-17.

Porter, D. W., Kerr, B. D., Flatt, P. R., Holscher, C. & Gault, V. A. (2010) Four weeks administration of Liraglutide improves memory and learning as well as glycaemic control in mice with high fat dietary-induced obesity and insulin resistance. *Diabetes Obes Metab 12*(10): 891-899.

Radde, R., Bolmont, T., Kaeser, S. A., Coomaraswamy, J., Lindau, D., Stoltze, L., Calhoun, M. E., Jaggi, F., Wolburg, H., Gengler, S., Haass, C., Ghetti, B., Czech, C., Holscher, C., Mathews, P. M. & Jucker, M. (2006) Abeta42-driven cerebral amyloidosis in transgenic mice reveals early and robust pathology. *EMBO Rep 7*(9): 940-946.

Reger, M. A., Watson, G. S., Green, P. S., Baker, L. D., Cholerton, B., Fishel, M. A., Plymate, S. R., Cherrier, M. M., Schellenberg, G. D., Frey, W. H., 2nd & Craft, S. (2008) Intranasal insulin administration dose-dependently modulates verbal memory and plasma amyloid-beta in memory-impaired older adults. *J Alzheimers Dis 13*(3): 323-331.

Reger, M. A., Watson, G. S., Green, P. S., Wilkinson, C. W., Baker, L. D., Cholerton, B., Fishel, M. A., Plymate, S. R., Breitner, J. C., DeGroodt, W., Mehta, P. & Craft, S. (2008) Intranasal insulin improves cognition and modulates beta-amyloid in early AD. *Neurology 70*(6): 440-448.

Ristow, M. (2004) Neurodegenerative disorders associated with diabetes mellitus. *J Mol Med 82*(8): 510-529.

Scheen, A. J. (2008) New therapeutic approaches in type 2 diabetes. *Acta Clin Belg 63*(6): 402-407.

Steen, E., Terry, B. M., Rivera, E., Cannon, J. L., Neely, T. R., Tavares, R., Xu, X. J., Wands, J. R. & de la Monte, S. M. (2005) Impaired insulin and insulin-like growth factor expression and signaling mechanisms in Alzheimer's disease - is this type 3 diabetes? *J Alzheimers Dis 7*(1): 63-80.

Stockhorst, U., de Fries, D., Steingrueber, H. J. & Scherbaum, W. A. (2004) Insulin and the CNS: effects on food intake, memory, and endocrine parameters and the role of intranasal insulin administration in humans. *Physiol Behav 83*(1): 47-54.

Strachan, M. W. (2005) Insulin and cognitive function in humans: experimental data and therapeutic considerations. *Biochem Soc Trans 33*(Pt 5): 1037-1040.

Sugaya, K., Kwak, Y., Ohmitsu, O., Marutle, A., Greig, N. & Choumrina, E. (2007) Practical issues in stem cell therapy for Alzheimer's disease. *Curr Alzheimer Res 4*: 370-377.

Townsend, M., Shankar, G. M., Mehta, T., Walsh, D. M. & Selkoe, D. J. (2006) Effects of secreted oligomers of amyloid beta-protein on hippocampal synaptic plasticity: a potent role for trimers. *J Physiol 572*(Pt 2): 477-492.

Trudeau, F., Gagnon, S. & Massicotte, G. (2004) Hippocampal synaptic plasticity and glutamate receptor regulation: influences of diabetes mellitus. *Eur J Pharmacol 490*(1-3): 177-186.

van Dam, P. & Aleman, A. (2004) Insulin-like growth factor-I, cognition and brain aging. *Eur J Pharmacol 490*(1-3): 87-95.

Wang, X. H., Li, L., Holscher, C., Pan, Y. F., Chen, X. R. & Qi, J. S. (2010) Val8-glucagon-like peptide-1 protects against Abeta1-40-induced impairment of hippocampal late-phase long-term potentiation and spatial learning in rats. *Neuroscience 170*(4): 1239-1248.

Watson, G. S. & Craft, S. (2004) Modulation of memory by insulin and glucose: neuropsychological observations in Alzheimer's disease. *Eur J Pharmacol 490*(1-3): 97-113.

Xie, L., Helmerhorst, E., Taddei, K., Plewright, B., Van, B. W. & Martins, R. (2002) Alzheimer's beta-amyloid peptides compete for insulin binding to the insulin receptor. *J Neurosci 22*(10): RC221.

Zhao, A. Z., Shinohara, M. M., Huang, D., Shimizu, M., Eldar-Finkelman, H., Krebs, E. G., Beavo, J. A. & Bornfeldt, K. E. (2000) Leptin induces insulin-like signaling that antagonizes cAMP elevation by glucagon in hepatocytes. *J Biol Chem 275*(15): 11348-11354.

Zhao, W. Q., Chen, H., Quon, M. J. & Alkon, D. L. w. (2004) Insulin and the insulin receptor in experimental models of learning and memory. *Eur J Pharmacol 490*(490): 71-81.

Zhao, W. Q., De Felice, F. G., Fernandez, S., Chen, H., Lambert, M. P., Quon, M. J., Krafft, G. A. & Klein, W. L. (2008) Amyloid beta oligomers induce impairment of neuronal insulin receptors. *Faseb J 22*: 246-260.

7

Metals Involvement in Alzheimer's Disease Pathogenesis

Rosanna Squitti[1,2] and Carlo Salustri[3]
[1]*Departement of Neuroscience, AFaR – Fatebenefratelli Hospital, Isola Tiberina, Rome*
[2]*Clinica Neurologica, Università Campus Biomedico, Rome*
[3]*Institute of Cognition Sciences and Technologies (CNR), Fatebenefratelli Hospital, Isola Tiberina, Rome,*
Italy

1. Introduction

When Auguste Deter died in 1906, Alois Alzheimer, who had closely followed her mental degradation over the previous 5 years, obtained her brain and performed a post-mortem study. By using a silver-staining method just developed by Bielschowsky, Alzheimer identified aggregations of fibrils and what he called 'miliary foci'. Alterations of that nature had been already observed by others in post-mortem brains, but Alzheimer was the first to relate them to his patient's dementia. He described the case a year later and Auguste Deter remained in medical history as the first clinical case of what has been ever since referred to as Alzheimer's disease. For an English translation of Alzheimer's 1907 paper, see (Alzheimer et al., 1995).

1.1 General description

Alzheimer's disease (AD) is an irreversible neurodegenerative disorder, characterized by a gradual loss of the cognitive functions inexorably leading to dementia. From an early stage characterized by a mild loss of recent memory, the disease advances to more devastating symptoms such as faulty judgments and even personality changes, to terminate in a complete loss of reasoning ability and self sufficiency. Death normally ensues 8 to 10 years after diagnosis.

AD is often referred to as early- or late-onset depending on whether it appears before or after age 65, and is normally distinguished in familial, i.e., inherited, and sporadic, which is caused by a combination of genetic, lifestyle and environmental factors.

About 75% of AD patients have the sporadic form, which has normally a late-onset. The familial form, which affects the remaining 25%, can have instead either an early-onset (about 5% of all familial cases) or a late-onset.

The early-onset familial AD is attributed to mutations in one of three genes: amyloid precursor protein (APP), Presenilin1 or Presenilin2. The genetic causes of the late-onset familial AD are not fully assessed, although the inheritance of the ε4 allele of the apolipoprotein E (*ApoE4*) has been recognized as a risk factor for both familial and sporadic late-onset AD. Carriers of this allele have a 90% statistical risk of contracting AD if they are heterozygote and a virtual certainty if homozygote (Corder et al., 1993).

All forms share the same alterations that include neuron loss, synapse loss, amyloid plaques, neurofibrillary tangles and microgliosis. However, although it is well established that AD symptoms are due to a compromised neurotransmission originating from these alterations, there is not yet full agreement on what actually initiates the neurodegeneration.

1.2 Diagnosis

Since no single test or biochemical measurement can securely lead to a diagnosis of AD, intellectual deterioration is diagnosed as possible or probable AD on the basis of a careful analysis of the symptoms, the medical history of both patient and his/her relatives, a variety of neuropsychological tests and from the exclusion of alternative conditions, generally attained via neuroimaging. Almost universally physicians today follow the NINCDS-ADRDA Criteria for diagnosis of Alzheimer's disease (McKhann et al., 1984), jointly published in 1984 by the National Institute of Neurological and Communicative Disorders and Stroke and the Alzheimer's Disease and Related Disorders Association, which specify eight cognitive domains that are compromised in AD - memory, language, perceptual skills, attention, constructive abilities, orientation, problem solving and functional abilities - and give guidelines for impairment assessment and diagnosis. NINCDS-ADRDA criteria have proven reliable over the years and have been extensively updated in 2007 to account for recent advances in neuroimaging (Dubois et al., 2007).

1.3 Symptoms

Symptom progression of AD			
Function	**Stage I (mild)**	**Stage II (moderate)**	**Stage III (severe)**
Memory	Mild amnesia (recent memory)	Amnesia (recent and remote)	Not measurable
Language	Quasi-normal, anomia	Sensory aphasia	Severely impaired
Perceptual skills	Mildly impaired	Moderately to severely impaired	Not measurable
Attention	Reduced	Impaired	Not measurable
Constructive abilities	Reduced	Impaired	Not measurable
Orientation	Mildly impaired	Impaired	Not measurable
Problem solving	Mildly impaired	Impaired	Not measurable
Functional abilities	Almost normal, some mistakes	Unreliable	Not measurable
Behavior	Mild changes, signs of withdrawal	Absent	Agitated, delusional
Gait	Normal	Normal	Impaired
Posture	Normal	Normal or flexed	Bedridden
MMSE	25-21	20-11	10-0

Table 1. Symptom progression of AD; MMSE: Mini-mental state examination (Folstein et al., 1975).

1.4 AD pathology

1.4.1 Macroscopic pathology

Atrophy is the major macroscopic characteristic of the AD brain. Ventricles are dilated, gyri appear narrower and sulci wider than in a normal brain. The loss of tissue, which roughly correlates with the degree of cognitive decline, is so severe that an AD brain can weigh less than 1000g. Frontal, parietal and temporal lobes are all involved, the hippocampus in particular being severely affected. The primary sensory-motor cortex appears affected with some delay, whereas the occipital lobe is relatively spared.

1.4.2 Microscopic pathology

The 'miliary foci' and fibril aggregations that Alzheimer observed are today normally referred to as senile plaques (SPs) and neurofibrillary tangles (NTFs), and remain the hallmarks of AD.

SPs are clusters of protein fibrils that form in the extracellular space, made of an amyloidal core, abnormal neurites and glial cells. The amyloidal core is mainly an aggregation of Amyloid-beta (Aβ), a 4 kDa peptide 39 to 43 amino acids long, which is produced by the proteolytic cleavage of the APP, a transmembrane protein present in many cell types and highly concentrated on neuron synapses. Usually, APP is cleaved on the extracellular side of the neuronal membrane by the enzyme α-secretase, but occasionally it can be cleaved by two other enzymes (β- and γ-secretase) at different sites. The result is anyway the production of Aβ segments that are released in the extracellular space and aggregate there in amyloidal plaques. The gene for APP is located on the long arm of chromosome 21.

SPs are roughly spherical with a diameter reaching up to 200 μm, and are normally distinguished in 'diffuse' and 'compact': Diffuse SPs are amorphous deposits of non-fibrillar 'pre-amyloid' Aβ, which produce no alteration of the neuropil. Compact SPs, more often referred to as 'neuritic', show instead an amyloid core surrounded by dystrophic neuritis. The latter appear as clusters of radially oriented neuronal processes.

There are at least 3 subtypes of neuritic SPs: Primitive, which lack the amyloidal core; Classical, in which a dense amyloid core is surrounded by dystrophic neuritis, which in turn appear interconnected by low density amyloidal fibrils; Burned-out, which have only the dense amyloidal core and at most a few neurites. This subdivision mirrors what researches believe is SPs' evolution: after being released, Aβ segments forms diffuse plaques in the extracellular space until elements such as cytokines, ApoE, proteoglycans and others become embedded with the complex causing it to degenerate into neuritic plaques. In other words, SPs start as diffuse and then evolve into neuritic, first primitive, then classical, and finally burned out.

SPs appear to have also an anatomical hierarchy: higher-order association areas have the highest density of SPs, whereas the primary sensory-motor cortex the lowest. Striatum and cerebellum show a rather high density of SPs, but they are all of the diffuse type. The hippocampus appears relatively spared.

Only neuritic SPs are specific to AD, whereas diffuse SPs are found also in the brains of non-demented elderly individuals.

NFTs are aggregates of modified protein tau in the intracellular space. In normal conditions, the protein tau binds to microtubules, contributes to the progress of their formation and is a key element in their stability. In AD, tau undergoes hyper-phosphorylation which causes the protein to aggregate. Moreover, upon hyper-phosphorylation, tau loses its binding capability so that the microtubules disintegrate. Each filament is made of two strands twisted around each other to form a helix, whose period is about 80 nm and diameter either 8 nm or 20 nm.

In AD, the areas most affected by NFTs are hippocampus, sibiculum, amygdala, entorhinal and transentorhinal corteces. In the neocortex, higher-order association areas are more affected than the unimodal association areas, and the primary sensory-motor cortex is relatively spared. NFTs are also numerous in the nucleus basalis, limbic nuclei of the thalamus, locus ceruleus, substantia nigra, and the raphe nuclei of the brainstem.

NFTs' shapes seem to be influenced by the shape of the neuron in which they are. In fact, they look like a flame in pyramidal neurons, as for example in the hippocampus, whereas they appear more globular in rounded neurons, such as those of the nucleus basalis.

NFT develop first into early and then into fully grown tangles. After the death of the neuron some NFTs (often referred to as 'ghost' tangles) are visible also in the extracellular space.

It is important to remember, though, that NFTs are not AD specific and are frequent also in non-demented elderly individuals.

Neuropil threads are another form of neurofibrillary degeneration that in AD is found widely distributed throughout the gray matter, especially in distal dendrites and axons. They owe their name to their appearance which resembles short threads.

As mentioned above, the ultimate result of the presence of plaques and tangles in AD is a severe neuronal loss that can reach 60% in the hippocampus and 80% in the nucleus basalis and in some frontal and temporal areas.

2. Hypotheses on the causes of AD

2.1 Classic hypotheses

There are three major classic hypotheses on the origin of AD. The cholinergic hypothesis (Francis et al., 1999, Rossor 1983), which is the oldest and the one on which the majority of currently available drug therapies are based, proposes that AD is caused by a reduced synthesis of the neurotransmitter acetylcholine. The amyloid hypothesis (Hardy & Allsop, 1991) postulates instead that the fundamental cause of the disease is the deposition of Aβ, which is supported by the evidence that mutations in the gene for APP, which is known to cause Aβ aggregation, are linked to AD. The tau hypothesis, based on a study demonstrating that deposition of Aβ plaques does not correlate well with neuron loss (Schmitz et al., 2004), proposes that abnormalities in the tau protein initiate the disease cascade.

Safety and efficacy of more than 500 pharmaceutical treatments are being investigated in clinical trials worldwide on the basis of these three hypotheses. In 2008, two separate clinical trials showed positive results in modifying the course of the disease in mild to moderate AD: one with the metal complexing agent PBT2 (Lannfelt et al., 2008) and one with methylthioninium chloride (Wischik, 2008), a drug that inhibits tau aggregation, which unfortunately failed to confirm the positive results in its phase III.

2.2 The metal hypothesis

Recently, researchers have uncovered an important role played in AD neurodegeneration by transition metals via their properties to cause oxidative stress. In fact, copper and iron are known to participate in Fenton-type reactions that generate uncontrollable reactive oxygen species (ROS) capable of damaging and destroying molecular and cellular compartments (Atwood et al., 2004).

Authors have widely reported enhanced metal concentrations in specific areas of AD patients' brains, in particular of iron, copper and zinc in cerebrospinal fluid (CSF) (Smith et al., 2010), of iron in the basal ganglia (Bartzokis et al., 2000, Bartzokis & Tishler, 2000), and of both iron and copper within SPs and NFTs (Good et al., 1992, Lovell et al., 1998). It has been also observed that APP possesses selective zinc and copper binding sites which mediate redox activity, causing precipitation of Aβ even at low concentrations (Bush et al., 1994). Also Aβ possesses selective high and low-affinity metal-binding sites. They can bind equimolar amounts of copper and zinc but, in conditions of acidosis, copper completely displaces zinc from Aβ (Atwood et al., 2000). Aβ reduces the metal ions by transferring electrons to O_2 and generating hydrogen peroxide in the process.

If on the one hand Aβ deposition in plaques is an age-dependent phenomenon, on the other hand Aβ production does not appear to increase with age. This seems to indicate that other age-dependent changes, as for example changes in metal homeostasis, may play a key role in Aβ transformation and neurotoxicity. Since copper and zinc are both modulators of the glutamatergic neurotransmission (Bush & Tanzi, 2008), abnormalities in metal homeostasis can have detrimental effects on synaptic processes, such as metal reuptake or storage in the synaptic cleft. All this evidence has eventually led to the proposal of a Metal Hypothesis of AD (Bush & Tanzi, 2008), which is based on the concept that it is the interaction of Aβ with specific metals, especially copper, that drives AD pathogenesis by promoting aggregation and neurotoxicity. By now, this view has become fully accepted and there is general agreement on the existence of a link between AD and oxidative stress phenomena triggered by transition metals. The Metal hypothesis of AD is now supported by the results of numerous clinical studies (Squitti et al., 2006, Squitti et al., 2002a, Squitti et al., 2003, Squitti et al., 2005).

3. Iron

3.1 Iron essentiality

Iron is essential for life. Of the 4-5 grams of iron normally present in a healthy body, about 2.5 g bind to hemoglobin and are used to promote respiration. Normally iron is absorbed from digested food or supplements. Average amounts are 1 mg/day for men, and 1.5–2 mg/day for women (Institute of Medicine Food and Nutrition Board, 2001). The majority is absorbed in the duodenum, where enterocytes of the duodenal lining reduce ferric Fe^{3+} to ferrous Fe^{2+}, which is then transported across the enterocyte's cell membrane into the cell by the divalent metal transporter 1 (DMT1). After completing a number of functions, available Fe^{+2} is transported back out of the cell by ferroportin, which is distributed throughout the duodenum enterocytes. Hephaestin, a ferroxidase found mainly in the small intestine, oxidizes Fe^{2+} back to ferric Fe^{3+}. At this point Fe^{+3} binds transferrin, a protein which takes it into circulation. Our body does not have a way to excrete iron in excess, so that the latter is stored inside another 450 kDa protein, ferritin, which can store up to 4500 atoms of iron per molecule (Fleming & Bacon, 2005).

3.2 Iron toxicity and the role of ceruloplasmin

Transported by transferrin, Fe^{3+} reaches the brain's capillaries and the Blood-Brain-Barrier (BBB), which is made of the brain capillary endothelial cells (BCECs) forming the wall of the capillaries. The luminal side of the BCECs presents transferrin receptors that pick up the iron-loaded transferrin protein. An endocytosis is initiated and the receptor-transferrin complex is internalized into an endosome. Iron remains inside the endosome while the latter crosses through the BCEC and reaches the abluminal side. Here the endosome fuses with the external membrane, exposing and then releasing Fe^{3+} to the extracellular interstitial space. The apo-transferrin remains attached to the receptor and the two undergo again an endocytosis to travel back to the BCEC luminal side, where apo-transferrin is released into the capillary blood for re-cycling.

In the extracellular space, two Fe^{3+} atoms bind to a passing transferrin molecule, which allows iron to reach the vicinity of a neuron. The neuron membrane displays transferrin receptors, an endocytosis is again initiated and the receptor-transferrin complex is engulfed in an endosome that sinks into the neuron. Differently from the BCECs, though, the neuron possesses DMT1s which allow Fe^{2+} to be released into the neuron's intracellular space, where iron can finally complete its nutritional function.

Unfortunately, a potentially dangerous outcome of this process is the reduction of iron back into Fe^{2+}. Iron is particularly dangerous in this oxidative state since it can easily enter Fenton reactions with H_2O_2:

$$Fe^{2+} + H_2O_2 \rightarrow Fe^{3+} + \bullet OH + OH^- \quad (1)$$

The hydroxyl radical $\bullet OH$ is the most reactive and vicious of all ROS species. Moreover, the above reaction easily proceeds as follows:

$$Fe^{3+} + H_2O_2 \rightarrow Fe^{2+} + \bullet OOH + H^+ \quad (2)$$

Fortunately, the neuron also displays ferroportin molecules on its membrane, which channel Fe^{2+} out into the extracellular space. At this point, a fundamental role in the neuron health is played by ceruloplasmin, a protein present on the astrocytic end-foot. In fact, ceruloplasmin catalyzes the oxidation of Fe2+ into Fe3+, by way of the following chemical reaction:

$$4\ Fe^{2+} + 4\ H^+ + O_2 \rightarrow 4\ Fe^{3+} + 2\ H_2O \quad (3)$$

Therefore, an unbalance of the ceruloplasmin content or efficiency induces iron-dependent oxidative damage to brain tissues (Patel et al., 2002).

Copper can enter exactly the same reactions, passing through Cu^{2+} to Cu^{1+} oxidative states. This confers to ceruloplasmin a special character as a 'crosstalk' factor linking copper to iron metabolism, which appears disarranged in AD.

4. Copper

4.1 Copper essentiality

Copper is also an essential nutrient for man and is normally ingested via food, although it has been recently proposed that varying degrees of intake originate from drinking water piped through copper plumbing (Brewer, 2010). Copper status in the body is regulated by both duodenal absorption (intestine) and biliary excretion (liver). After crossing the intestinal lumen, copper is transported to the liver via portal circulation. Here, copper is partly stored and partly redistributed to other organs. In the hepatocytes, in particular, copper is incorporated into ceruloplasmin and into low-molecular-weight compounds, and then routed into peripheral circulation or secreted into the bile for excretion. Absorption and excretion interplay in such a way that an occasional over-ingestion in healthy adults normally results in a down-regulation of copper uptake in the duodenum and an up-regulation of biliary excretion.

4.2 Bound and free copper

About 85-95% of copper tightly binds to ceruloplasmin, whereas the remainder loosely binds to and is exchanged among albumin, α2 macroglobulin, amino acids, peptides and several micronutrients. We will refer to the portion that binds to ceruloplasmin as 'bound' copper, and to the portion that binds to the loose compounds as 'free' copper (Linder et al., 1979), following a custom of Wilson's Disease clinical care.

A key difference between bound and free copper lies in the fact that the limited size of the low-molecular-weight compounds and the labile nature of their binding allow free copper to easily cross the BBB (Chutkow, 1978). A recent study (Choi & Zheng, 2009) has in fact shown that the bulk of copper transport into the brain is achieved by free copper ions travelling through the BBB, whereas ceruloplasmin-bound copper represents less than 1% of the brain bound copper. Normal ranges, within which 95% of the normal population falls and which are normally taken as reference values, are 11-22.4 μmol/L for serum copper (corresponding to 70-142.7 μg/dL), 20-60 mg/dL for ceruloplasmin, and 0-1.6 μmol/L for free copper (corresponding to 10 μg/dL) (Jacobs, 2002).

It is generally assumed that normal values are 'healthy', although some authors suggest caution in this regard considering that natural selection works to optimize health and survival only during the reproductive period. Consequently, 'normal' values may not be necessarily optimal after age 50 (Brewer, 2007). In fact, ranges of plasma/serum copper values of healthy elderly individuals reported in the literature are very heterogeneous, adding complexity in the interpretation of their results (Squitti, 2011).

4.3 Copper toxicity

Although copper is an essential nutrient for man, it becomes extremely toxic when its levels loose balance. It is a transition metal and as such takes part in a variety of biological reduction and oxidation (redox) reactions, which make it an important cofactor of many redox enzymes. As mentioned above, copper can easily go into Haber-Weiss and Fenton reactions producing •OH (1), against which the body has no defenses (Gutteridge & Halliwell, 1990). An overload of this metal can easily lead to oxidative reactions resulting in cell damage and death.

Moreover, copper absorption and excretion is regulated by mechanisms controlled by genetic as well as environmental factors. Therefore, a copper toxicosis is generally the result of a failure of one or more of those mechanisms, although sometimes, but infrequently, a copper excess may be due to a clinical disease, such a liver cirrhosis. The genetic origin of copper toxicosis manifests itself most clearly in the failure to express a specific copper transporter, particularly in the liver (see below). Sheep, for example, are easily subject to copper toxicosis since they are not able to increase biliary copper excretion in response to an increased intake. Conversely, pigs are known to tolerate even severe increases of copper intake very well for the opposite reason (Bremner, 1979). However, toxicity per se ultimately stems from copper's ability to catalyze the production of compounds that generate oxidative stress, as expressed in reactions (1), (2), (3) detailed above.

The disruption of the system controlling copper homeostasis has serious consequences for the health and development of the brain. This is well exemplified by two genetic disorders, showing either shortage - Menkes' disease - or excess - Wilson's disease - of systemic copper, but both resulting in neurodegeneration. In these diseases, the genes coding for the two membrane copper transport proteins ATPase7A and ATPase7B are mutated. These two proteins are highly homologous, but with different patterns of tissue expression: ATPase7A (Menkes' protein) is mainly expressed in the intestine and in the BBB, while ATPase7B (Wilson's protein) is primarily found in the liver (Harris, 2000). The mutation impairs the function of the ATPase7A pump and prevents copper absorption at the intestinal level. This causes copper deficiency and reduces the levels of cuproenzymes (Harris, 2000). The location of ATPase7A at the choroid plexes makes this pump crucial for controlling the copper flux into the ventricles of the brain (Qian et al., 1998). Indeed, the copper deficiency in the brain of Menkes' patients is particularly severe because of a decrease in the activity of ATPase7A at the BBB. Defects of ATPase7B in Wilson's disease cause impairment of copper incorporation into ceruloplasmin, with consequent failure of copper release into the bile canalicula for excretion (Iyengar et al., 1988). This produces a copper overload into the hepatocytes, inducing liver cirrhosis as well as slight increased levels of free copper. At the death of the cirrhotic hepatocytes, copper – actually free copper - is released into general circulation in huge amounts and reaches all organs and tissues, including the brain (Choi & Zheng, 2009, Hartter & Barnea, 1988, Iyengar et al., 1988). The holo-active form of ceruloplasmin depends on the ATPase7B activity, which mediates the incorporation of copper atoms into ceruloplasmin during its biosynthesis (Bielli & Calabrese, 2002). ATPase7B absence or impairment prevents copper translocation to the secretory pathway, resulting in 1) secretion of unstable apo-ceruloplasmin which is rapidly degraded in the blood (Bielli & Calabrese, 2002); 2) alteration of copper excretion through the bile via ceruloplasmin (Iyengar et al., 1988); 3) severe hypo-function, which can even cause death, of hepatocytes; 4) release of free copper in general circulation and tissue copper overload or intoxication (Bielli & Calabrese, 2002). During aging, control over copper homeostasis can undergo progressive failure and even "normal" copper values could result in an altered copper burden in the aged brain (Deibel et al., 1996).

4.4 Copper chaperones

Besides the obvious function as means of transportation, chaperones are also the main defense system against copper excess. Copper import into the intestinal epithelial cells is mediated by the membrane protein Copper transporter protein 1 (Ctr1) (Figure 1) (Kim et al., 2008).

Based on its structural and biochemical properties, Ctr1 could be thought of as a Cu^{+1}-specific pore. In hepatocytes, intracellular copper is carried by specific chaperone proteins to Cu-dependent enzymes. So far, researchers have identified three copper chaperones, although new candidates are being investigated: the Human Atox 1 Homologue (HAH1), homologous to the yeast Antioxidant protein 1 (Atox1); the Copper Chaperone for Superoxide Dismutase (CCS); the Cytochrome C Oxidase Assembly Homologue (COX17). HAH1 delivers copper to the two mammalian P-type Cu-transporting ATPases, ATPase7A and ATPase7B. CCS delivers copper to the metal-binding site of Copper-Zinc superoxide dismutase (Cu,Zn SOD). COX17 delivers copper to the mitochondria, where it is ultimately incorporated into the Cytochrome C Oxidase. In a healthy physiological environment, virtually no copper remains unbound (Fig. 1) (Kim, et al., 2008). The chaperone system also includes metallothioneins, a family of proteins, whose expression is regulated by copper and other metals (Palmiter, 1994) and which are active in trapping metals in excess. It has been reported that Metallothionein-3, a member of the family expressed exclusively in the central nervous system and involved in neuronal damage repair through its neuro-inhibitory activity, is significantly down-regulated in AD (Durand et al.,2010 , Meloni et al., 2008, Yu et al., 2001). It was recently proven that this protein protects cultured neurons from toxicity generated by Aβ. A metal swap between Metallothionein-3 and soluble aggregated Aβ 1–40-Cu^{2+} avoids ROS production and consequent cellular toxicity. Finally, Cu,Zn SOD, beside its primary antioxidant function of superoxide dismutation, also plays a role as a buffer of intracellular free copper, since it is stable in its copper-free form (Rossi et al., 1994).

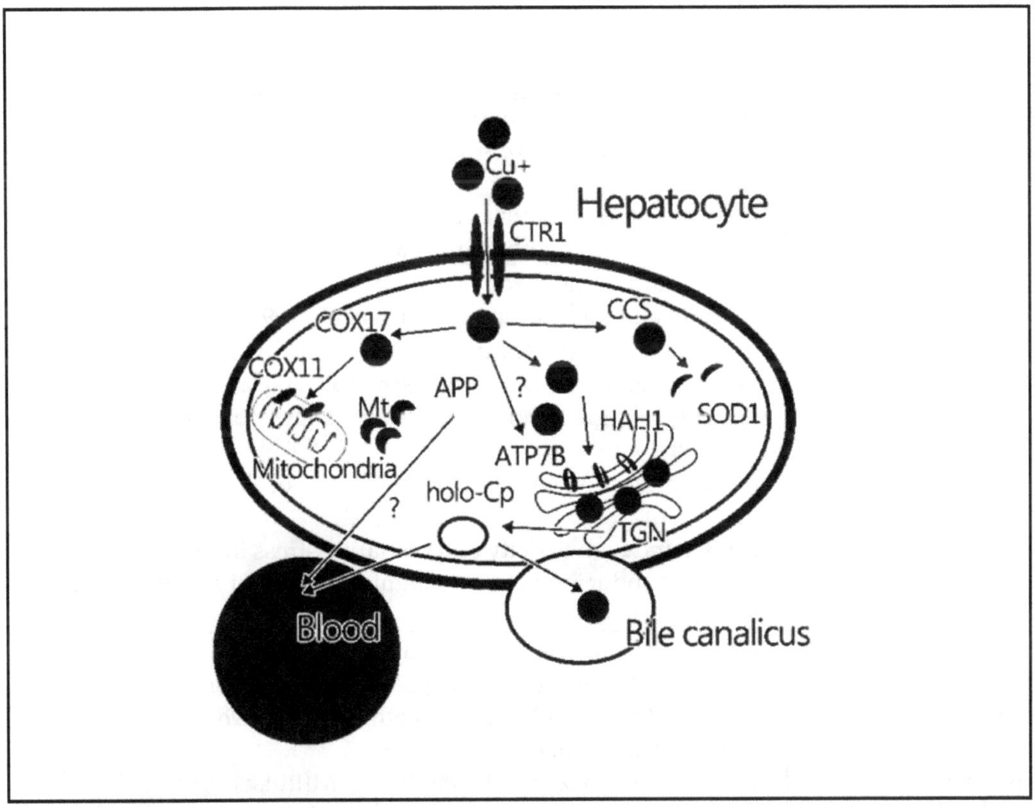

Fig. 1. Copper is metabolically finely regulated by the organism. Once copper crosses the intestinal lumen, it is transported into the liver via portal circulation. In the hepatocytes copper is incorporated into ceruloplasmin, other copper proteins and compounds and then routed into peripheral circulation or secreted into the bile for excretion. Copper in excess from general circulation is excreted through the kidney, in urine. In the hepatocytes, intracellular copper is carried by specific chaperone proteins to Cu-dependent enzymes. Three copper chaperones have been identified to date: the Human Atox 1 Homologue (HAH1), homologous to the yeast Antioxidant protein 1 (Atox1); the Copper Chaperone for Superoxide Dismutase (CCS); the Cytochrome C Oxidase assembly homologue (COX17). The amyloid precursor protein (APP) is deemed to be a new copper chaperone.

4.5 Copper and Aβ

Neurodegenerative metallochemistry has developed on the observation that APP possesses selective zinc and copper binding sequences (Table 1). These sites mediate redox activity and can cause the precipitation of Aβ under mildly acidic conditions, even at very low concentrations (Atwood et al., 1998). Researchers believe that this is what happens in the AD brain (Atwood et al., 1998). Moreover, Aβ reduces the metal ions, producing hydrogen peroxide by transferring electrons to O_2 (Huang et al., 1999a, Huang et al., 1999b). This reduction is the key of Aβ-induced oxidative stress and toxicity, since hydrogen peroxide is a well known pro-oxidant molecule as it triggers Fenton's like reactions (1) (2) that generate hydroxyl radicals (see formulas in iron paragraph).

Milestones	Key Findings
The amyloid precursor protein (APP) is a copper protein	APP has a copper binding domain which reduces Cu(II) to Cu(I) and produces oxidative stress (Barnham et al., 2003b, Multhaup et al., 1996) Depletion of intracellular copper results in a reduction of APP gene expression (Bellingham et al., 2004b)
Zinc and copper interactions with Aβ	Zinc rapidly destabilized human Aβ40 solutions, inducing tinctorial amyloid formation (Bush et al., 1994) Aβ peptide with the sulfur atom of Met-35 oxidized to a sulfoxide is toxic to neuronal cells (Barnham et al., 2003a) Aβ peptide aggregation is induced by copper binding (Atwood et al., 2000) Aβ-Cu interaction generates ROS (Huang et al., 1999b, Multhaup et al., 1996) APP-Cu induced toxicity and oxidative stress in primary neuronal cultures, producing neuronal demise (Huang et al., 1999a, White et al., 1999a)
Solubilization of native Aβ from AD brain, transgenic mice and cell models by metal complexing agents	Solubilization of Aβ from post-mortem brain tissue was significantly increased by the presence of chelators, EGTA, N,N,N*,N*-tetrakis(2-pyridyl-methyl) ethylene diamine, and bathocuproine (Cherny et al., 1999) bis(thiosemicarbazonato) complexes - MII(btsc) examined in chinese hamster ovary cells overexpressing APP increased levels of bioavailable intracellular copper and zinc but also resulted in a dose-dependent reduction of Aβ levels (Donnelly et al., 2008)
Cu-dependent catalytic conversion of dopamine, cholesterol, and biological reducing agents to neurotoxic H_2O_2 *in vitro* and animal models	Aβ binds copper and cholesterol, facilitating copper oxidation of cholesterol to 7–OH cholesterol and to 4-cholestenone, which are extremely toxic to neurons. Cholesterol can catalyse copper-Aβ redox cycling (Opazo et al., 2002, Puglielli et al., 2005) Trace amounts of copper given to cholesterol-fed rabbits induced accumulation of Aβ in senile plaques and impaired the animals' learning capability (Sparks et al., 2006, Sparks & Schreurs, 2003)

Table 2. Milestones of the Evidence of Metal Implication in AD

APP binds copper in two domains, one located in the extracellular N-terminal region and the other in the C-terminal region within the Aβ peptide (review in Squitti & Zito, 2009). It has been proposed that APP reduces Cu^{2+} to Cu^{1+} upon coordination, thus promoting the non-amyloidogenic cleavage pathway (Barnham et al., 2003b). The ablation of APP, which is normally expressed both in the brain and in a limited number of non-neural tissues as platelets, liver, kidney, and heart (Duce et al., 2010, White et al., 1999b) in knockout mice models produces metal dishomeostasis in these organs and tissues. APP-depleted knockout mice have shown a stunning 80% increase of copper concentrations in the liver and a 40% increase in the brain. Recently, Duce et al., (2010) reported that APP ablation causes an iron increase of 26% in the brain, 31% in the liver and 15% in the kidney.

As mentioned above, Aβ is generated from APP cleavage by α-, β- and γ-secretases. β-secretase (BACE1) cleaves at the N terminus, while γ-secretase cleaves at the C terminus of the Aβ sequence. BACE1 is an aspartic protease and may function as a dimer, whereas γ-secretase is a complex of presenilin-1/2, Aph1, Pen2, and Nicastrin (Edbauer et al., 2003). It was reported that BACE1 modulates APP processing and the release of Aβ by interacting with CCS. The concept that copper content can modulate BACE1, i.e. the rate-limiting enzyme in the production of Aβ (Angeletti et al., 2005), is supported by the recent evidence that copper (Cu^{2+}) and manganese (Mn^{2+}) potently increase the expression of both APP and BACE1 in a time- and concentration-dependent manner, whereas zinc (Zn^{2+}), iron (Fe^{2+}) and aluminum (Al^{3+}) do not (Lin et al., 2008). *In vitro* studies have demonstrated that different variants of Aβ (1-40, 1-42) have different affinity for copper, and that higher affinity generates higher toxicity (Crouch et al., 2007). The results of recent *in vitro* studies suggest that Cytochrome C Oxidase, and therefore the energy production of the cell, may be one of the targets of the Cu-Aβ toxic effect (Crouch et al., 2005). Conversely, copper plays a role in the basal regulation of the APP gene. This has been shown in human fibroblasts over-expressing ATPase7A, a condition that causes copper intracellular depletion. Depletion of intracellular copper in these cells results in significant reduction of APP gene expression (Bellingham et al., 2004a, Bellingham et al., 2004b). Moreover, a study of cDNA microarray technology demonstrated an up-regulation of APP and of the normal cellular prion protein (PrPC) in two genetic models of chronic copper overload mutants - fibroblasts from C57BL/6-Atp7aMobr and C57BL/6-Atp7aModap - and in a nutritional model of chronic copper overload (Armendariz et al., 2004).

Overall, this evidence shows that the APP gene harbours a copper response element within its promoter, such that copper depletion leads to a marked decrease in APP expression and supports the evidence that APP is involved in copper homeostasis as a copper detoxification/efflux protein.

Another line of evidence is the effectiveness of copper and iron chelators in hindering redox and toxic activities of Aβ and NTFs, whereas a replacement with those metals fully restores those activities (Sayre et al., 2000).

Regarding genetic risk factors, the *ApoE4*, which is the only well established risk factor for AD, has been demonstrated to interact with copper metabolism at different levels. It has been shown that ApoE protein possesses antioxidant properties which depend on 'bound' copper (Miyata & Smith, 1996, Moir et al., 1999, Sanan et al., 1994). ApoE4 isoform has a lower antioxidant power than ApoE2 or ApoE3, and is therefore the least effective in protecting neurons from the oxidative damage caused by Aβ. In fact, absolute and free copper concentrations are higher in carriers of the *ApoE4* allele than in non-carriers

(Gonzalez et al., 1999, Squitti et al., 2002a, Squitti et al., 2007). In addition, the correlation between typical electroencephalographic (EEG) spectral abnormalities of the AD brain and higher-than-normal serum levels of free copper is stronger in *ApoE4* carriers than in non-carriers (Babiloni et al., 2007b, Zappasodi et al., 2008).

The level of plasma homocysteine is a risk factor for AD (Babiloni et al., 2007a, Gorgone et al., 2009), and it's known that copper mediates Low-Density Lipoprotein (LDL) oxidation by homocysteine (Nakano et al., 2004).

Aβ binds copper and cholesterol, facilitating copper oxidation of cholesterol to 7-0H cholesterol and to 4-cholestenone (Puglielli et al., 2005), which are extremely toxic to neurons (Nelson & Alkon, 2005).

Trace amounts of copper, well below the levels considered safe for humans, given to cholesterol-fed rabbits have induced accumulation of Aβ in senile plaques and impaired the animals' learning capability (Sparks & Schreurs, 2003). Thus, it appears that cholesterol increases Aβ formation and copper promotes Aβ aggregation and toxicity. Furthermore, cholesterol can catalyze copper-Aβ redox cycling (Opazo et al., 2002). The results from the cholesterol-fed rabbit model have been confirmed in transgenic mice (Sparks et al., 2006) and provided the rational for the results of a large community prospective study showing a strong correlation between copper intake from a diet rich in saturated and trans fats and mental decline (Morris et al., 2006). As a result, serious concerns have been raised about a possible relationship between copper overexposure from vitamins or drinking water and cognitive disturbances (Brewer, 2010, Bush et al., 2003). The belief that copper toxicity is involved in the evolution of cognitive disturbances is also supported by recent investigations demonstrating an inverse correlation between cognitive performance and serum copper levels in cohorts of healthy aged individuals (Lam et al., 2008, Salustri et al., 2010a).

5. Metals in AD: A systemic view

The link between metals and AD has been traditionally investigated focusing on local metal accumulations in specific areas of the brain critical for AD. In this frame, authors have reported enhanced iron concentrations in AD brains, both in autopsy brain tissues and in CSF (Smith et al., 2010), in the basal ganglia (Bartzokis et al., 2000, Bartzokis & Tishler, 2000), and around SPs and NFTs (Good et al., 1992, Lovell, et al., 1998). Altered local concentrations of copper (Adlard & Bush, 2006), ceruloplasmin (Castellani et al., 1999, Loeffler et al., 1996), transferrin and ferritin (Connor et al., 1992) have been also reported.

We believe instead that the issue should be approached from the different perspective of systemic, rather than local, alterations. Results of many *in vivo* studies demonstrating correlations between abnormalities in metal homeostasis and specific deficits and markers of AD suggest that local accumulations should be viewed in a wider systemic alteration.

5.1 Iron

Besides of course its own levels in general circulation, typical markers of iron status are the levels of transferrin, ceruloplasmin, ferritin, transferrin saturation, together with the H63D and C282Y mutations of the HFE gene and transferrin's C2 polymorphism (TfC2). Since these gene variants are often associated with a distress of the liver, the classic liver function panel, i.e., albumin, transaminases (aspartate transaminase, AST; alanine transaminase, ALT) and prothrombin time, contribute to the picture.

In a study of 160 AD patients and 79 healthy elderly controls performed by our laboratory (Giambattistelli et al., 2011), we evaluated whether and how all the above listed markers of iron and liver status are interconnected. Our study revealed that AD patients have lower albumin, longer prothrombin time and higher AST/ALT values than controls, indicating a liver distress. Also, transferrin was lower and ferritin higher in AD patients. A multiple logistic regression backward analysis performed to evaluate the effects of these biochemical variables upon the probability to develop AD revealed that a simple one-unit decrease in serum transferrin increases the probability of AD by 80%. A one-unit albumin serum-decrease reduces the AD probability by 20%, while a one-unit increase of AST/ALT ratios generates a fourfold probability increase. The role of genetic mutations is well described by the fact that while healthy controls carriers of the H63D mutation showed a normal iron status, AD patients carriers of the same mutation showed a panel resembling hemochromatosis, i.e., higher levels of iron, lower levels of transferrin and ceruloplasmin. This picture was not found in non-carrier AD patients. These results suggest that carrying the H63D mutation is not itself sufficient to increase the risk of AD. Rather, it is a synergy between iron increase, a condition of liver dysfunction and the genetic mutation that appears to increase the probability of developing AD (Giambattistelli et al., 2011).

In another study, we measured serum levels of iron, ceruloplasmin and transferrin, calculated the transferrin saturation and evaluated the activation of the ceruloplasmin-transferrin (Cp-Tf) system, expressed by the Cp/Tf ratio, in relation to the main cognitive and anatomical deficit of AD, namely MMSE and medial temporal lobe atrophy (Squitti et al., 2010c). Results demonstrated that the values of ceruloplasmin, peroxides and Cp/Tf, besides being elevated, inversely correlated with MMSE scores, while medial temporal lobe atrophy positively correlated with Cp/Tf and negatively with serum iron levels. All these findings demonstrate that the alterations of iron metabolism that accompany the disease are systemic rather than local, and indicate that the role attributed by existing literature to local metal accumulations in brain areas critical for AD should be rather viewed in the frame of a wider systemic alteration, which could be approached taking into account both circulating biochemical markers variations and their genetic makeup. In this line, we recently explored the hypothesis that polymorphisms of ATP7B, the gene encoding the protein that controls the levels of free copper in the body and whose defects cause Wilson's disease, have higher frequencies in AD than in healthy individuals. Two groups of 190 AD patients and 164 controls were studied in order to compare the frequency of alleles for these two polymorphisms using a 'case-control' design. Two polymorphisms previously associated with Wilson's disease - GG genotype in the SNP 2495 A>G (Lys832Arg) (exon 10) and GG in c.1216T>G (Ser406Ala) (exon 2) – showed an association with susceptibility to AD (Bucossi et al., 2010). These polymorphisms also show a link to non-ceruloplasmin copper levels.

5.2 Copper

The existence of systemic copper dysfunctions in AD has been a controversial issue for many years. In fact, many studies have reported an increase of circulating copper in AD patients with respect to healthy controls (Arnal et al., 2010, Bocca et al., 2005, Gonzalez et al., 1999, Smorgon et al., 2004, Squitti et al., 2006, Squitti et al., 2009, Squitti et al., 2002a, Squitti, et al., 2003, Squitti et al., 2007, Zappasodi, et al., 2008), many others no variation (Basun et al., 1991, Baum et al., 2010, Gerhardsson et al., 2008, Jeandel et al., 1989, Kapaki et al., 1989, Molina et al., 1998, Ozcankaya & Delibas, 2002, Snaedal et al., 1998), and two very recent studies even a decrease of copper in plasma (Vural et al., 2010) and serum (Brewer et al., 2010) of AD patients. Moreover, the latter two studies are in line with two older studies showing that low plasma copper concentrations correlate with clinical worsening in AD, one reporting a copper plasma-decrease in more severe vs. less severe patients (Kessler et al., 2006), and the other a direct correlation between low plasma copper concentrations and cognitive decline (Pajonk et al., 2005).

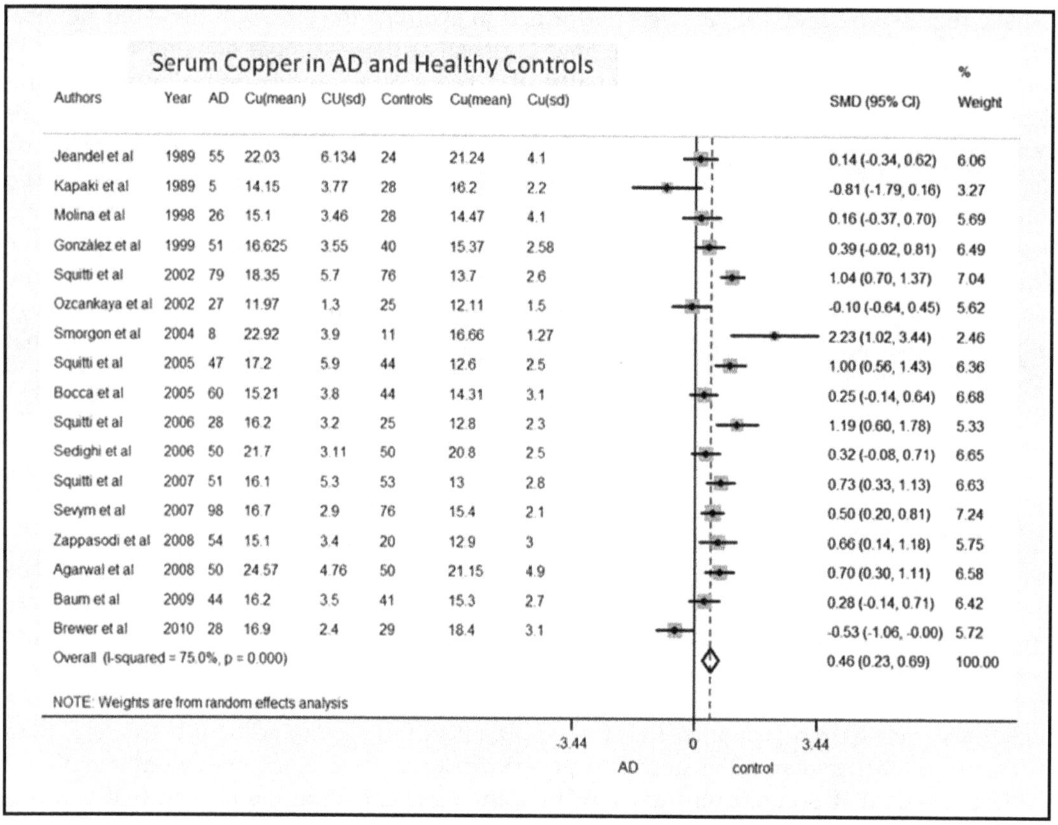

Fig. 2. Standardized mean difference (SMD) in copper serum level. The square represents the SMD between patients and controls. The size of the squares is proportional to the sample size of the study, the whiskers represents the 95% confidence interval. The diamond represents the pooled estimate based one random effects model, with the centre representing the point estimate and the width the associated 95% confidential intervals.

Recently, we have evaluated these heterogeneous results in a meta-analysis, which has analyzed data from all the serum, plasma and CSF studies published since 1983 on AD patients, to gain an objective evaluation of whether systemic copper variation are associated or not with AD. Meta-analysis is a quantitative method that combines the results of independent reports to distinguish between small effects and no effects, random variations, variations in sample used or in different analytical approaches. After an initial selection based on statistical criteria, data from 21 studies on serum copper and 5 studies on plasma copper were merged for a pooled total of 966 AD patients and 831 controls (Bucossi et al., 2010). The analysis concluded that AD patients have actually higher levels of serum copper than healthy controls (Fig. 2). Even though moderate, the assessed copper increase is sufficient to unambiguously distinguish AD patients from healthy controls.

Plasma data did not allow conclusions because of extremely high heterogeneity, but the meta-analysis of the combined serum and plasma studies confirmed higher copper levels in AD. The analysis of CSF data, instead, revealed no difference between AD patients and controls. Previous results from our laboratory are in line with the meta-analysis outcome. When we measured copper, iron, transferrin and copper-enzymes as ceruloplasmin and Cu,Zn SOD, together with total hydro-peroxides and total radical-trapping antioxidant potential (TRAP) levels in the sera of diverse AD patients cohorts (Rossi et al., 2002, Squitti et al., 2006, Squitti et al., 2004, Squitti et al., 2002a, Squitti et al., 2005, Squitti et al., 2007), we found that copper, peroxides and Cu,Zn SOD activity (Rossi et al., 2002) were higher, TRAP was lower and ceruloplasmin and iron did not differ between AD patients and healthy controls. These changes appeared to be specifically referred to the AD patients since they were not present in vascular dementia (VAD) patients, with the exception of TRAP that was lower in VAD patients in comparison to healthy controls (Squitti et al., 2003).
Diverse explanations can be advocated to account for the systemic copper abnormalities in AD. Inflammation can be one reason. In fact, ceruloplasmin, which accounts for 85-95% of circulating copper, is an acute phase reactant, whose levels increase during the inflammatory response. In a previous study (Squitti et al., 2005), our laboratory investigated whether markers of inflammation in general circulation were abnormal in AD, and showed that levels of ceruloplasmin were higher in AD than in healthy controls, though close to the significance threshold. However, it was clear that the level of ceruloplasmin increase could not account for the pronounced rise of serum copper estimated in the patient sample analyzed in that study. In fact, when we performed a deeper analysis by distinguishing between bound and free copper, results revealed that the copper increase in our AD patients was attributable to this latter fraction (Squitti et al., 2006, Squitti et al., 2009, Squitti et al., 2005). It must be remembered, though, that free copper abnormalities should be considered as an additional rather than alternative explanatory variable of copper disturbances in AD (Althaus, 2008, Arnal et al., 2010, Brewer et al., 2010, Hoogenraad, 2007).

5.3 The role of free copper

The considerations above support the notion of a fundamental distinction between the biochemical properties of bound and free copper.
The levels of free copper are higher in AD patients than in healthy individuals. One ultrafiltration study, aimed at finding filterable free copper in AD sera, has also revealed concentrations of free copper 3.7 times higher in AD patients than in controls (Squitti et al., 2006). Free copper levels correlate with AD main cognitive deficits (Squitti et al., 2006, Squitti et al., 2009, Squitti et al., 2004, Squitti et al., 2002a, Squitti et al., 2003, Squitti et al., 2005), with neuro-anatomical (Squitti et al., 2002a) and electrophysiological changes (Babiloni et al., 2007b, Zappasodi et al., 2008), with accepted AD markers (Squitti et al., 2006) and with known genetic risk factors, such as *ApoE4* (Squitti et al., 2002a, Zappasodi et al., 2008). Copper systemic abnormalities in AD resemble those observed in Wilson's disease, where the free fraction transported by micronutrients plays a fundamental role, while ceruloplasmin appears fragmented. Ceruloplasmin fragmentation, revealed by fragments <50 KDa, has been reported in AD patients showing higher-than-normal levels of free copper (Squitti et al., 2008). This suggests impairment in the incorporation of copper into the protein during the biosynthesis (see the "copper chaperones" section). It must be noted, though, that in Wilson's disease the free copper percentage is much higher than the one estimated in AD (Siotto et al., 2010) (Fig. 3).

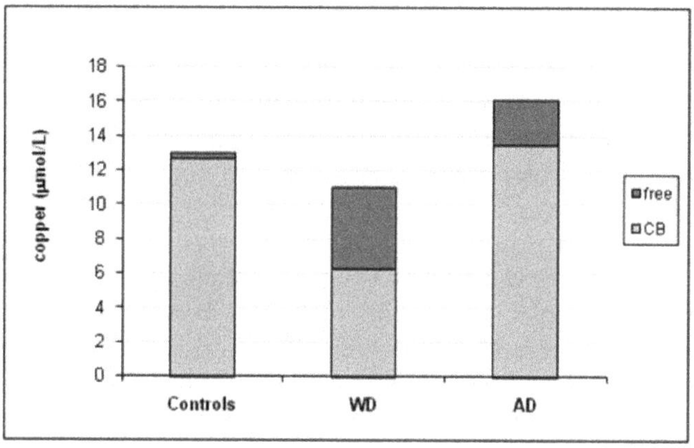

Fig. 3. Free copper in Alzheimer's disease (AD). The figure shows copper distribution its two serum pool - copper bound to ceruloplasmin (CB) and free copper - in healthy controls, Wilson's disease (WD) and AD patients.

Ceruloplasmin fragmentation, together with the free copper rise in AD, is a copper systemic abnormality that could be the cause or the result of a disturbed hepatocyte function, possibly resulting in liver hypo-metabolism. This notion is supported by the results of a clinical study by our laboratory which demonstrated that AD patients with no evidence of additional pathological conditions - including liver diseases - have higher free copper, longer prothrombin time and lower albumin levels than controls matched for age, sex and risk factors for cardiovascular diseases and medication intake (Squitti et al., 2007). Very recently, we reproduced the same evidence in a bigger cohort of AD associated with iron abnormalities (Giambattistelli et al., 2011). The hypothesis that copper, as well as iron (see below) in AD, might be related to liver hypofunction linked to APP metabolism at the hepatocyte level is strongly supported by the evidence that, in the APP knock-out mouse model, the APP ablation causes a massive (80%) copper increase in the liver (White et al., 1999b). More precisely, it could be speculated that, in this mouse model, a perturbation of copper efflux linked to APP at the liver level disrupts normal copper transport, producing a reduction of the liver's efficiency to excrete copper through the bile. This would explain the elevated (40%) copper level found in the brain (White et al., 1999b). A hint towards this interpretation comes from another study of ours, in which we estimated - via a clearance measure - that about 3% of serum free copper is related to CSF copper increase in AD patients, possibly interacting with Aβ (Squitti et al., 2006). This evidence fits very well with previous results in a mouse model of brain uptake of radiocopper [^{67}Cu(II)], as also confirmed by data of a recent study (Choi & Zheng, 2009). In the [^{67}Cu(II)] mouse model, a net brain copper uptake occurs and parallels the free copper increase in the injectate, starting from a concentration of Cu(II) of 3.2 ng/mL, corresponding to 0.05 µmol/L, much lower than the 2.5 µmol/L value that we evaluated in clinical studies on AD patients (Squitti & Salustri, 2009).

The belief that there is a direct interaction between copper and Aβ, based on the strong negative correlation between free copper in serum and Aβ in the CSF (Squitti et al., 2006), is sustained by the negative correlation between copper and Aβ in the CSF found by other authors (Strozyk et al., 2009). This evidence is also supported by the fact that copper detectable in the CSF is not ceruloplasmin-bound, but is bound to a not yet identified ligand (Que et al., 2008).

The occurrence of copper increase or decrease in the brain is a debated issue. Some authors suggested that there is a decrease in bulk tissue levels in AD brains, and particularly in the neocortex (Adlard & Bush, 2006). Loeffer and coworkers (Loeffler et al., 1996) reported instead that ceruloplasmin and copper are actually increased in AD. Deibel and coworkers (Deibel et al., 1996) and Platin and coworkers (Platin et al., 1987) reported lower levels of copper in the amygdala and in the hippocampus of AD brains than controls, however the authors determined nanograms of copper on micrograms of weight tissue, instead of nanograms of copper on micrograms of proteins present in the sample, and it is known that the AD brain tissue has plenty of plaques and not of proteins, so their evaluation at least arises some concerns. Religa's and Squitti's groups (Religa et al. 2006, Squitti et al., 2007) did not find a copper decrease in AD. Also our recent meta-analysis of copper-related literature (Bucossi et al., 2010) revealed no difference in CSF copper between AD patients and healthy controls. So caution is needed when facing this issue. Seminal studies indicate that copper dyshomeostasis in the brain, present in normal aging (Maynard et al., 2002), is substantially more pronounced in the aged AD brain (Lovell et al., 1998). In fact, copper levels in the plaque-free neuropil of an AD brain are approximately 4 times higher than in the neuropil of a healthy brain, and approximately 30% higher in the Aβ plaques than in plaque-free regions.

Our laboratory has started investigating metal involvement in AD as revealed by systemic markers detectable in general circulation, and clinical indices of prognosis or AD conversion. In particular, in order to evaluate whether information on iron or copper abnormalities can help in the AD prognosis, we assessed levels of copper, iron, zinc, transferrin, ceruloplasmin, peroxides, TRAP, free copper and *ApoE4* genotype in 81 mild or moderate AD patients (Squitti et al., 2009). We studied the association of these wide set of parameters with the patients' scores in the MMSE (primary outcome), in the Activities of Daily Living (ADL) and Instrumental of Daily Living (IADL) tests (secondary outcomes), performed at study entry and after 1 year. Our study revealed that free copper can predict the annual change in MMSE, adjusted for the baseline MMSE: it raised the explained variance from 2.4% (with only sex, age and education) to 8.5% ($p = 0.026$). When the annual change in MMSE was divided into <3 or >=3 points, free copper was the only predictor of a more severe decline (predicted probability of MMSE worsening 23%). In other words, this study showed an association between systemic copper deregulation and unfavorable evolution of cognitive function in AD patients, demonstrating that free copper identify those patients at higher risk for a more severe decline (Squitti et al., 2009).

In a very recent study we tested the hypothesis that free copper was increased significantly enough to distinguish also individuals affected by mild cognitive impairment (MCI) from healthy controls (Squitti et al., 2011). To verify this hypothesis a sample of 83 MCI subjects were compared with 100 elderly controls in terms of levels of serum copper, free copper, ceruloplasmin, *ApoE4*, iron, transferrin, and TRAP. The groups were compared also in terms of demographic and cardiovascular risk factors. The comparison with an additional group of 105 mild to moderate AD patients was also evaluated. A multinomial logistic regression analysis demonstrated that *ApoE4* and free copper differentiated MCI from healthy subjects. Chances to acquire MCI increased about 24% for each free copper unit (μmol/L) increment. *ApoE4* and free copper differentiated the MCI group also from the AD group. *ApoE4* and free copper appeared associated to

MMSE worsening, as did age and sex (Squitti et al., 2011). A follow-up study is in progress on MCI subjects, which will test whether free copper can provide information about who, within the MCI subjects, will progress to AD.

In another study we have investigated normal women over age 50 (Salustri et al., 2010a). We studied their free and ceruloplasmin bound copper, and measured MMSE and several other measures of memory and cognition (19 neuropsychological test battery). We found that free (but not ceruloplasmin bound) copper levels correlated inversely with MMSE and certain other measures of memory, that is, the higher the free copper, the poorer the performance on these measures of cognition.

Subsequently, we investigated the relationship between depression, which is advocated as a risk factor of AD, markers of oxidative stress and neurotransmission, as expressed by sensory cortex excitability (Dal Forno et al., 2005, Salustri et al., 2010b). Serum levels of oxidative stress markers and somatosensory magnetic fields, evoked by external galvanic stimulation, were measured in 13 depressed patients and 13 controls. Depressives had higher levels of total and free copper than controls and lower levels of transferrin. They also showed lower sensory cortex excitability, which correlated with copper levels in controls, but not in depressed patients. Transferrin correlated with sensory cortex excitability in both patients and controls, although in opposite ways. Copper level results associated with the patients' clinical status. Pro-oxidant compounds appear to affect neuronal excitability and clinical state of depressed patients, as free copper excess alters their cortical glutamatergic neurotransmission (Salustri et al., 2010a).

6. Treatment of AD with metal complexing agents

Since the '90s, researchers have cultivated the idea that a tuned redistribution of metals (aluminum, iron, selenium, zinc, copper) via metal complexing or ligand agents may positively affect the natural progression of AD. Numerous studies have been published reporting on tests with metal complexing agents as potential therapeutics for AD (Duce & Bush, 2010, Liu et al., 2010, Price et al., 2007), and their pros and cons, as well as the challenges associated with their usage, are under debate (Hegde et al., 2009, Squitti & Salustri, 2009, Squitti & Zito, 2009). The following is a summary of the most promising molecules with metal redistribution properties developed so far, together with a description of their potential or proven applications.

Zinc-induced aggregation of Aβ can be reversed by the divalent metal ion chelator ethilendiamine tetra acetic acid (EDTA)(Huang et al., 1999a). Solubilisation of Aβ derived from AD brains was achieved with N,N,N′,N′-tetrakis (2-pyridylmethyl) ethylene diamine (TPEN) and 2,9-dimethyl-4,7-diphenyl-1,10-phenanthroline (bathocuproine) (Cherny et al., 1999). Bathocuproine, bathophenahtroline and diethylenetriamine penta-acetic acid (DTPA) halted Aβ redox activity complexing copper (Atwood et al., 2004).

Another metal ligand molecule [1,2-bis(2-aminophenyloxy)ethane-N,N,N′,N′-bis (2-octadecyloxyethyl) ester,N,N′-disodiumsalt] DP-109 (Lee et al., 2004), was found to reduce amyloid plaques and cerebral amyloid angiopathy in Tg2576 mice.

XH1, a lipophilic amyloid-targeting metal chelator designed with amyloid-binding and metal chelating moieties, reduced APP protein expression in human cells and Aβ pathology in APP transgenic mice (Dedeoglu et al., 2004). Similar results were achieved with the lipophilic metal chelator DP-109, which markedly decreased Aβ plaques in APP transgenic mice (Lee et al., 2004).

Ammonium tetrathiomolybdate forms a stable tripartite complex with copper and proteins (Squitti & Salustri, 2009). Given with food, tetrathiomolybdate can complex food copper with food proteins, making all copper, including the endogenously secreted copper in saliva, gastric juice and intestinal secretion completely unabsorbable and thus causing an immediate negative copper unbalance. Given instead separate from food, tetrathiomolybdate is absorbed into the blood, where it forms the tripartite complex, bridging the freely available, and potentially toxic, copper with albumin. This complexed copper cannot be taken up by cells, and is therefore non-toxic, it has no known biological activity, and is largely cleared in the bile (Squitti & Salustri, 2009). A recent study tested the ability of tetrathiomolybdate to reduce Aβ pathology and spatial memory impairment in both a prevention and a treatment paradigm in Tg2576 mice. The study demonstrated that tetrathiomolybdate lowered brain copper concentrations and reduced Aβ levels in the prevention paradigm, but not in the treatment paradigm, suggesting that lowering systemic copper may achieve anti-amyloid effects if initiated early in the disease process (Quinn et al., 2010).

Metal bis(thiosemicarbazonato) complexes - MII(btsc), where M stands for either Copper (II) or Zinc (II) - can affect extracellular levels of Aβ. Treating Chinese hamster ovary cells overexpressing APP with engineered MII(btsc) increased levels of bioavailable intracellular copper and zinc but also resulted in a dose-dependent reduction of Aβ levels (Donnelly et al., 2008).

Iron-regulated APP in Aβ peptide in cell cultures were decreased by (-)-epigallocatechin-3-gallate, the main poliphenol constituent of green tea (Reznichenko et al., 2006). It was demonstrated that this molecule has metal-chelating and radical-scavenging properties that have an effect on iron metabolism in AD.

Nanoparticles conjugated to chelators were shown to easily cross the BBB, chelate metals, and exit through the BBB with their corresponding complexed metal ions (Liu et al., 2010). Early studies from this group (Liu et al., 2005) showed that these nanochelators can effectively remove iron from tissue of AD brain and also from ferritin.

Some studies (Lim et al., 2001, Lin et al., 2008) recently demonstrated the potential application of curcumin, a commonly used spice extracted by turmeric, as an anti-inflammatory and anti-oxidant molecule with neuroprotective properties. Some authors (Cole et al., 2007) demonstrated its metal chelating and neuroprotectant (Jiao et al., 2006) effects. In particular, Lin and coworkers (Lin et al., 2008) demonstrated in PC12 cells that this compound has strong effects on APP and BACE1 transcription up-regulation mediated by copper. The authors suggest that curcumin might have a combined effect on suppressing APP and BACE1 transcriptions, blocking the effect of copper. Due to its multi-functional effect new derivates have been created to improve curcumin brain bioavailability. Clinical studies are currently in progress to verify whether the use of this natural, non-toxic, neuroprotective compound with brain access could offer potential therapeutic benefits against neuronal damage.

Clioquinol (see also below) has been found to reverse the aggregation and redox activity of Aβ (49%) by its low affinity for copper in Tg2576 mice (Cherny et al., 2001).

6.1 Desferrioxamine

Desferrioxamine is a hexadentate chelator that does not cross the BBB. This chelator was tested for AD efficacy in a single-blinded study and it was reported to slow the clinical progression of dementia (Crapper McLachlan et al., 1991). The target metal of the study was aluminum. Iron was administered together with desferrioxamine throughout the whole trial period, with the aim of attenuating the bioavailability of aluminum, but not of iron. A generalized decrease of metal concentration was observed which, together with a decoppering effect, might have been at the basis of the positive clinical outcome.

Rationale	Agent	Type of study	Outcome
Induction of a negative metal balance throughout the whole body, as it happens with D-penicillamine or Zinc compounds in the treatment of Wilson's disease.	Desferrioxamine	One single-blinded study (Crapper McLachlan et al., 1991).	The clinical progression of dementia was reported to slow down.
	D-penicillamine	Prospective, randomized, double blind, parallel, placebo controlled phase II clinical trial (Squitti et al., 2002b).	H_2O_2 levels decreased in a group of AD patients with respect to both their own levels before the treatment and the levels of the AD patients who had taken the placebo
Studies based on the hypothesis that solubilization of Aβ plaques could be achieved by stripping them of their metal content or by facilitating the delivery of metals into the cell	Clioquinol	Prospective, randomized, double blind, parallel, placebo controlled phase II clinical trial (125-375 mg/BID over 36 weeks) (Ritchie et al., 2003).	Slowing of the rate of clinical decline in a subset of AD patients with moderate dementia
	PBT2	Prospective, randomized, double blind, parallel, placebo controlled phase II clinical trial (12-week treatment) (Lannfelt et al., 2008).	Dose-dependent reduction of Aβ concentrations in the CSF and positive impact on two executive functions.
Studies based on the hypothesis that copper supplementation can slow AD progression	Copper	Prospective, randomized, double-blind, placebo-controlled phase II clinical trial. Sixty-eight AD patients were given oral copper supplementation [Cu-(II)-orotate-dihydrate; 8 mg Cu daily, for 12 months (Kessler et al., 2008).	Cu supplementation did not change the rate of clinical decline.
Studies based on the hypothesis that aluminium could cause AD	Zinc aspartate	Preliminary trial with zinc aspartate administrated *per os* and i.v. for three to twelve months to 10 AD patients (Constantinidis, 1992).	Improved memory, understanding and communication in 8 of the 10 patients treated. The 2 patients who did not respond to the treatment had been given zinc aspartate only *per os*.

Table 3. Milestones in the Treatment of AD Patients with Metals or Metal Complexing Agents

The fact that desferrioxamine showed such an effect without crossing the BBB could be explained by the induction of a negative metal balance throughout the whole body, as it happens with D-penicillamine, Zinc compoundsor ammonium tetrathiomolybdate in the treatment of Wilson's disease.

6.2 D-penicillamine

D-penicillamine has been widely used for treatment of Wilson's disease. It functions as a copper chelator, controlling both the reactivity and bioavailability of that metal, ultimately facilitating its disposal through the urine. However, adverse events have been reported which have drastically limited its use.

A study of D-penicillamine tolerability and efficacy in the treatment of AD had to be interrupted before finishing recruitment, due to a number of serious adverse events (Squitti et al., 2002b). Some conclusions were drawn from the patients who had completed the treatment at the moment of interruption (18 patients out of 34). Serum and urine copper were measured together with red blood cells Cu,Zn SOD (Squitti et al., 2002b, Rossi et al., 2002). While serum copper had remained stable, urine copper levels were drastically elevated, indicating that large amounts of copper were indeed being removed from the tissues. Cu,Zn SOD activity was drastically reduced, revealing that this enzyme could be used as an indicator of general depletion of bioavailable copper. A significant reduction was also observed in the hydroperoxide levels.

Despite the positive effect in decreasing the bioavailable copper and the content of hydroperoxides, the clinical relevance of those results could not be fully assessed because of the short duration (24 weeks) of the observation, during which patients in the placebo arm did not worsen, precluding the detection of cognitive differences between the treated and the placebo groups. Crapper McLachlan and colleagues (Crapper McLachlan, et al., 1991) have shown a positive effect of chelation therapy in AD by treating patients for a 24-month period, and Ritchie and coworkers (Ritchie et al., 2003) reported some positive results with clioquinol (see below) after 36 weeks.

6.3 Iodochlorhydroxyquin (clioquinol) drug class

In the early 2000s, clioquinol was tested in man revealing that a treatment of just 21 days resulted in a significant improvement of patients' cognitive performance (Regland et al., 2001). This study was followed by a case report on two AD patients showing that clioquinol could ameliorate focal cerebral glucose metabolism and halt clinical deterioration (Ibach et al., 2005), and by a double-blind placebo-controlled clinical trial, in which 36 patients were treated with 125 mg/day for the first 12 week, then 250 mg/day between week 13 and 24 and finally 375 mg/day in the latest period of weeks 25-36 (Ritchie et al., 2003). The trial revealed that clioquinol slowed the rate of clinical decline in a subset of AD patients having more severe dementia. However, in the subgroup of patients with moderate dementia the difference between clioquinol and placebo did not reach statistical significance. In addition, in this subgroup the drug had no significant effects on the plasma Aβ levels.

As stated by the authors, the results of the clioquinol study supported a proof of concept in humans that a drug targeting Aβ-metal interaction can have a significant effect on slowing the progression of AD.

Clioquinol is capable of crossing the BBB, and it is believed that it solubilizes Aβ plaques by stripping them of their metal content. However, after *in vitro* investigations, it is unclear whether the positive results shown by the clinical trial were related to an attenuated Aβ-metal ion interaction or to some other mechanisms.

In the end, the relevance of the clioquinol conclusions has been severely questioned (Hegde et al., 2009). Arguments against the chelating effectiveness of clioquinol referred mostly to the evidence coming from a study by Treiber and co-workers (Treiber et al., 2004), who, by using a yeast model system, demonstrated that the addition of clioquinol to the culture drastically increased copper concentration within the yeast cells. Thus, they attributed the positive effects of clioquinol on AD patients to an increase of copper uptake into the neural cell, instead of an attenuated Aβ-metal ion interaction outside the cell. However, the authors (Treiber et al., 2004) did not report information about the bioavailability of the intracellular copper-clioquinol complex.

Some information to this regard could be found in a subsequent study demonstrating a decreased intracellular metal bioavailability linked to the accumulation of soluble Aβ outside the cell (White et al., 2006). Clioquinol, by facilitating the delivery of metals (copper and zinc, but not iron) into the cell, seemed to activate the phosphoinositol 3-kinase mediated protein kinase pathways, ultimately leading to an increase in the secretion of matrix metalloproteinases, which can degrade Aβ outside the cell. This is why molecules of the clioquinol drug class have been defined as metal protein attenuating compounds (MPAC), and have been attributed both chelating and ionophoretic properties.

Establishing the exact localization of clioquinol within the cell, or the copper biovailability of the putative clioquinol derivates-copper-complex, could be of help to define the molecular mechanisms either triggered or prevented by this class of molecules. Further clioquinol phase II/III studies were stalled by difficulties in preventing di-iodo 8-hydroxy quinoline contamination upon large-scale chemical synthesis, as well as its citotoxicity profile. In the end, clioquinol was withdrawn from human experimentation.

New compounds were then developed, such as PBT-2, a second-generation compound of the clioquinol drug class, that lacks iodine. PBT-2 has been recently tested on AD patients in a phase II, double-blind, randomized, placebo-controlled 12 week trial. 74 patients completed the trial and well tolerated the 250 mg of PBT-2 daily dosage. This study revealed that PBT2 induced a significant dose-dependent reduction of Aβ concentrations in the CSF, even though no drug effects on either Aβ40 or Aβ42 plasma levels were detected. Moreover, PBT-2 was found to preserve two executive functions, as evaluated via category fluency and trail making tests (Adlard et al., 2008, Lannfelt et al., 2008). This promising MPAC is now been tested in a phase III clinical trial.

6.4 Zinc therapy

Some agents used in anti-copper therapies are specifically aimed at maintaining a state of copper malabsorption (Squitti & Zito, 2009). Zinc acetate and other zinc salts, such as zinc carbonate, zinc sulfate, zinc gluconate, zinc oxide, zinc chloride and zinc stearate, are currently used in the treatment of Wilson's disease (Squitti & Zito, 2009). Zinc antagonizes the absorption of copper in the gut by increasing metallothioneins concentrations in the mucosa up to 25 times. The liver is the main human storage place for copper and metallothioneins are the major copper binding proteins in this organ. Diffusible free copper present in the blood is sequestered in a non-toxic form in the mucosal cells lining the intestine by metallothioneins. In this form copper is then excreted with the stools. The copper body balance becomes negative within 2 weeks when zinc sulphate is administrated in a dose of 600 mg/day. The safety and positive effects shown by zinc compounds, such as zinc sulphate or aspartate, in treating Wilson's disease strongly recommend the testing of these compounds in AD. Encouraging results in this direction were obtained in a preliminary study by Constantinidis (Constantinidis, 1992), who reported improvements in memory, understanding, communication, and social contact in eight out of ten AD patients treated with zinc compounds.

6.5 Side effects of anti-copper complexing agents

The side effects of anti-copper complexing agents and MPAC are primarily limited to anemia and leucopenia, due to bone marrow depletion of copper, and occasionally to liver toxicity. The frequency of occurrence of these effects shows a correlation with dose strength and frequency of drug assumption. For ammonium tetrathiomolybdate, a relatively new copper-lowering agent, these events have been associated with the reduction of serum ceruloplasmin levels, which is assumed to be a marker of copper defective bioavailability. For example, at ceruloplasmin concentrations of 5 mg/dL or less, bone marrow suppression is common; it is somewhat frequent at concentrations between 5 and 10 mg/dL, it is only occasional between 10-18 mg/dL, and very rare above 18.

Clioquinol usage in humans has been halted as it has been related with subacute myelo-optic neuropathy.

Zinc compounds have only minor adverse events, limited to gastrointestinal troubles.

7. Conclusion

The results of the studies described in this chapter should be regarded as single pieces of a complex mosaic of systemic disarrangements which result in severe neurodegeneration via a variety of biochemical phenomena, among which oxidative stress plays a leading role. In this view, systemic metal abnormalities, even if mild but over a long period of time, have disrupting effects on central processes controlling the defenses against metal-induced damage. Glutamatergic synapses definitely represent focal sites where the metal-Aβ toxic action can be promoted resulting in Aβ precipitation (Bush et al., 2003, Bush & Tanzi, 2008). The identification in AD of a free copper serum-level increase, as well as of disturbances of iron homeostasis and the activation of the antioxidant Cp-Tf system, appear coherent with this picture. Not only can free copper cross the BBB and enter reactions promoting Aβ toxicity, but it can systemically activate the Cp-Tf system, promoting iron subtraction from general circulation and its consequent internalization into neural cells. Both pathways converge towards neurodegeneration and neuronal death. In this framework, properly tuning the redistribution of metals via molecules which induce or maintain a state of copper malabsorption, such as zinc compounds or metal complexing agents, may possibly have a positive effect on the natural progression of AD.

8. Acknowledgement

This study was partially supported by the following grants:

Italian Health Department: "Profilo Biologico e Genetico della Disfunzione dei Metalli nella Malattia di Alzheimer e nel 'Mild Cognitive Impairment" [RF 2006 conv.58].

Programma Strategico 2007 conv. PS39; "Ricerca Corrente" grants IRCCS Brescia, Italy.

ERA-Net NEURON (JTC 2008 nEUROsyn), AFaR Foundation - Osp. Fatebenefratelli "AAMS l gioco sicuro".

The author have no conflict of interest.

9. References

Adlard, P.A. & Bush, A.I. (2006). Metals and Alzheimer's disease. *J Alzheimers Dis*. Vol. 10, No. 2-3, pp. 145-63.

Adlard, P.A., Cherny, R.A., Finkelstein, D.I., Gautier, E., Robb, E., Cortes, M., Volitakis, I., Liu, X., Smith, J.P., Perez, K., Laughton, K., Li, Q.X., Charman, S.A., Nicolazzo, J.A., Wilkins, S., Deleva, K., Lynch, T., Kok, G., Ritchie, C.W., Tanzi, R.E., Cappai, R., Masters, C.L., Barnham, K.J. & Bush, A.I. (2008). Rapid restoration of cognition in Alzheimer's transgenic mice with 8-hydroxy quinoline analogs is associated with decreased interstitial Abeta. *Neuron*. Vol. 59, No. 1, pp. 43-55.

Althaus, J., Quinn, J.F. Kaye, J.A., Newsome, D.A., Bisgaier C.L., Kanzer, S.H. (2008). Free copper measured directly in serum using a novel device is elevated in Alzheimer's disease. *Invest Ophthalmol Vis Sci*. Vol. 49(E-abstract), 5218.

Alzheimer, A., Stelzmann, R.A., Schnitzlein, H.N. & Murtagh, F.R. (1995). An English translation of Alzheimer's 1907 paper, "Uber eine eigenartige Erkankung der Hirnrinde". *Clin Anat*. Vol. 8, No. 6, pp. 429-31.

Angeletti, B., Waldron, K.J., Freeman, K.B., Bawagan, H., Hussain, I., Miller, C.C., Lau, K.F., Tennant, M.E., Dennison, C., Robinson, N.J. & Dingwall, C. (2005). BACE1 cytoplasmic domain interacts with the copper chaperone for superoxide dismutase-1 and binds copper. *J Biol Chem*. Vol. 280, No. 18, pp. 17930-7.

Armendariz, A.D., Gonzalez, M., Loguinov, A.V. & Vulpe, C.D. (2004). Gene expression profiling in chronic copper overload reveals upregulation of Prnp and App. *Physiol Genomics*. Vol. 20, No. 1, pp. 45-54.

Arnal, N., Cristalli, D.O., de Alaniz, M.J. & Marra, C.A. (2010). Clinical utility of copper, ceruloplasmin, and metallothionein plasma determinations in human neurodegenerative patients and their first-degree relatives. *Brain Res*. Vol. 1319, No., pp. 118-30.

Atwood, C.S., Moir, R.D., Huang, X., Scarpa, R.C., Bacarra, N.M., Romano, D.M., Hartshorn, M.A., Tanzi, R.E. & Bush, A.I. (1998). Dramatic aggregation of Alzheimer abeta by Cu(II) is induced by conditions representing physiological acidosis. *J Biol Chem*. Vol. 273, No. 21, pp. 12817-26.

Atwood, C.S., Perry, G., Zeng, H., Kato, Y., Jones, W.D., Ling, K.Q., Huang, X., Moir, R.D., Wang, D., Sayre, L.M., Smith, M.A., Chen, S.G. & Bush, A.I. (2004). Copper mediates dityrosine cross-linking of Alzheimer's amyloid-beta. *Biochemistry*. Vol. 43, No. 2, pp. 560-8.

Atwood, C.S., Scarpa, R.C., Huang, X., Moir, R.D., Jones, W.D., Fairlie, D.P., Tanzi, R.E. & Bush, A.I. (2000). Characterization of copper interactions with alzheimer amyloid beta peptides: identification of an attomolar-affinity copper binding site on amyloid beta1-42. *J Neurochem*. Vol. 75, No. 3, pp. 1219-33.

Babiloni, C., Bosco, P., Ghidoni, R., Del Percio, C., Squitti, R., Binetti, G., Benussi, L., Ferri, R., Frisoni, G., Lanuzza, B., Cassetta, E., Anello, G., Gurzi, M., Bartesaghi, S., Lizio, R., Tombini, M. & Rossini, P.M. (2007a). Homocysteine and electroencephalographic rhythms in Alzheimer disease: a multicentric study. *Neuroscience*. Vol. 145, No. 3, pp. 942-54.

Babiloni, C., Squitti, R., Del Percio, C., Cassetta, E., Ventriglia, M.C., Ferreri, F., Tombini, M., Frisoni, G., Binetti, G., Gurzi, M., Salinari, S., Zappasodi, F. & Rossini, P.M. (2007b). Free copper and resting temporal EEG rhythms correlate across healthy, mild cognitive impairment, and Alzheimer's disease subjects. *Clin Neurophysiol*. Vol. 118, No. 6, pp. 1244-60.

Barnham, K.J., Ciccotosto, G.D., Tickler, A.K., Ali, F.E., Smith, D.G., Williamson, N.A., Lam, Y.H., Carrington, D., Tew, D., Kocak, G., Volitakis, I., Separovic, F., Barrow, C.J., Wade, J.D., Masters, C.L., Cherny, R.A., Curtain, C.C., Bush, A.I. & Cappai, R. (2003a). Neurotoxic, redox-competent Alzheimer's beta-amyloid is released from lipid membrane by methionine oxidation. *J Biol Chem*. Vol. 278, No. 44, pp. 42959-65.

Barnham, K.J., McKinstry, W.J., Multhaup, G., Galatis, D., Morton, C.J., Curtain, C.C., Williamson, N.A., White, A.R., Hinds, M.G., Norton, R.S., Beyreuther, K., Masters, C.L., Parker, M.W. & Cappai, R. (2003b). Structure of the Alzheimer's disease amyloid precursor protein copper binding domain. A regulator of neuronal copper homeostasis. *J Biol Chem*. Vol. 278, No. 19, pp. 17401-7.

Bartzokis, G., Sultzer, D., Cummings, J., Holt, L.E., Hance, D.B., Henderson, V.W. & Mintz, J. (2000). In vivo evaluation of brain iron in Alzheimer disease using magnetic resonance imaging. *Arch Gen Psychiatry*. Vol. 57, No. 1, pp. 47-53.

Bartzokis, G. & Tishler, T.A. (2000). MRI evaluation of basal ganglia ferritin iron and neurotoxicity in Alzheimer's and Huntingon's disease. *Cell Mol Biol (Noisy-le-grand)*. Vol. 46, No. 4, pp. 821-33.

Basun, H., Forssell, L.G., Wetterberg, L. & Winblad, B. (1991). Metals and trace elements in plasma and cerebrospinal fluid in normal aging and Alzheimer's disease. *J Neural Transm Park Dis Dement Sect*. Vol. 3, No. 4, pp. 231-58.

Baum, L., Chan, I.H., Cheung, S.K., Goggins, W.B., Mok, V., Lam, L., Leung, V., Hui, E., Ng, C., Woo, J., Chiu, H.F., Zee, B.C., Cheng, W., Chan, M.H., Szeto, S., Lui, V., Tsoh, J., Bush, A.I., Lam, C.W. & Kwok, T. (2010). Serum zinc is decreased in Alzheimer's disease and serum arsenic correlates positively with cognitive ability. *Biometals*. Vol. 23, No. 1, pp. 173-9.

Bellingham, S.A., Ciccotosto, G.D., Needham, B.E., Fodero, L.R., White, A.R., Masters, C.L., Cappai, R. & Camakaris, J. (2004a). Gene knockout of amyloid precursor protein and amyloid precursor-like protein-2 increases cellular copper levels in primary mouse cortical neurons and embryonic fibroblasts. *J Neurochem*. Vol. 91, No. 2, pp. 423-8.

Bellingham, S.A., Lahiri, D.K., Maloney, B., La Fontaine, S., Multhaup, G. & Camakaris, J. (2004b). Copper depletion down-regulates expression of the Alzheimer's disease amyloid-beta precursor protein gene. *J Biol Chem*. Vol. 279, No. 19, pp. 20378-86.

Bielli, P. & Calabrese, L. (2002). Structure to function relationships in ceruloplasmin: a 'moonlighting' protein. *Cell Mol Life Sci*. Vol. 59, No. 9, pp. 1413-27.

Bocca, B., Forte, G., Petrucci, F., Pino, A., Marchione, F., Bomboi, G., Senofonte, O., Giubilei, F. & Alimonti, A. (2005). Monitoring of chemical elements and oxidative damage in patients affected by Alzheimer's disease. *Ann Ist Super Sanita*. Vol. 41, No. 2, pp. 197-203.

Bremner, I., Ed. (1979). Copper toxicity studies using domestic and laboratory animals. In *Copper in the environment*. New York, John Wiley & Sons.

Brewer, G.J. (2007). Iron and copper toxicity in diseases of aging, particularly atherosclerosis and Alzheimer's disease. *Exp Biol Med (Maywood)*. Vol. 232, No. 2, pp. 323-35.

Brewer, G.J. (2010). Toxicity of copper in drinking water. *J Toxicol Environ Health B Crit Rev*. Vol. 13, No. 6, pp. 449-52; author reply 53-9.

Brewer, G.J., Kanzer, S.H., Zimmerman, E.A., Celmins, D.F., Heckman, S.M. & Dick, R. (2010). Copper and ceruloplasmin abnormalities in Alzheimer's disease. *Am J Alzheimers Dis Other Demen*. Vol. 25, No. 6, pp. 490-7.

Bucossi, S., Ventriglia, M., Panetta, V., Salustri, C., Pasqualetti, P., Mariani, S., Siotto, M., Rossini, P.M. & Squitti, R. (2011). Copper in Alzheimer's Disease: A Meta-Analysis of Serum,Plasma, and Cerebrospinal Fluid Studies. *J Alzheimers Dis*. Vol. 24, No, 1, pp. 175-85.

Bush, A.I., Masters, C.L. & Tanzi, R.E. (2003). Copper, beta-amyloid, and Alzheimer's disease: tapping a sensitive connection. *Proc Natl Acad Sci U S A*. Vol. 100, No. 20, pp. 11193-4.

Bush, A.I., Pettingell, W.H., Multhaup, G., d Paradis, M., Vonsattel, J.P., Gusella, J.F., Beyreuther, K., Masters, C.L. & Tanzi, R.E. (1994). Rapid induction of Alzheimer A beta amyloid formation by zinc. *Science*. Vol. 265, No. 5177, pp. 1464-7.

Bush, A.I. & Tanzi, R.E. (2008). Therapeutics for Alzheimer's disease based on the metal hypothesis. *Neurotherapeutics*. Vol. 5, No. 3, pp. 421-32.

Castellani, R.J., Smith, M.A., Nunomura, A., Harris, P.L. & Perry, G. (1999). Is increased redox-active iron in Alzheimer disease a failure of the copper-binding protein ceruloplasmin? *Free Radic Biol Med*. Vol. 26, No. 11-12, pp. 1508-12.

Cherny, R.A., Atwood, C.S., Xilinas, M.E., Gray, D.N., Jones, W.D., McLean, C.A., Barnham, K.J., Volitakis, I., Fraser, F.W., Kim, Y., Huang, X., Goldstein, L.E., Moir, R.D., Lim, J.T., Beyreuther, K., Zheng, H., Tanzi, R.E., Masters, C.L. & Bush, A.I. (2001). Treatment with a copper-zinc chelator markedly and rapidly inhibits beta-amyloid accumulation in Alzheimer's disease transgenic mice. *Neuron*. Vol. 30, No. 3, pp. 665-76.

Cherny, R.A., Legg, J.T., McLean, C.A., Fairlie, D.P., Huang, X., Atwood, C.S., Beyreuther, K., Tanzi, R.E., Masters, C.L. & Bush, A.I. (1999). Aqueous dissolution of Alzheimer's disease Abeta amyloid deposits by biometal depletion. *J Biol Chem*. Vol. 274, No. 33, pp. 23223-8.

Choi, B.S. & Zheng, W. (2009). Copper transport to the brain by the blood-brain barrier and blood-CSF barrier. *Brain Res*. Vol. 1248, No., pp. 14-21.

Chutkow, J.G. (1978). Evidence for uptake of nonceruloplasminic copper in the brain: effect of ionic copper and amino acids. *Proc Soc Exp Biol Med*. Vol. 158, No. 1, pp. 113-6.

Cole, G.M., Teter, B. & Frautschy, S.A. (2007). Neuroprotective effects of curcumin. *Adv Exp Med Biol*. Vol. 595, No., pp. 197-212.

Connor, J.R., Snyder, B.S., Beard, J.L., Fine, R.E. & Mufson, E.J. (1992). Regional distribution of iron and iron-regulatory proteins in the brain in aging and Alzheimer's disease. *J Neurosci Res*. Vol. 31, No. 2, pp. 327-35.

Constantinidis, J. (1992). Treatment of Alzheimer's disease by zinc compounds. *Drug Dev. Res*. Vol. 27, No 1, pp. 1-14.

Corder, E.H., Saunders, A.M., Strittmatter, W.J., Schmechel, D.E., Gaskell, P.C., Small, G.W., Roses, A.D., Haines, J.L. & Pericak-Vance, M.A. (1993). Gene dose of apolipoprotein E type 4 allele and the risk of Alzheimer's disease in late onset families. *Science*. Vol. 261, No. 5123, pp. 921-3.

Crapper McLachlan, D.R., Dalton, A.J., Kruck, T.P., Bell, M.Y., Smith, W.L., Kalow, W. & Andrews, D.F. (1991). Intramuscular desferrioxamine in patients with Alzheimer's disease. *Lancet*. Vol. 337, No. 8753, pp. 1304-8.

Crouch, P.J., Blake, R., Duce, J.A., Ciccotosto, G.D., Li, Q.X., Barnham, K.J., Curtain, C.C., Cherny, R.A., Cappai, R., Dyrks, T., Masters, C.L. & Trounce, I.A. (2005). Copper-dependent inhibition of human cytochrome c oxidase by a dimeric conformer of amyloid-beta1-42. *J Neurosci*. Vol. 25, No. 3, pp. 672-9.

Crouch, P.J., White, A.R. & Bush, A.I. (2007). The modulation of metal bio-availability as a therapeutic strategy for the treatment of Alzheimer's disease. *Febs J*. Vol. 274, No. 15, pp. 3775-83.

Dal Forno, G., Palermo, M.T., Donohue, J.E., Karagiozis, H., Zonderman, A.B. & Kawas, C.H. (2005). Depressive symptoms, sex, and risk for Alzheimer's disease. *Ann Neurol*. Vol. 57, No. 3, pp. 381-7.

Dedeoglu, A., Cormier, K., Payton, S., Tseitlin, K.A., Kremsky, J.N., Lai, L., Li, X., Moir, R.D., Tanzi, R.E., Bush, A.I., Kowall, N.W., Rogers, J.T. & Huang, X. (2004). Preliminary studies of a novel bifunctional metal chelator targeting Alzheimer's amyloidogenesis. *Exp Gerontol*. Vol. 39, No. 11-12, pp. 1641-9.

Deibel, M.A., Ehmann, W.D. & Markesbery, W.R. (1996). Copper, iron, and zinc imbalances in severely degenerated brain regions in Alzheimer's disease: possible relation to oxidative stress. *J Neurol Sci*. Vol. 143, No. 1-2, pp. 137-42.

Donnelly, P.S., Caragounis, A., Du, T., Laughton, K.M., Volitakis, I., Cherny, R.A., Sharples, R.A., Hill, A.F., Li, Q.X., Masters, C.L., Barnham, K.J. & White, A.R. (2008). Selective intracellular release of copper and zinc ions from bis(thiosemicarbazonato) complexes reduces levels of Alzheimer disease amyloid-beta peptide. *J Biol Chem*. Vol. 283, No. 8, pp. 4568-77.

Dubois, B., Feldman, H.H., Jacova, C., Dekosky, S.T., Barberger-Gateau, P., Cummings, J., Delacourte, A., Galasko, D., Gauthier, S., Jicha, G., Meguro, K., O'Brien, J., Pasquier, F., Robert, P., Rossor, M., Salloway, S., Stern, Y., Visser, P.J. & Scheltens, P. (2007). Research criteria for the diagnosis of Alzheimer's disease: revising the NINCDS-ADRDA criteria. *Lancet Neurol*. Vol. 6, No. 8, pp. 734-46.

Duce, J.A. & Bush, A.I. Biological metals and Alzheimer's disease: implications for therapeutics and diagnostics. *Prog Neurobiol*. Vol. 92, No. 1, pp. 1-18.

Duce, J.A., Tsatsanis, A., Cater, M.A., James, S.A., Robb, E., Wikhe, K., Leong, S.L., Perez, K., Johanssen, T., Greenough, M.A., Cho, H.H., Galatis, D., Moir, R.D., Masters, C.L., McLean, C., Tanzi, R.E., Cappai, R., Barnham, K.J., Ciccotosto, G.D., Rogers, J.T. & Bush, A.I. (2010). Iron-export ferroxidase activity of beta-amyloid precursor protein is inhibited by zinc in Alzheimer's disease. *Cell*. Vol. 142, No. 6, pp. 857-67.

Durand, J., Meloni, G., Talmard, C., Vasak, M. & Faller, P. (2010). Zinc release of Zn-metallothionein-3 induces fibrillar type amyloid-beta aggregates. *Metallomics*. Vol. 2, No. 11, pp. 741-4.

Edbauer, D., Winkler, E., Regula, J.T., Pesold, B., Steiner, H. & Haass, C. (2003). Reconstitution of gamma-secretase activity. *Nat Cell Biol*. Vol. 5, No. 5, pp. 486-8.

Fleming, R.E. & Bacon, B.R. (2005). Orchestration of iron homeostasis. *N Engl J Med*. Vol. 352, No. 17, pp. 1741-4.

Folstein, M.F., Folstein, S.E. & McHugh PR. (1975) "Mini-mental state". A practical method for grading the cognitive state of patients for the clinician. *J Psychiatr Res* Vol. 12, No 3, pp. 189-198.

Francis, P.T., Palmer, A.M., Snape, M. & Wilcock, G.K. (1999). The cholinergic hypothesis of Alzheimer's disease: a review of progress. *J Neurol Neurosurg Psychiatry*. Vol. 66, No. 2, pp. 137-47.

Gerhardsson, L., Lundh, T., Minthon, L. & Londos, E. (2008). Metal concentrations in plasma and cerebrospinal fluid in patients with Alzheimer's disease. *Dement Geriatr Cogn Disord*. Vol. 25, No. 6, pp. 508-15.

Giambattistelli, F., Bucossi, S., Salustri, C., Panetta, V., Mariani, S., Siotto, M., Ventriglia, M., Vernieri, F., Dell'Acqua, M., Cassetta, E., Rossini, P.M. & Squitti, R. (2011). Effects of Hemochromatosis (HFE) and Transferrin gene mutations on iron dyshomeostasis, liver dysfunction and on the risk of Alzheimer's disease. *Neurobiology of Aging, Epub ahead of print.*

Gonzalez, C., Martin, T., Cacho, J., Brenas, M.T., Arroyo, T., Garcia-Berrocal, B., Navajo, J.A. & Gonzalez-Buitrago, J.M. (1999). Serum zinc, copper, insulin and lipids in Alzheimer's disease epsilon 4 apolipoprotein E allele carriers. *Eur J Clin Invest.* Vol. 29, No. 7, pp. 637-42.

Good, P.F., Perl, D.P., Bierer, L.M. & Schmeidler, J. (1992). Selective accumulation of aluminum and iron in the neurofibrillary tangles of Alzheimer's disease: a laser microprobe (LAMMA) study. *Ann Neurol.* Vol. 31, No. 3, pp. 286-92.

Gorgone, G., Ursini F., Altamura C., Bressi F., Tombini M., Curcio G., Chiovenda P., Squitti R., Silvestrini M., Ientile R., Pisani F., Rossini PM. & Vernieri F. (2009). Hyperhomocysteinemia, intima-media thickness and C677T MTHFR gene polymorphism: a correlation study in patients with cognitive impairment. *Atherosclerosis, Vol.* 206, No 1, pp 309-13.

Gutteridge, J.M. & Halliwell, B. (1990). The measurement and mechanism of lipid peroxidation in biological systems. *Trends Biochem Sci.* Vol. 15, No. 4, pp. 129-35.

Hardy, J. & Allsop, D. (1991). Amyloid deposition as the central event in the aetiology of Alzheimer's disease. *Trends Pharmacol Sci.* Vol. 12, No. 10, pp. 383-8.

Harris, E.D. (2000). Cellular copper transport and metabolism. *Annu Rev Nutr.* Vol. 20, No., pp. 291-310.

Hartter, D.E. & Barnea, A. (1988). Evidence for release of copper in the brain: depolarization-induced release of newly taken-up 67copper. *Synapse.* Vol. 2, No. 4, pp. 412-5.

Hegde, M.L., Bharathi, P., Suram, A., Venugopal, C., Jagannathan, R., Poddar, P., Srinivas, P., Sambamurti, K., Rao, K.J., Scancar, J., Messori, L., Zecca, L. & Zatta, P. (2009). Challenges associated with metal chelation therapy in Alzheimer's disease. *J Alzheimers Dis.* Vol. 17, No. 3, pp. 457-68.

Hoogenraad, T. (2007). Measuring hypercupremia in blood of patients with Alzheimer's disease is logical, but the utility of measuring free-copper has to be proven. *Neurologie,* Frijns CJM, Kappelle LJ, Klijn CJM, Wokke JHJ. (Utrechts) Tijdschrift voor, pp. 111-112

Huang, X., Atwood, C.S., Hartshorn, M.A., Multhaup, G., Goldstein, L.E., Scarpa, R.C., Cuajungco, M.P., Gray, D.N., Lim, J., Moir, R.D., Tanzi, R.E. & Bush, A.I. (1999a). The A beta peptide of Alzheimer's disease directly produces hydrogen peroxide through metal ion reduction. *Biochemistry.* Vol. 38, No. 24, pp. 7609-16.

Huang, X., Cuajungco, M.P., Atwood, C.S., Hartshorn, M.A., Tyndall, J.D., Hanson, G.R., Stokes, K.C., Leopold, M., Multhaup, G., Goldstein, L.E., Scarpa, R.C., Saunders, A.J., Lim, J., Moir, R.D., Glabe, C., Bowden, E.F., Masters, C.L., Fairlie, D.P., Tanzi, R.E. & Bush, A.I. (1999b). Cu(II) potentiation of Alzheimer abeta neurotoxicity. Correlation with cell-free hydrogen peroxide production and metal reduction. *J Biol Chem.* Vol. 274, No. 52, pp. 37111-6.

Ibach, B., Haen, E., Marienhagen, J. & Hajak, G. (2005). Clioquinol treatment in familiar early onset of Alzheimer's disease: a case report. *Pharmacopsychiatry.* Vol. 38, No. 4, pp. 178-9.

Institute of Medicine Food and Nutrition Board (2001). *Dietary Reference Intakes for Vitamin A, Vitamin K, Arsenic, Boron, Chromium, Copper, Iodine, Iron, Manganese, Molybdenum, Nickel, Silicon, Vanadium, and Zinc*, National Academy Press, Washington, DC.

Iyengar, V., Brewer, G.J., Dick, R.D. & Chung, O.Y. (1988). Studies of cholecystokinin-stimulated biliary secretions reveal a high molecular weight copper-binding substance in normal subjects that is absent in patients with Wilson's disease. *J Lab Clin Med*. Vol. 111, No. 3, pp. 267-74.

Jacobs, D., Oxley, DK, DeMott, WR (2002). *Laboratory Test Handbook: Concise with Disease Index, 2nd ed.*, Hudson (Cleveland), OH: Lexi-Comp.

Jeandel, C., Nicolas, M.B., Dubois, F., Nabet-Belleville, F., Penin, F. & Cuny, G. (1989). Lipid peroxidation and free radical scavengers in Alzheimer's disease. *Gerontology*. Vol. 35, No. 5-6, pp. 275-82.

Jiao, Y., Wilkinson, J.t., Christine Pietsch, E., Buss, J.L., Wang, W., Planalp, R., Torti, F.M. & Torti, S.V. (2006). Iron chelation in the biological activity of curcumin. *Free Radic Biol Med*. Vol. 40, No. 7, pp. 1152-60.

Kapaki, E., Segditsa, J. & Papageorgiou, C. (1989). Zinc, copper and magnesium concentration in serum and CSF of patients with neurological disorders. *Acta Neurol Scand*. Vol. 79, No. 5, pp. 373-8.

Kessler, H., Pajonk, F.G., Meisser, P., Schneider-Axmann, T., Hoffmann, K.H., Supprian, T., Herrmann, W., Obeid, R., Multhaup, G., Falkai, P. & Bayer, T.A. (2006). Cerebrospinal fluid diagnostic markers correlate with lower plasma copper and ceruloplasmin in patients with Alzheimer's disease. *J Neural Transm*. Vol. 113, No. 11, pp. 1763-9.

Kessler H, Bayer TA, Bach D, Schneider-Axmann T, Supprian T, Herrmann W, Haber M, Multhaup G, Falkai P & Pajonk F.G. (2008). Intake of copper has no effect on cognition in patients with mild Alzheimer's disease: a pilot phase 2 clinical trial. *J Neural Transm*. Vol. 115, No 8, pp. 1181-7.

Kim, B.E., Nevitt, T. & Thiele, D.J. (2008). Mechanisms for copper acquisition, distribution and regulation. *Nat Chem Biol*. Vol. 4, No. 3, pp. 176-85.

Lam, P.K., Kritz-Silverstein, D., Barrett Connor, E., Milne, D., Nielsen, F., Gamst, A., Morton, D. & Wingard, D. (2008). Plasma trace elements and cognitive function in older men and women: the Rancho Bernardo study. *J Nutr Health Aging*. Vol. 12, No. 1, pp. 22-7.

Lannfelt, L., Blennow, K., Zetterberg, H., Batsman, S., Ames, D., Harrison, J., Masters, C.L., Targum, S., Bush, A.I., Murdoch, R., Wilson, J. & Ritchie, C.W. (2008). Safety, efficacy, and biomarker findings of PBT2 in targeting Abeta as a modifying therapy for Alzheimer's disease: a phase IIa, double-blind, randomised, placebo-controlled trial. *Lancet Neurol*. Vol. 7, No. 9, pp. 779-86.

Lee, J.Y., Friedman, J.E., Angel, I., Kozak, A. & Koh, J.Y. (2004). The lipophilic metal chelator DP-109 reduces amyloid pathology in brains of human beta-amyloid precursor protein transgenic mice. *Neurobiol Aging*. Vol. 25, No. 10, pp. 1315-21.

Lim, G.P., Chu, T., Yang, F., Beech, W., Frautschy, S.A. & Cole, G.M. (2001). The curry spice curcumin reduces oxidative damage and amyloid pathology in an Alzheimer transgenic mouse. *J Neurosci*. Vol. 21, No. 21, pp. 8370-7.

Lin, R., Chen, X., Li, W., Han, Y., Liu, P. & Pi, R. (2008). Exposure to metal ions regulates mRNA levels of APP and BACE1 in PC12 cells: blockage by curcumin. *Neurosci Lett*. Vol. 440, No. 3, pp. 344-7.

Linder, M.C., Houle, P.A., Isaacs, E., Moor, J.R. & Scott, L.E. (1979). Copper regulation of ceruloplasmin in copper-deficient rats. *Enzyme*. Vol. 24, No. 1, pp. 23-35.

Liu, G., Garrett, M.R., Men, P., Zhu, X., Perry, G. & Smith, M.A. (2005). Nanoparticle and other metal chelation therapeutics in Alzheimer disease. *Biochim Biophys Acta*. Vol. 1741, No. 3, pp. 246-52.

Liu, G., Men, P., Perry, G. & Smith, M.A. (2010). Nanoparticle and iron chelators as a potential novel Alzheimer therapy. *Methods Mol Biol*. Vol. 610, No., pp. 123-44.

Loeffler, D.A., LeWitt, P.A., Juneau, P.L., Sima, A.A., Nguyen, H.U., DeMaggio, A.J., Brickman, C.M., Brewer, G.J., Dick, R.D., Troyer, M.D. & Kanaley, L. (1996). Increased regional brain concentrations of ceruloplasmin in neurodegenerative disorders. *Brain Res*. Vol. 738, No. 2, pp. 265-74.

Lovell, M.A., Robertson, J.D., Teesdale, W.J., Campbell, J.L. & Markesbery, W.R. (1998). Copper, iron and zinc in Alzheimer's disease senile plaques. *J Neurol Sci*. Vol. 158, No. 1, pp. 47-52.

Maynard, C.J., Cappai, R., Volitakis, I., Cherny, R.A., White, A.R., Beyreuther, K., Masters, C.L., Bush, A.I. & Li, Q.X. (2002). Overexpression of Alzheimer's disease amyloid-beta opposes the age-dependent elevations of brain copper and iron. *J Biol Chem*. Vol. 277, No. 47, pp. 44670-6.

McKhann, G., Drachman, D., Folstein, M., Katzman, R., Price, D. & Stadlan, E.M. (1984). Clinical diagnosis of Alzheimer's disease: report of the NINCDS-ADRDA Work Group under the auspices of Department of Health and Human Services Task Force on Alzheimer's Disease. *Neurology*. Vol. 34, No. 7, pp. 939-44.

Meloni, G., Sonois, V., Delaine, T., Guilloreau, L., Gillet, A., Teissie, J., Faller, P. & Vasak, M. (2008). Metal swap between Zn7-metallothionein-3 and amyloid-beta-Cu protects against amyloid-beta toxicity. *Nat Chem Biol*. Vol. 4, No. 6, pp. 366-72.

Miyata, M. & Smith, J.D. (1996). Apolipoprotein E allele-specific antioxidant activity and effects on cytotoxicity by oxidative insults and beta-amyloid peptides. *Nat Genet*. Vol. 14, No. 1, pp. 55-61.

Moir, R.D., Atwood, C.S., Romano, D.M., Laurans, M.H., Huang, X., Bush, A.I., Smith, J.D. & Tanzi, R.E. (1999). Differential effects of apolipoprotein E isoforms on metal-induced aggregation of A beta using physiological concentrations. *Biochemistry*. Vol. 38, No. 14, pp. 4595-603.

Molina, J.A., Jimenez-Jimenez, F.J., Aguilar, M.V., Meseguer, I., Mateos-Vega, C.J., Gonzalez-Munoz, M.J., de Bustos, F., Porta, J., Orti-Pareja, M., Zurdo, M., Barrios, E. & Martinez-Para, M.C. (1998). Cerebrospinal fluid levels of transition metals in patients with Alzheimer's disease. *J Neural Transm*. Vol. 105, No. 4-5, pp. 479-88.

Morris, M.C., Evans, D.A., Tangney, C.C., Bienias, J.L., Schneider, J.A., Wilson, R.S. & Scherr, P.A. (2006). Dietary copper and high saturated and trans fat intakes associated with cognitive decline. *Arch Neurol*. Vol. 63, No. 8, pp. 1085-8.

Multhaup, G., Schlicksupp, A., Hesse, L., Beher, D., Ruppert, T., Masters, C.L. & Beyreuther, K. (1996). The amyloid precursor protein of Alzheimer's disease in the reduction of copper(II) to copper(I). *Science*. Vol. 271, No. 5254, pp. 1406-9.

Nakano, E., Williamson, M.P., Williams, N.H. & Powers, H.J. (2004). Copper-mediated LDL oxidation by homocysteine and related compounds depends largely on copper ligation. *Biochim Biophys Acta*. Vol. 1688, No. 1, pp. 33-42.

Nelson, T.J. & Alkon, D.L. (2005). Oxidation of cholesterol by amyloid precursor protein and beta-amyloid peptide. *J Biol Chem*. Vol. 280, No. 8, pp. 7377-87.

Opazo, C., Huang, X., Cherny, R.A., Moir, R.D., Roher, A.E., White, A.R., Cappai, R., Masters, C.L., Tanzi, R.E., Inestrosa, N.C. & Bush, A.I. (2002). Metalloenzyme-like activity of Alzheimer's disease beta-amyloid. Cu-dependent catalytic conversion of dopamine, cholesterol, and biological reducing agents to neurotoxic H(2)O(2). *J Biol Chem*. Vol. 277, No. 43, pp. 40302-8.

Ozcankaya, R. & Delibas, N. (2002). Malondialdehyde, superoxide dismutase, melatonin, iron, copper, and zinc blood concentrations in patients with Alzheimer disease: cross-sectional study. *Croat Med J*. Vol. 43, No. 1, pp. 28-32.

Pajonk, F.G., Kessler, H., Supprian, T., Hamzei, P., Bach, D., Schweickhardt, J., Herrmann, W., Obeid, R., Simons, A., Falkai, P., Multhaup, G. & Bayer, T.A. (2005). Cognitive decline correlates with low plasma concentrations of copper in patients with mild to moderate Alzheimer's disease. *J Alzheimers Dis*. Vol. 8, No. 1, pp. 23-7.

Palmiter, R.D. (1994). Regulation of metallothionein genes by heavy metals appears to be mediated by a zinc-sensitive inhibitor that interacts with a constitutively active transcription factor, MTF-1. *Proc Natl Acad Sci U S A*. Vol. 91, No. 4, pp. 1219-23.

Patel, B.N., Dunn, R.J., Jeong, S.Y., Zhu, Q., Julien, J.P. & David, S. (2002). Ceruloplasmin regulates iron levels in the CNS and prevents free radical injury. *J Neurosci*. Vol. 22, No. 15, pp. 6578-86.

Plantin, L.O., Lying-Tunell, U., & Kristensson, K. (1987). Trace elemnts in the human central nervous system studied with neutron activation analysis. *Biochem. Trace Element Research*. Vol 13, pp. 69-75

Price, K.A., Crouch, P.J. & White, A.R. (2007). Therapeutic treatment of Alzheimer's disease using metal complexing agents. *Recent Pat CNS Drug Discov*. Vol. 2, No. 3, pp. 180-7.

Puglielli, L., Friedlich, A.L., Setchell, K.D., Nagano, S., Opazo, C., Cherny, R.A., Barnham, K.J., Wade, J.D., Melov, S., Kovacs, D.M. & Bush, A.I. (2005). Alzheimer disease beta-amyloid activity mimics cholesterol oxidase. *J Clin Invest*. Vol. 115, No. 9, pp. 2556-63.

Qian, Y., Tiffany-Castiglioni, E., Welsh, J. & Harris, E.D. (1998). Copper efflux from murine microvascular cells requires expression of the menkes disease Cu-ATPase. *J Nutr*. Vol. 128, No. 8, pp. 1276-82.

Que, E.L., Domaille, D.W. & Chang, C.J. (2008). Metals in neurobiology: probing their chemistry and biology with molecular imaging. *Chem Rev*. Vol. 108, No. 5, pp. 1517-49.

Quinn, J.F., Harris, C.J., Cobb, K.E., Domes, C., Ralle, M., Brewer, G. & Wadsworth, T.L. A copper-lowering strategy attenuates amyloid pathology in a transgenic mouse model of Alzheimer's disease. *J Alzheimers Dis*. Vol. 21, No. 3, pp. 903-14.

Regland, B., Lehmann, W., Abedini, I., Blennow, K., Jonsson, M., Karlsson, I., Sjogren, M., Wallin, A., Xilinas, M. & Gottfries, C.G. (2001). Treatment of Alzheimer's disease with clioquinol. *Dement Geriatr Cogn Disord*. Vol. 12, No. 6, pp. 408-14.

Religa, D., Strozyk, D., Cherny, R.A., Volitakis, I., Haroutunian, V., Winblad, B., Naslund, J. & Bush, A.I. (2006). Elevated cortical zinc in Alzheimer disease. *Neurology*. Vol. 67, No. 1, pp. 69-75.

Reznichenko, L., Amit, T., Zheng, H., Avramovich-Tirosh, Y., Youdim, M.B., Weinreb, O. & Mandel, S. (2006). Reduction of iron-regulated amyloid precursor protein and beta-amyloid peptide by (-)-epigallocatechin-3-gallate in cell cultures: implications for iron chelation in Alzheimer's disease. *J Neurochem*. Vol. 97, No. 2, pp. 527-36.

Ritchie, C.W., Bush, A.I., Mackinnon, A., Macfarlane, S., Mastwyk, M., MacGregor, L., Kiers, L., Cherny, R., Li, Q.X., Tammer, A., Carrington, D., Mavros, C., Volitakis, I., Xilinas, M., Ames, D., Davis, S., Beyreuther, K., Tanzi, R.E. & Masters, C.L. (2003). Metal-protein attenuation with iodochlorhydroxyquin (clioquinol) targeting Abeta amyloid deposition and toxicity in Alzheimer disease: a pilot phase 2 clinical trial. *Arch Neurol*. Vol. 60, No. 12, pp. 1685-91.

Rossi, L., Ciriolo, M.R., Marchese, E., De Martino, A., Giorgi, M. & Rotilio, G. (1994). Differential decrease of copper content and of copper binding to superoxide dismutase in liver, heart and brain of copper-deficient rats. *Biochem Biophys Res Commun*. Vol. 203, No. 2, pp. 1028-34.

Rossi, L., Squitti, R., Pasqualetti, P., Marchese, E., Cassetta, E., Forastiere, E., Rotilio, G., Rossini, P.M. & Finazzi-Agro, A. (2002). Red blood cell copper, zinc superoxide dismutase activity is higher in Alzheimer's disease and is decreased by D-penicillamine. *Neurosci Lett*. Vol. 329, No. 2, pp. 137-40.

Rossor, M.N. (1983). Focal changes in Alzheimer's disease and cholinergic hypothesis. *Lancet*. Vol. 2, No. 8347, pp. 465.

Salustri, C., Barbati, G., Ghidoni, R., Quintiliani, L., Ciappina, S., Binetti, G. & Squitti, R. (2010a). Is cognitive function linked to serum free copper levels? A cohort study in a normal population. *Clin Neurophysiol*. Vol. 121, No. 4, pp. 502-7.

Salustri, C., Squitti, R., Zappasodi, F., Ventriglia, M., Bevacqua, M.G., Fontana, M. & Tecchio, F. (2010b). Oxidative stress and brain glutamate-mediated excitability in depressed patients. *J Affect Disord*. Vol. 127, No. 1-3, pp. 321-5.

Sanan, D.A., Weisgraber, K.H., Russell, S.J., Mahley, R.W., Huang, D., Saunders, A., Schmechel, D., Wisniewski, T., Frangione, B., Roses, A.D. & et al. (1994). Apolipoprotein E associates with beta amyloid peptide of Alzheimer's disease to form novel monofibrils. Isoform apoE4 associates more efficiently than apoE3. *J Clin Invest*. Vol. 94, No. 2, pp. 860-9.

Sayre, L.M., Perry, G., Harris, P.L., Liu, Y., Schubert, K.A. & Smith, M.A. (2000). In situ oxidative catalysis by neurofibrillary tangles and senile plaques in Alzheimer's disease: a central role for bound transition metals. *J Neurochem*. Vol. 74, No. 1, pp. 270-9.

Schmitz, C., Rutten, B.P., Pielen, A., Schafer, S., Wirths, O., Tremp, G., Czech, C., Blanchard, V., Multhaup, G., Rezaie, P., Korr, H., Steinbusch, H.W., Pradier, L. & Bayer, T.A. (2004). Hippocampal neuron loss exceeds amyloid plaque load in a transgenic mouse model of Alzheimer's disease. *Am J Pathol*. Vol. 164, No. 4, pp. 1495-502.

Siotto, M., Bucossi, S. & Squitti, R. Copper status abnormalities and how to measure them in neurodegenerative disorders. *Recent Pat CNS Drug Discov*. Vol. 5, No. 3, pp. 182-94.

Smith, M.A., Zhu, X., Tabaton, M., Liu, G., McKeel, D.W., Jr., Cohen, M.L., Wang, X., Siedlak, S.L., Dwyer, B.E., Hayashi, T., Nakamura, M., Nunomura, A. & Perry, G. (2010). Increased iron and free radical generation in preclinical Alzheimer disease and mild cognitive impairment. *J Alzheimers Dis*. Vol. 19, No. 1, pp. 363-72.

Smorgon, C., Mari, E., Atti, A.R., Dalla Nora, E., Zamboni, P.F., Calzoni, F., Passaro, A. & Fellin, R. (2004). Trace elements and cognitive impairment: an elderly cohort study. *Arch Gerontol Geriatr Suppl*. Vol., No. 9, pp. 393-402.

Snaedal, J., Kristinsson, J., Gunnarsdottir, S., Olafsdottir, Baldvinsson, M. & Johannesson, T. (1998). Copper, ceruloplasmin and superoxide dismutase in patients with Alzheimer's disease. A case-control study. *Dement Geriatr Cogn Disord*. Vol. 9, No. 5, pp. 239-42.

Sparks, D.L., Friedland, R., Petanceska, S., Schreurs, B.G., Shi, J., Perry, G., Smith, M.A., Sharma, A., Derosa, S., Ziolkowski, C. & Stankovic, G. (2006). Trace copper levels in the drinking water, but not zinc or aluminum influence CNS Alzheimer-like pathology. *J Nutr Health Aging*. Vol. 10, No. 4, pp. 247-54.

Sparks, D.L. & Schreurs, B.G. (2003). Trace amounts of copper in water induce beta-amyloid plaques and learning deficits in a rabbit model of Alzheimer's disease. *Proc Natl Acad Sci U S A*. Vol. 100, No. 19, pp. 11065-9.

Squitti, R. (2011). Metals In Alzheimer's Disease: A Systemic Perspective. *Frontiers in Bioscience, in press.*

Squitti, R., Barbati, G., Rossi, L., Ventriglia, M., Dal Forno, G., Cesaretti, S., Moffa, F., Caridi, I., Cassetta, E., Pasqualetti, P., Calabrese, L., Lupoi, D. & Rossini, P.M. (2006). Excess of nonceruloplasmin serum copper in AD correlates with MMSE, CSF [beta]-amyloid, and h-tau. *Neurology*. Vol. 67, No. 1, pp. 76-82.

Squitti, R., Bressi, F., Pasqualetti, P., Bonomini, C., Ghidoni, R., Binetti, G., Cassetta, E., Moffa, F., Ventriglia, M., Vernieri, F. & Rossini, P.M. (2009). Longitudinal prognostic value of serum "free" copper in patients with Alzheimer disease. *Neurology*. Vol. 72, No. 1, pp. 50-5.

Squitti, R., Cassetta, E., Dal Forno, G., Lupoi, D., Lippolis, G., Pauri, F., Vernieri, F., Cappa, A. & Rossini, P.M. (2004). Copper perturbation in 2 monozygotic twins discordant for degree of cognitive impairment. *Arch Neurol*. Vol. 61, No. 5, pp. 738-43.

Squitti, R., Ghidoni, R., Scrascia, F., Benussi, L., Panetta, V., Pasqualetti, P., Moffa, F., Bernardini, S., Ventriglia, M., Binetti, G. & Rossini, P.M. (2011). Free copper distinguishes mild cognitive impairment subjects from healthy elderly individuals. *J Alzheimers Dis*. Vol. 23, No. 2, pp. 239-48.

Squitti, R., Lupoi, D., Pasqualetti, P., Dal Forno, G., Vernieri, F., Chiovenda, P., Rossi, L., Cortesi, M., Cassetta, E. & Rossini, P.M. (2002a). Elevation of serum copper levels in Alzheimer's disease. *Neurology*. Vol. 59, No. 8, pp. 1153-61.

Squitti, R., Pasqualetti, P., Cassetta, E., Dal Forno, G., Cesaretti, S., Pedace, F., Finazzi-Agro, A. & Rossini, P.M. (2003). Elevation of serum copper levels discriminates Alzheimer's disease from vascular dementia. *Neurology*. Vol. 60, No. 12, pp. 2013-4.

Squitti, R., Pasqualetti, P., Dal Forno, G., Moffa, F., Cassetta, E., Lupoi, D., Vernieri, F., Rossi, L., Baldassini, M. & Rossini, P.M. (2005). Excess of serum copper not related to ceruloplasmin in Alzheimer disease. *Neurology*. Vol. 64, No. 6, pp. 1040-6.

Squitti R, Q.C., Forno GD, Antuono P, Wekstein DR, Capo CR, Salustri C, Rossini PM. (2007). Ceruloplasmin (2-D PAGE) Pattern and Copper Content in Serum and Brain of Alzheimer Disease Patients. *Biomark Insights*. Vol. 7, No. 1, pp. 205-13.

Squitti, R., Quattrocchi, C.C., Salustri, C. & Rossini, P.M. (2008). Ceruloplasmin fragmentation is implicated in 'free' copper deregulation of Alzheimer's disease. *Prion*. Vol. 2, No. 1, pp. 23-7.

Squitti, R., Rossini, P.M., Cassetta, E., Moffa, F., Pasqualetti, P., Cortesi, M., Colloca, A., Rossi, L. & Finazzi-Agro, A. (2002b). d-penicillamine reduces serum oxidative stress in Alzheimer's disease patients. *Eur J Clin Invest*. Vol. 32, No. 1, pp. 51-9.

Squitti, R. & Salustri, C. (2009). Agents complexing copper as a therapeutic strategy for the treatment of Alzheimer's disease. *Curr Alzheimer Res*. Vol. 6, No. 6, pp. 476-87.

Squitti, R., Salustri, C., Siotto, M., Ventriglia, M., Vernieri, F., Lupoi, D., Cassetta, E. & Rossini, P.M. (2010c). Ceruloplasmin/Transferrin ratio changes in Alzheimer's disease. *Int J Alzheimers Dis*. Vol. 2011, No., pp. 231595.

Squitti, R., Ventriglia, M., Barbati, G., Cassetta, E., Ferreri, F., Dal Forno, G., Ramires, S., Zappasodi, F. & Rossini, P.M. (2007). 'Free' copper in serum of Alzheimer's disease patients correlates with markers of liver function. *J Neural Transm*. Vol. 114, No. 12, pp. 1589-94.

Squitti, R. & Zito, G. (2009). Anti-copper therapies in Alzheimer's disease: new concepts. *Recent Pat CNS Drug Discov*. Vol. 4, No. 3, pp. 209-19.

Strozyk, D., Launer, L.J., Adlard, P.A., Cherny, R.A., Tsatsanis, A., Volitakis, I., Blennow, K., Petrovitch, H., White, L.R. & Bush, A.I. (2009). Zinc and copper modulate Alzheimer Abeta levels in human cerebrospinal fluid. *Neurobiol Aging*. Vol. 30, No. 7, pp. 1069-77.

Treiber, C., Simons, A., Strauss, M., Hafner, M., Cappai, R., Bayer, T.A. & Multhaup, G. (2004). Clioquinol mediates copper uptake and counteracts copper efflux activities of the amyloid precursor protein of Alzheimer's disease. *J Biol Chem*. Vol. 279, No. 50, pp. 51958-64.

Vural, H., Demirin, H., Kara, Y., Eren, I. & Delibas, N. (2010). Alterations of plasma magnesium, copper, zinc, iron and selenium concentrations and some related erythrocyte antioxidant enzyme activities in patients with Alzheimer's disease. *J Trace Elem Med Biol*. Vol. 24, No. 3, pp. 169-73.

White, A.R., Du, T., Laughton, K.M., Volitakis, I., Sharples, R.A., Xilinas, M.E., Hoke, D.E., Holsinger, R.M., Evin, G., Cherny, R.A., Hill, A.F., Barnham, K.J., Li, Q.X., Bush, A.I. & Masters, C.L. (2006). Degradation of the Alzheimer disease amyloid beta-peptide by metal-dependent up-regulation of metalloprotease activity. *J Biol Chem*. Vol. 281, No. 26, pp. 17670-80.

White, A.R., Multhaup, G., Maher, F., Bellingham, S., Camakaris, J., Zheng, H., Bush, A.I., Beyreuther, K., Masters, C.L. & Cappai, R. (1999a). The Alzheimer's disease amyloid precursor protein modulates copper-induced toxicity and oxidative stress in primary neuronal cultures. *J Neurosci*. Vol. 19, No. 21, pp. 9170-9.

White, A.R., Reyes, R., Mercer, J.F., Camakaris, J., Zheng, H., Bush, A.I., Multhaup, G., Beyreuther, K., Masters, C.L. & Cappai, R. (1999b). Copper levels are increased in the cerebral cortex and liver of APP and APLP2 knockout mice. *Brain Res*. Vol. 842, No. 2, pp. 439-44.

Wischik, C., Bentham, P, Wischik, DJ, Seng, KM (2008). O3-04-07: Tau aggregation inhibitor (TAI) therapy with rember™ arrests disease progression in mild and moderate Alzheimer's disease over 50 weeks. *Alzheimer's & Dementia*. Vol. 4, No. 4, Supplement, pp. T167.

Yu, W.H., Lukiw, W.J., Bergeron, C., Niznik, H.B. & Fraser, P.E. (2001). Metallothionein III is reduced in Alzheimer's disease. *Brain Res*. Vol. 894, No. 1, pp. 37-45.

Zappasodi, F., Salustri, C., Babiloni, C., Cassetta, E., Del Percio, C., Ercolani, M., Rossini, P.M. & Squitti, R. (2008). An observational study on the influence of the APOE-epsilon4 allele on the correlation between 'free' copper toxicosis and EEG activity in Alzheimer disease. *Brain Res*. Vol. 1215, No., pp. 183-9.

8

Glucose Metabolism and Insulin Action in Alzheimer's Disease Pathogenesis

Domenico Bosco[1], Massimiliano Plastino[1], Antonio Spanò[1], Caterina Ermio[2] and Antonietta Fava[3]
[1]*Department of Neuroscience, "S. Giovanni di Dio" Hospital, Crotone*
[2]*Department of Neuroscience, "S. Giovanni Paolo II" Hospital, Lamezia Terme*
[3]*Clinical Nutrition Unit, Medical School, University of Catanzaro*
Italy

1. Introduction

Alzheimer's disease (AD) is a neurological disorder characterized by profound memory loss and progressive dementia. The pathological and histological hallmarks of AD include amyloid plaques, neurofibrillary tangles and amyloidal angiopathy, accompanied by diffuse loss of neurons and synapses [1]. Environmental and genetic factors interact in the development of disease. Type 2 diabetes mellitus (DM) appears to be a significant risk factor for vascular dementia and AD in several epidemiological studies [2, 3]. Recent longitudinal studies have shown that AD and disorder of glucose metabolism are related [4, 5]. One explanation could be that vascular complications of diabetes result in neurodegenerative disease [6]. On the other hand, in addition to its peripheral metabolic effects, insulin also appears have important outcome on brain functions. A recent commentary offers two models of the link between type-2 DM and AD, 1. "central insulin resistance" and 2. inflammation. Both mechanisms influence insulin sensitivity in the brain, finally leading to β-amyloid accumulation and, consequently, to AD [7]. Complex molecular mechanisms, referring to insulin and/or insulin like growth factor-1 (IGF-1) signaling could link DM and AD [8]. In fact, there is evidence that altered insulin and/or IGF-1 signaling to brain cells is probably responsible of amyloid accumulation in AD [9] and several independent effects of insulin on brain functions and cognitive performance have been described [10]. Insulin resistance with associated hyperinsulinemia are the mechanisms suggested to explain the increased AD risk in diabetes [11]. Subsequent investigations demonstrated reduced blood glucose levels and increased insulin levels in patients with late onset AD compared to aged controls or patients with vascular dementia. Although the authors concluded that these findings did not support an association between diabetes and AD [12], the same data were reinterpreted as an increased prevalence of insulin resistance in AD. The latter conclusion contradicts the finding that glucose administration could both increase plasma insulin levels and improve cognition in AD. Working under the assumption that increased insulin rather than glucose was responsible for the improvement in memory, further studies were used to demonstrate that the administration of insulin significantly improved memory performance in AD [8, 13]. Hyperinsulinemic euglycemic clamp studies in humans showed improvement of attention in AD patients and neuroelectric changes in evoked potential induced by insulin [14]. In contrast, increases in plasma glucose that were not accompanied by increases in insulin levels did not influence cognitive performances [15]. The Rotterdam Study was one of the first epidemiology surveys to provide convincing evidence on a relationship between DM and dementia based on a significantly higher prevalence of dementia in patients with insulin-dependent (Type 1) DM compared to non diabetic aged controls [3]. In addition, the possible association between DM-insulin resistance and degree of hippocampal and amygdala atrophy was investigated in vivo by magnetic resonance imaging [16]. The study showed that: 1. Individuals with DM had greater degree of hippocampal and amygdala atrophy compared with subjects who did not have DM; 2. Severity of insulin resistance associated with degree of amygdala atrophy. The inability to convincingly demonstrate a correlation between DM and AD, or find evidence that DM causes neuropathology, led to the alternative hypothesis that diabetes may serve as a co-factor in the pathogenesis of dementia and possibly AD. In this regard, epidemiological studies showed that hyperinsulinemia in patients with APO E_4-negative genotype was correlated with AD-type dementia, whereas in the absence of diabetes, APO E_4+ genotype was also correlated with AD [17], suggesting that APO E_4 genotype and DM contribute independently to the pathogenesis of AD. Correspondingly, post-mortem studies have shown that individuals with DM and APO E_4 genotype had significantly more abundant Aβ deposits and neurofibrillary tangles compared with diabetics who did not have an APO E_4 allele [18]. In this review, we will summarize current evidences supporting the association between insulin action, insulin receptors, IGF-1 and AD, and we will describe the underlying mechanisms.

2. Insulin, IGF-1: Secretion, transport and distribution in human brain

Insulin is almost exclusively synthesized and secreted into the plasma by pancreatic β-cells and has important role in metabolic homeostasis. Although accumulated evidence indicate that insulin is derived from peripheral insulin and transferred by a transporter regulated way through the blood-brain-barrier (BBB), [19, 20] there is also evidence consistent with local synthesis of insulin in the brain. In fact, Schechter et al. demonstrated that insulin can be produced locally in rabbit neuronal cells from culture [21]. besides, Devaskar et al. revealed localization of insulin expressing neurons involved in associative areas of limbic system and areas regulating olfaction [22]. On the other hand, it is now generally thought that insulin synthesis in the brain is restricted is not synthesized to any significant amount in adult developed brain [20]. Over the past few years, it has become clear that insulin and IGF-1 also have intense effects in the central nervous system (CNS), regulating key processes such as energy homeostasis, neuronal survival, longevity, as well as learning and memory. Insulin and IGF-1 bind to tyrosine kinase receptors, the insulin receptor (IR) and IGF-1 receptor (IGF-1R), which share a high degree of identity in their structure and function. Insulin and IR are abundant but selectively distributed in the brain. Rodent studies have shown that insulin binding is highest in the olfactory bulb, cerebral cortex, hippocampus, hypothalamus, amygdala and septum [23, 24]. In the adult mammalian brain, two types of IR were found: a peripheral type and a neuron-specific type [25]. Insulin signaling within the cell is mediated, in general, by two functional cascades, one acting through the phosphatidylinositol-3 (PI3) kinase pathway, and other acting through the mitogen-activated protein kinase pathway [26]. Binding of insulin or IGF-1 induces a conformational change of the receptor and activates tyrosine-kinase which leads to auto-phosphorylation of the intracellular β-subunit [27]. Tyrosine-phosphorylate IR and IGF-1R β-subunits recruit and subsequently phosphorylate tyrosine residues of the intracellular insulin receptor substrates (IRS). The IRS protein family has at least four members, IRS-1 to -4 [28]. IRS proteins are homologue in structure and function but show distinct tissue distribution: IRS-1 and IRS-2 are widely distributed throughout different tissues and the brain, whereas IRS-3 is only expressed in rodent adipose tissue, and IRS-4 is predominantly localized in hypothalamus, thymus, skeletal muscle, heart, kidney, and liver [29]. IR and IGF-1R are also expressed on brain capillaries and mediate the high efficiency translocation of insulin and IGF-1 into the brain across the BBB [30, 31]. Several studies have shown the highest IR density in olfactory bulb, hippocampal formation, hypothalamus, and cerebral cortex [32, 33]. In fact, in postmortem studies in adult humans, Adem et al. showed the highest IGF-1R density in hippocampus, amygdala and parahippocampal gyrus [33]. Whereas the density of brain IR decreases during age, IGF-1R increases, suggesting that specific insulin mediated signals are involved in aging and possibly cause age associated cognitive decline [34, 35]. Insulin has been shown to cross the BBB by different mechanisms: extracellular pathways, non-saturable transmembrane diffusion or saturable active transport [36]. Currently, the majority of studies suggests that the largest proportion of insulin crosses the BBB by receptor-mediated transport [37]. In contrast, insulin IGF-1 is formed within the CNS during the development and, to a lesser extent, in the mature brain [38]. However, Rotwein suggests that IGF-1 might cross the BBB via an analogous mechanism like insulin [39].

3. Insulin and IGF-1 signaling in Alzheimer's disease

In normal physiology, insulin facilitates memory as demonstrated when administration at optimal doses and in contrast of sufficient glucose availability [15]. Type-2-diabetic patients are insulin resistant and have chronic hyperinsulinemia. The peripheral utilization of insulin reduces insulin transport into the brain, ultimately producing brain insulin deficiency [40], and abrogating the beneficial influences of insulin on the brain functions [15]. Different insulin levels have been observed in different brain regions [30, 41], probably linked to multiple insulin actions in CNS. Studies on type-2-DM animal models have shown a reduced uptake of insulin into the brain. It was observed that obese diabetic Zucker rats have a decreased insulin transport into the brain, reduced brain levels of insulin and peripheral hyperglycemia [30, 36, 41]. Recent studies linked diabetes with AD [8, 9, 18] and suggested that the brain may be influenced by changes in insulin levels and sensitivity. The observations that insulin, insulin receptors and C-peptide levels in cerebrospinal fluid (CSF) appears to be reduced in aging [42], along with the finding that AD patients have lower levels of insulin in the CSF, suggest impaired transport of insulin into the brain [43]. However the salutary effect of insulin on brain functions are reserved under conditions that impair its functioning, such as insulin resistance [44]. Frolich et al. found that neuronal tyrosine-kinase activity is decreased in AD patients compared to age-matched controls [35]. The overall expression of IGF-1R is reduced in AD brains dependent on the severity of the disease. Brain IGF-1 mRNA levels diminish in severe AD, whereas IGF-1 serum levels are increased in early stages of the disease, suggesting that IGF-1 resistance plays a role in the pathogenesis of AD [35]. IRS-1/2 protein expression is reduced in AD brains, and inactivating Serine-phosphorylation of IRS-^{312} and Ser^{616} is improved, leading to impaired insulin resistance and IGF-1R signaling [45]. Given that IRS are widely expressed in the hippocampus, the most studied brain region for learning and memory, it seems to be plausible that decline of insulin resistance signaling leads to cognitive impairment [46]. Experiments with adult mice lacking liver IGF-1 production with an up of 85% reduction in circulating IGF-1 showed impaired spatial memory in the Morris water maze task compared to wild type litter mates [46]. These findings might explain the reduction of cognitive functions during aging, since IGF-1 serum levels diminish under physiological conditions [47]. Unpredictably, studies in neuronal-IR-knockout mice (NIRKO) did not provide evidence for impairment in learning and memory, proposing that insulin resistance alone is not a key feature in dementia and neurodegeneration [17].

3.1 Glucose metabolism and Alzheimer's disease

Some of the earliest work on senile dementia, which probably corresponded to AD, vascular dementia, or a combination of both, documented the development of altered brain metabolism soon after the onset of clinical symptoms [48, 49]. The metabolic abnormalities consisted of impaired glucose utilization and energy metabolism, with features that resemble type-2 DM [48]. In addition, several studies confirmed that cerebral metabolism declined prior to the deterioration of cognitive functions, suggesting that energy failure is one of the earliest reversible hallmarks of AD. These observations led to the hypothesis that AD-associated abnormalities in energy metabolism are caused by IR action in the brain, i.e. brain diabetes [49].

3.2 Insulin therapy and Alzheimer's disease

There are conflicting findings regarding the effects of antidiabetic therapy on clinical and neuropathology of AD. The Honolulu-Asia Aging Study demonstrated improvement of cognitive function and memory following induced hyperinsulinemia in patients with AD [2]. Conversely, the Rotterdam Study [3] observed increased risk of dementia in subjects with diabetes treated with insulin. In fact, in this prospective study, DM almost doubled the risk of dementia [Relative Risk (RR) 1.9] and patients treated with insulin were at higher risk of dementia [RR 4.3]. In opposition, recent studies suggest that the combination of insulinic therapy with other diabetes medications is associated to a lower neuritic plaques [50] and to slower cognitive decline in patients with AD [13]. Besides, studies in animals have revealed the beneficial effects of peripheral and cerebroventricular injections of insulin on memory and learning [51]. Several studies have recognized that increasing plasma glucose levels improves memory in patients with AD [14, 15, 30]. Increasing plasma glucose levels also increases endogenous insulin levels, raising the query whether memory improvement is due to changes in insulin, independently of hyperglycemia [14], although the exact mechanism remains unclear. Dense IR distributions have been documented in the dentate gyros, CA1, and CA3 fields of the hippocampus [52]. These regions are known to play a role in declarative memory and they are affected earlier and most severely by the neuropathologic changes of AD [53]. Increased plasma insulin levels result in amplified insulin binding in hippocampus. In turn, increased brain insulin levels results in enlarged glucose utilization in the entorhinal cortex [54]. In contrast to the traditional notion that the brain is not an insulin-sensitive organ, insulin-promoted glucose utilization also results in glycolytic production of acetyl-CoA and subsequent increase in acetylcholine [55], a neurotransmitter closely linked to memory function and severely reduced in AD. Craft et al. confirm that elevated insulin without hyperglycaemia enhances memory in adults with AD, when endogenous insulin was suppressed by concomitant infusion of somatostatin analogues [14]. Moreover, the beneficial effect of insulin appears to be reduced when insulin resistance is present [17]. Craft et al. showed acute effect of hyperinsulinemia in older adults and in patients with AD using a hyperinsulinemic-euglycemic clamps [15]. Low doses of insulin improve memory in normal subjects; AD patients with insulin resistance required higher insulin doses to obtain memory improvement. To date, no genetic risk factors have been identified for these patients, raising the possibility that factors relating to insulin resistance may be important for AD pathogenesis [15].

3.3 Insulin and oxidative stress mechanisms in Alzheimer's disease

Insulin promotes cell membrane expression of N-methyl-D-aspartate (NMDA) receptors, with increased neuronal Ca^{2+} influx [56]. Ca^{2+} influx presumably activates Ca^{2+}dependent enzymes, including α-dependent enzymes and strengthens neuronal synaptic association [10]. A recent study identified a molecular mechanism that protects CNS neurons against β-amyloid-derived-diffusible ligands (ADDL), responsible for synaptic deterioration underlying AD memory failure. The authors found ADDL binding to particular synaptic sites, and the resulting oxidative stress on synapses loss are markedly decreased by the presence of insulin. The protection mechanism does not involve simple competition between ADDLs and insulin, but rather is signaling-dependent down regulation of ADDL binding sites [57]. Another metabolic disturbance of emerging importance in AD involves insulin signaling in the brain. Levels of insulin receptors, glucose-transport proteins, and other insulin pathway components are reduced in some studies of AD brain (central resistance) [30]. Han et al. proposed a central insulin resistance together with decreased brain insulin levels might lead to accumulation of β-amyloid and consequently AD [7]. Insulin and brain derived IGF-1 instigate signals in the brain by activating the phosphatidylinositol-3-kinase-Akt pathway and the mitogen-activated protein kinase-extracellular signal-regulated kinase pathway [58], but it is unclear whether signaling is up-regulated (compensatory) or down-regulated (pathologic) in AD. Aging and life span are also influenced by insulin. Both in AD and in normal aging process mtDNA sustains high levels of oxidative damage **(Figure 1)** [59]. In fact, it was observed the accumulation of Aβ within structural damaged mitochondria isolated from the brains of AD patients [59, 60] and transgenic brains [61], which impair critical mitochondrial enzymes. Dysfunctional mitochondria release oxidizing free radicals, with peroxidation of membrane lipids and output of toxic aldehydes that cause considerable oxidative stress in AD and in normal aging brains [62]. Other essential proteins resulted oxidized, yielding carbonyl and nitrated derivatives, in neuronal cytoplasm in cerebral regions of neurodegeneration, in human brain affected by AD [63]. Subsequently, increased membrane permeability to calcium, and impaired glucose transport aggravate the energy imbalance [64]. Experimental model show that markers of oxidative damage precede pathological changes [65]. Destruction of mitochondria by the oxidation of a dynamic like transporter protein may cause synapse loss in AD [66]. The "receptor for advanced glycation end products" (RAGE) mediates Aβ's pro-oxidant effects on neural, microglial, and cerebrovascular cells [67]. The RAGE receptor is a multi-ligand receptor, and one of its ligands is Aβ [67]. RAGE regulates several intracellular pathways [68], such stimulates expression of b-site Amyloid Precursor Protein (APP)-cleaving enzyme 1 (BACE1) [69], an enzyme that is necessary for Aβ production. Moreover RAGE seems to negatively affect the long term potentiation (LTP) synaptic process of learning and memory [70]. RAGE also exists in a soluble form, structured by alternative splicing [71] or proteolytic cleavage by the metalloprotease 10 (ADAM 10) [72]. Soluble

RAGE (sRAGE) contains the ligand-binding site, but does not have the signaling properties of full-length RAGE (flRAGE). It was observed that flRAGE is engaged in positive feedback mechanisms, enhancing its own production, and limiting sRAGE proposed protective actions. This notion is supported by the finding that flRAGE expression is increased in AD brains [73]. Indeed, studies have shown that sRAGE can inhibit the accumulation and aggregation of Aβ in mice brains [74]. In addition, it has been shown that sRAGE is present at lower levels in the blood and brain of AD patients [75]. Abnormal expression of RAGE in AD brain suggests that it is relevant to the pathogenesis of neuronal dysfunction and death.

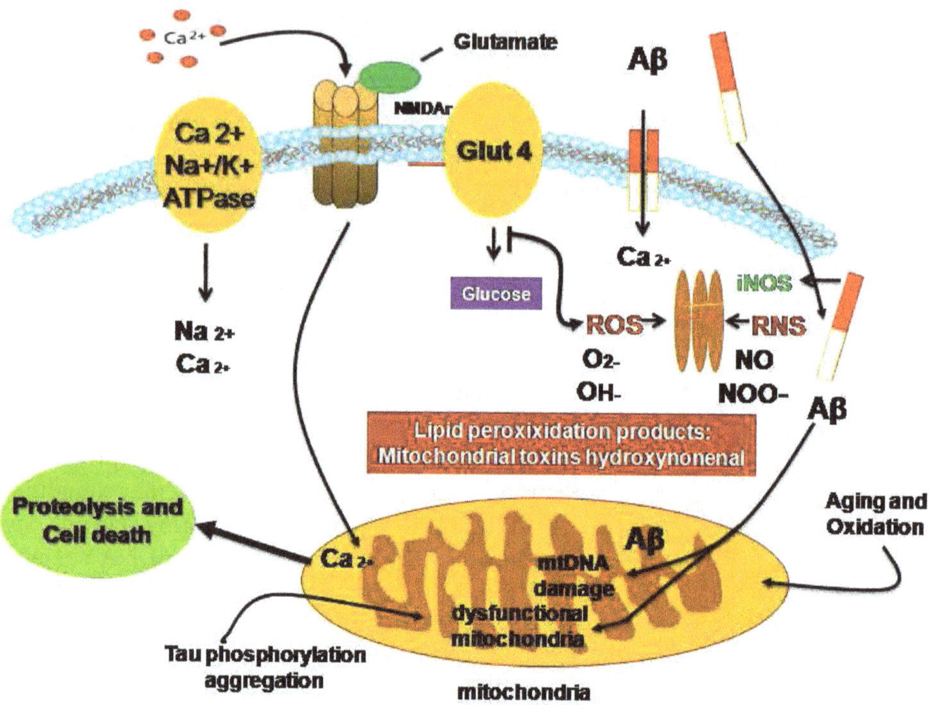

Fig. 1. Oxidative distress

Dysfunctional mitochondria release oxidizing free radicals, and in Alzheimer's disease (AD), they cause significant oxidative stress. Oxidative damage precede pathological changes. Aβ, a strong generator of reactive oxygen species (ROS) and reactive nitrogen species (RNS), is a prime author of this damage. The receptor for advanced glycation end products (RAGE) mediates Aβ's pro-oxidant effects on neural, microglial and cerebrovascular cells. Mitochondrial hydrogen peroxide readily diffuses into the cytosol to contribute in metal-ion-catalyzed hydroxyl radical development. Moved microglia are a major source of the highly diffusible nitric oxide radical. These reactive oxygen species and reactive nitrogen species damage several molecular targets. Peroxidation of membrane lipids yields toxic aldehydes, which impair critical mitochondrial enzymes. Other essential proteins are directly oxidized, yielding carbonyl and nitrated derivates. Consequently, increases in membrane permeability to calcium, other ionic imbalances, and impaired glucose transportation worsen the energy imbalance.

4. The insulin and IGF-1R signaling and Tau phosphorylation

Soluble tau proteins assemble with tubulin to constitute cross bridge between adjacent microtubule and promote stability of microtubules and vesicle transport [76]. Hyperphosphorylation of tau induces abnormal insoluble tau protein [77]. Neurofibrillary tangles are hyperphosphorilated, intracellular polymers of tau proteins. Neurofibrillary tangles are intracellular polymers of tau proteins, observed in cytoplasm of neurons [76] in AD and in other neurodegenerative disorders, such as frontotemporal dementia, Pick's disease, corticobasal degeneration, supranuclear palsy. Several studies [78, 79] supposed that the interaction between Aβ and tau proteins is necessary to cause neuronal loss. When hyperphosphorylated, tau aggregates and interferes with intraneuronal metabolism and transport, leading to neurodegeneration. IR/IGF1 R mediated might be involved in regulation of tau phosphorilation, amyloid precursor protein cleavage, β amyloid transport and degradation, in memory and aging [8]. The phosphorilation of tau is mainly promoted by glycogen syntase kinase (GSK)3β and cyclin dependent kinase(Cdk5).GSK3β is a serine-treonine kinase,regulated by insulin/IGF-1 signaling pathway. GSK-3β is functionally main for regulating glycogen metabolism, proliferation survival, and cell migration [77]. When the IR/IGF-1cascade is activated, GSKβ is phoshorilated by protein kinase AKT at serin leading to its inactivation [80-82] **(Figure 2).** PP2A dephosphorylates tau maintaining an equilibrium of phosphorylation and dephosphorilation of tau [82, 83]. Protein phosphatases 2A (PP2A) is the major phosphatases with 70% activity in human brains [84]. This implies a protective role of PP2A in neurodegeneration which is consistent with the finding that PP2A activity is reduced in AD brains [85]. In vitro studies it was found that insulin influences a regulatory interaction between PP2A and GSK 3β, inducing in activity of both enzymes change in the same direction. This balanced response seemed to preserve equilibrated tau phosphorilation [86, 87]. Several studies on different animal models of insulin resistance showed that impaired IR /IGF-1 signaling and hyperinsulinemia increased tau phosphorylation.[88-89]. In streptozotocina treated mice, model of type 1 diabetes, hyperphosphorilation of tau has be shown, which was reversible after peripheral insulin treatment [90]. Another important physiological role of insulin and IGF-1 in the brain is the regulation of gene transcription by MAP kinase cascade. This pathway leads to activation of extracellular signal-regulated kinase (ERK)-1/-2, involved in long lasting neuronal plasticity, memory consolidation and apoptotic neuronal death [91-93]. Thus, altered IR/IGF-1 signaling as well as lack of insulin might lead to hyperphosphorylation of tau protein and an increased formation of neurofibrillary tangles. These findings suggest that hyperphosphorylation of tau follows an imbalance of insulin regulated tau kinases and phosphatases [94].

Protein phosporylation/dephosphorylation imbalance is generate, at least in part, by a decrease in the activities of tau phosphatases (PP2A), and increase the activities of tau kinase (i.e. cdk5, GSK-3, etc.) affected by insulin. Impaired insulin signaling stimulates GSK-3β activity that increases oxidative stress and tau hyper-phosphorylation, by Cdk-5. Severe or sustained oxidative injury leads to mithocondrial DNA damage, mithocondrial dysfunction, apoptosis and the attendant cell loss and impaired neuronal function lead to dementia. Age reduces membrane fluidity inducing mutations in transmembrane proteins, (i.e. PS1, PS2,..), and vulnerability of the cell membrane to variation in pathological signal transduction.

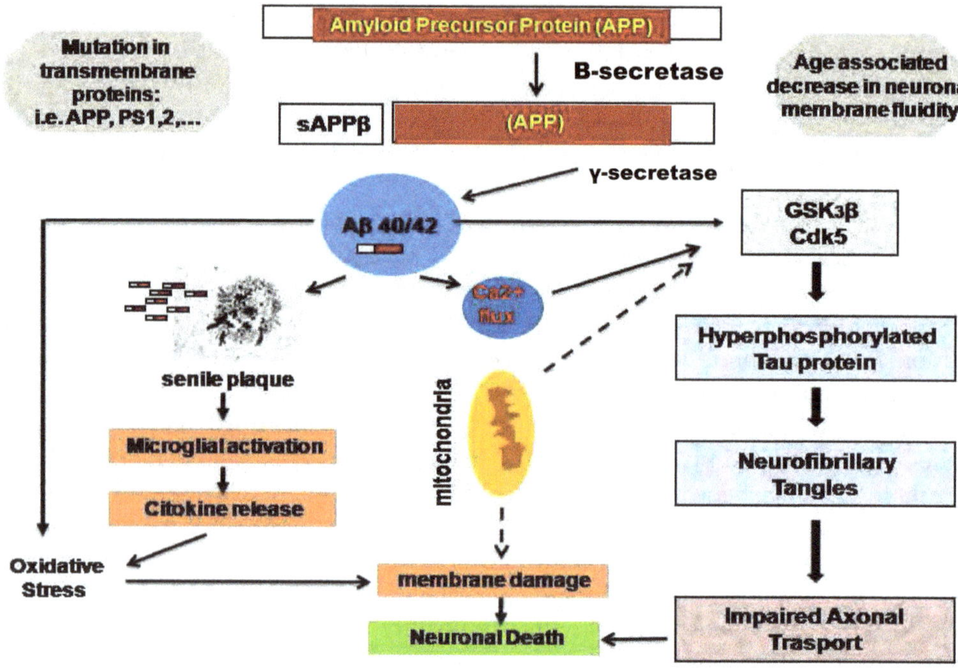

Fig. 2. Dementia and anomalous hyperphosphorylation of tau

4.1 Protein phosphatases A (PPA) processing in Alzheimer's disease

The amyloid plaques is formed by amyloid β (Aβ) peptides organized in fibrils intermixed with non fibrillar forms of this peptide and are surrounded by dystrophic dendrites, axons, reactive astrocytes and activated microglia. Aβ consists of small hydrophobic peptides with N- and C-terminal heterogeneity, i.e. $A\beta_{1\text{-}40}$ and $A\beta_{1\text{-}42}$ which are proteolytically released from a large type 1 integral membrane glycoprotein, the APP, via sequential cleavage by two aspartyl proteases, the β- and γ-secretases [enzymatic complex, containing nicastrina, presenilina, preselin enhancer-2 (PEN-2), CD_{147}] [95]. Initial β-secretase cleavage generates a soluble fragment from the NH_2-terminus of APP, while the c-terminal fragment (β-CTF) stays membrane bound. Full-length APP can undergo alternative processing by α-secretase, generating a soluble APPsα ectodomain and a membrane-bound carboxy-terminal fragment, APP-CTFα. Processing of APP by α-secretase is postulated to be protective in the context of AD, because the enzyme cleaves within the Aβ-sequence, thereby preventing the production of Aβ. APP, αCTF and βCTF are further cleaved by γ-secretase to generate p83 fragment and Aβ respectively [96]. Multiple lines of biochemical evidence have shown γ-secretases activity to reside in a high molecular weight complex, consisting of at least four components: presenilin (PS, PS1, PS2), nicastrin, anterior pharynx-defective (APH-1) and PEN-2 [97]. The p83 fragment is rapidly degraded and widely believed to possess no important function, if any. γ-secretase-mediated cleavage is unique in that the cleavage takes place within the membrane domain, though the exact site can vary. γ-cleavage can yield both $A\beta_{1\text{-}40}$ and to a lesser extent $A\beta_{1\text{-}42}$ [96]. Aβ are toxic, and their accumulation is currently seen as a key step in the pathogenesis of AD **(Figure 3).** Closer examination of the amyloidogenic β- and γ-secretates discovered the membrane-anchored aspartyl protease β-site BACE-1, which acts as β-secretase and presenelin 1-2, transmembrane proteins involved in formation of the γ-secretase complex, as the responsible cleavage enzymes. Thus, alteration of their activity might be a possible target for AD treatment [98]. It has been shown that BACE-1 levels are increased in post-mortem brain sections from AD patients [99]. During aging changes in the cerebral expression levels of the neurotrophin receptors, TrkA (tyrosine kinase receptor A) and $p75^{NTR}$ (p75 neurotrophin receptor) have been described. In the human neuroblastoma cell line SHSY5Y as well as primary cultured neurons, chronic treatment with IGF-1 leads to a switch from TrkA to $p75^{NTR}$ expression as seen in aging brains [100]. This switch causes increased β-secretase activity indirectly by activation of neuronal sphingomyelinase which is responsible for hydrolysis of sphingomyelin and active liberation of the second messenger ceramide [101]. Ceramide is responsible for the molecular stabilization of BACE-1, the β-secretase which is rate-limiting for generation of Aβ [102]. This process leads to accumulation of Aβ, connecting IGF-1R signaling to neurotrophin action. These data might provide a molecular link between aging, pathogenesis of AD and neuronal insulin-IGF-1 signaling. Lots of research has been done on the formation and accumulation of Aβ, however, in the last years the mechanisms of amyloid clearance came into focus.

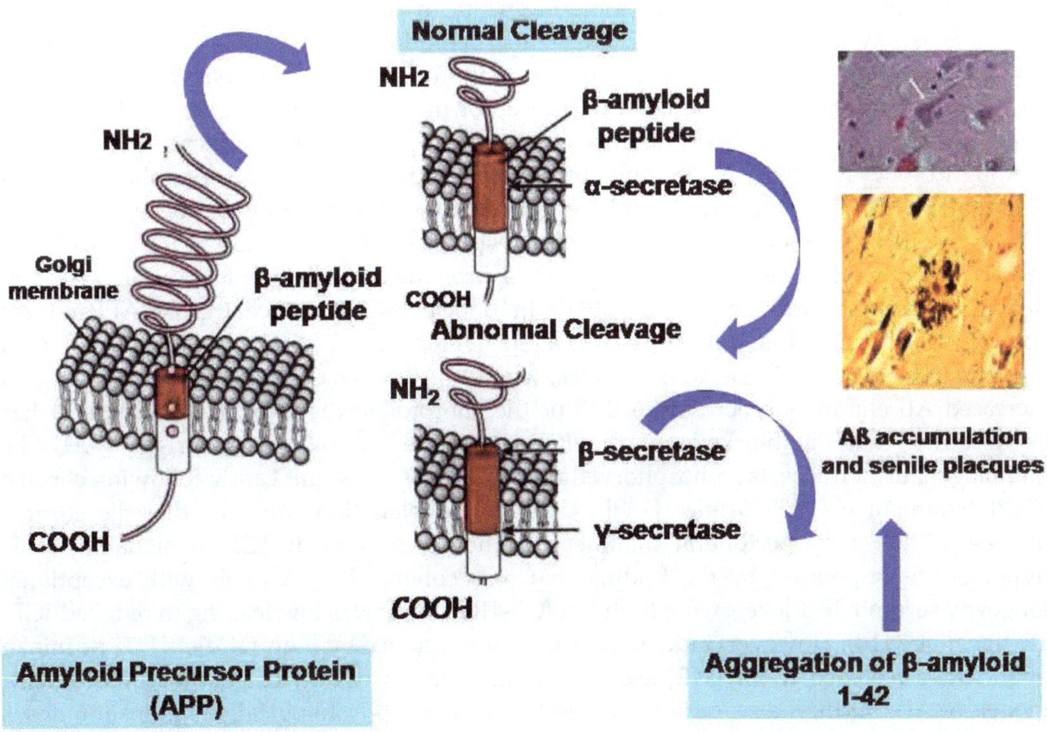

Fig. 3. Amyloid placque formation.

The histological and pathological features of AD are amyloid plaques, neurofibrillary tangles and amyloid angiopathy. The dominant component of the placque core is the the amyloid beta-peptide (Aβ) organized in fibrils of approximately 7-10 nm intermidex with non fibrillar forms of this peptide. Aβ is a a 39-43 aminoacid peptide proteolytically released from a much larger precursor, tha amyloid precursor protein (APP). The generation of Aβ from APP requires the sequential recruitment of two enzymatic activities: β-secretase, also called BACE1 (for beta side APP cleaving enzyme), and γ-secretase , a multicentric protein complex containing presenelin, nicastrina,..Aβ spontaneously self-aggregates into multiple coexisting physical forms, such as oligomers (2 to 6 peptides), transitional assemblies, fibrils that coalesce into β pleated sheets to form insoluble fibers and amyloid plaques. While monomeric Aβ is not neurotoxic, the Aβ oligomers exhibits a marked toxicity (Adapte from Martin JB; 1999).

4.2 Insulin, IGF-1 signaling and β-amyloid in Alzheimer's disease

β-amyloid spontaneously self-aggregates into multiple coexisting physical forms, such as oligomers (2 to 6 peptides), intermediate assemblies, fibrils that coalesce into β pleated sheets to form insoluble fibers and amyloid plaques [103]. While monomeric Aβ is not neurotoxic, the Aβ oligomers exhibits a marked toxicity [104]. Neuronal activation rapidly increase Aβ secretion at the synapse, during the process of neurotransmitters release. Normal levels of Aβ at this site may modulate neuronal transmission and prevent hyperactivity [105]. It was assumed that imbalance between production, aggregation and clearance of peptides, is considered initiating factor in AD [106]. For Aβ clearance several mechanisms have been described: 1. enzymatic degradation by activated microglia or by insulin degrading enzyme (IDE), neprilysin, endothelin converting enzyme (ECE), and angiotensin converting enzyme (ACE); 2. receptor-mediated transport across the BBB by binding to the low-density lipoprotein receptor-related protein (LRP), either directly or after binding to APO E and/or α2-macroglobulin (α2M), to be delivered to peripheral sites of degradation, e.g., liver and kidney [41]. Concerning insulin resistance it has been shown that IDE expression is stimulated by the insulin resistance-IGF-1R cascade [107]. It has been recently reported that membrane associated G protein-coupled receptor kinase-5 (GRK5) deficiency occurs during early AD [108]. In deficient GRK5 mice (tg2576-APPsw) Aß accumulation resulted significantly increased [108]. IGF-1 administration resulted in reduction of cerebral Aβ load in these mice, whereas Aβ was elevated in CSF suggesting an increased Aβ elimination across the BBB or the choroid plexus [109]. Furthermore, it has been shown that the blockade of the IGF-1R in the choroid plexus triggers AD-like pathology. Furthermore, tau phosphorylation did not change significantly following chronic IGF-1 treatment in Tg2576 mice [109]. A possible explanation could be that the chronic increase of IGF-1 by peripheral treatment might down regulate IGF-1R signaling. This hypothesis is supported by the finding that in a cohort of individuals with exceptional longevity serum IGF-1 levels were high but IGF-1R activity was low leading to reduced IGF-1R signaling [110]. However, induction of insulin resistance by high fat diet [111] or intake of sucrose-sweetened water [112] leads to an aggravation of amyloid pathology in mouse models of AD. Furthermore, peripheral injection of supra physiologically high insulin doses but not of physiological doses leads to transient cerebral tau phosphorylation [113], leading to the proposal that there is a dose dependent effect of insulin resistance-IGF-1R signaling in the pathogenesis of AD.

5. Insulin, inflammation and Alzheimer's disease

In recent years inflammatory pathway have been linked to type 2 diabetes mellitus, metabolic syndrome (MS) and neurodegenerative diseases, including AD. Inflammation as able to accelerates the development type2 DM, through its influence on peripheral insulin sensitivity and pancreatic islet function; on the other hand, in addition to impaired insulin signaling, diabetes accelerated the appearance of cerebrovascular inflammation and Aβ deposition, as evidenced by increased levels of proinflammatory cytokines IL6 and TNFα, as well as dense amyloid deposits in blood vessels. [7, 114]. Cerebrovascular and central inflammation, along with increased accumulation of β amyloid, disrupts normal synaptic function, a starting point of AD progression. It was hypothesized the mutual interaction between AD and DM. Takaeda observed increased severity of diabetic phenotype in AD animal models. The reciprocal actions between AD and type-2 DM thus form a vicious cycle, further illustrating the possibility that AD and type-2 DM may share common cellular and molecular mechanisms [114] **(Figure 4).** Peripheral and central inflammation might affect pathogenesis of DM and AD. Elevated concentrations of interleukin (IL) 6 E_2-isoprostane have been observed in CFS of patients with AD [115]. Furthermore, in vitro and animal studies suggest that inflammation interacts with processing and deposit of Aβ [116]. Insulin exerts multiple effects involved in inflammation. In peripheral tissues insulin modulates many aspects of inflammatory network. Low doses of insulin exert anti-inflammatory effects [117]; however, during chronic hyperinsulinemia, insulin may exacerbate inflammatory responses and increase markers of oxidative stress [118]. In human, co administration of insulin and lipopolysaccharide produces a synergist increase in plasma concentrations of C-reactive protein and proinflammatory cytokines IL-1β, IL-6, TNFα [119]. TNFα has both neurotoxic and neuroprotective effects mediated respectively by two receptor subtypes, TNF-R1 and TNF-R2. TNF-R1 contains a death receptor domain, and has been implicated in pro-apoptotic events, whereas TNF-R2 promotes cell survival. Increased levels of TNF-R1 and decreased levels of TNF-R2 have been observed in AD brain [120]. Abnormal levels of soluble TNF-R1 and R2 have been documented in adults with diabetes and impaired glucose tolerance [121], which reportedly normalize after a 3-weeks low calorie diet [122]. Insulin may also modulate levels of eicosanoids such as F2-isoprostane via regulation of prostaglandin production in adypocites [123]. For example, elevated eicosanoid concentrations have been observed in hyperisulinemic Zucker rats [41]. Furthermore, excessive or chronic hyperinsulinemia inhibits degradation of protein damaged by oxidation and leads to formation of superoxide anions [124]. Insulin may also contribute to inflammation in the CNS, partially through effects on Aβ. In fact, $A\beta_{42}$ interacts with inflammatory agents in a cyclically reinforcing manner, such that Aβ elevations increase pro-inflammatory cytokines [125]. In vitro, soluble Aβ oligomers rapidly increase IL-1β and TNFα levels [126]. Conversely, IL-6 and IL-1β can regulate processing of the APP from which Aβ is derived and increase production of $A\beta_{42}$ [127]. The mutually reinforcing effects of Aβ, TNFα, IL-1β and IL-6 may thus create a "cytokine cycle" [125]. In the periphery, insulin reduces hepatic production of Apo E and regulates its uptake by low-density lipoprotein receptor-related protein [128]. Fishel et al. showed that insulin reduced plasma Apo E levels, an effect that increased with age. In contrast, insulin increased CSF Apo E concentrations for older subjects [129]. Increased brain APO E levels have been reported in AD in association with polymorphisms in the promoter region of the APO E gene that influence protein expression [130]. Recent studies showed that insulin-induced elevations of CSF APO E levels were associated with attenuated increase IL6 and TNFα levels and with higher anti-inflammatory cytokine, IL-1α concentration. This pattern suggests multiple insulin effects that modulate the role of APO E in response to inflammation in CNS [129] .Insulin can regulate CNS norepinephrine [131], an endogenous anti-inflammatory neuromodulator that blocks IL-1β expression [132]. Increased Aβ plaque load in AD has been linked to neuronal loss in the locus coeruleus, the primary source of brain norepinephrine [133]. In human, raising plasma insulin levels while maintain euglycemia increases CSF norepinephine levels [134].Thus, these findings support the notion that insulin action is involved in neutrasmitter modulation and insulin abnormalities might contribute to CNS inflammation.

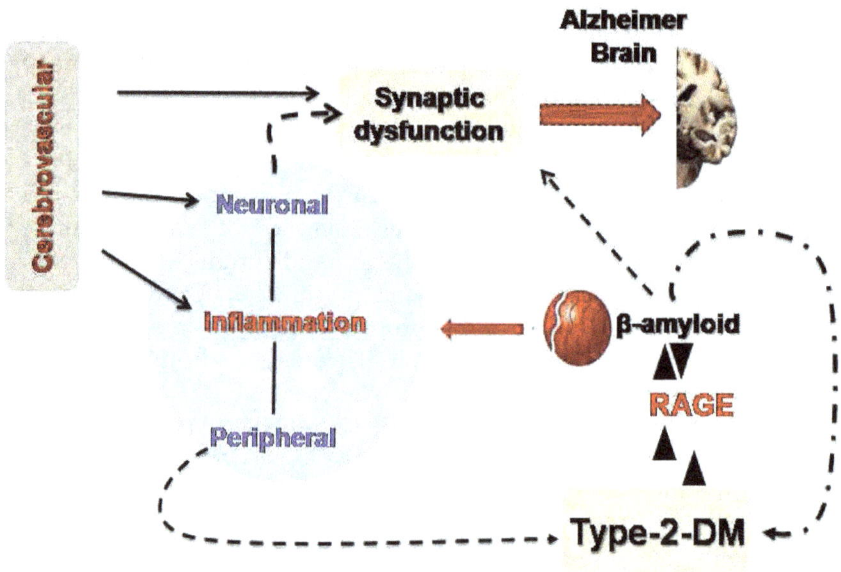

Fig. 4. The underlying link between Alzheimer's disease (AD) and type-2 Diabetes Mellitus (DM).
Inflammation influences islet function and peripheral insulin sensitivity. Besides, inflammation accelerates the development of type-2 DM. Cerebrovascular and central inflammation, along with increased accumulation of β-amyloid, disrupts normal synaptic function, a starting point of AD pathological progression.

6. Conclusion

Mild to moderate impairments of cognitive functioning has been reported both in patients with DM-type1 and in patients with DM-type2. The potential impact of DM on cognitive functions in the elderly is further emphasized by several large epidemiological surveys that report an increased incidence of dementia among DM patients. Several mechanisms may be involved in accelerated cognitive decline in patients with DM. Insulin may affect the metabolism of Aβ and tau, two proteins that represent the building blocks of amyloid plaques and neurofibrillary tangles, the neuropathological hallmarks of AD. Moreover, insulin and its receptor are widely distributed throughout the brain, with particular abundance in defined areas, such as the hypothalamus and the hippocampus. In addition, insulin appears to act as "neuromodulator", that influences the release and reuptake of neurotransmitters, and improves learning and memory. These findings could provide insights to develop a strategy for prevention and treatment of AD. Insulin therapy plays an important role in cognitive processes and could slow dementia in patients with AD and DM. This could be explained by: 1.*molecular mechanisms*, insulin promotes cell membrane expression of NMDA receptors, which increases neuronal Ca2+ influx [56], that activates Ca^{2+}-dependent enzymes, including α-dependent enzymes and strengthens neuronal synaptic association [10]; 2. *glucose metabolism,* low concentrations of exogenous insulin may increase cerebral glucose metabolism and then modulate brain functions such as memory [135]. In fact, insulin has shown a significant effect on global brain glucose metabolism and this effect is mainly expressed in the cerebral cortex; 3. *neurotransmitter modulation,* low doses of insulin can reverse the amnestic effects of cholinergic blockade [136]. Although the concepts of "Cerebral Insulin Resistance" and "insulin-induced amyloid pathology" are an attractive explanation for some of the effects of DM2 on the brain, there are still many loose ends. It is important to point out that definitive conclusions about the value of insulinic treatment in course of AD cannot be established at this time.

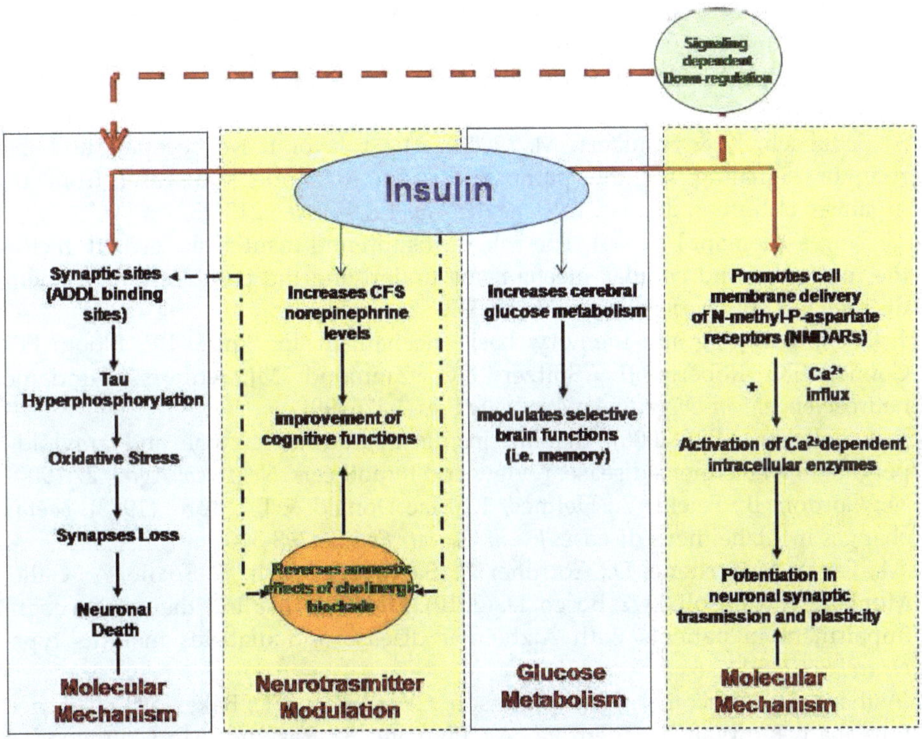

Fig. 5. Schematic representation of molecular mechanism, glucose metabolism and neurotransmitter modulation

Insulin promotes cell membrane expression of NMDA receptors, which increases neuronal Ca^{2-} influx, that activates Ca^{2-} dependent enzymes and strengthens neuronal synaptic association. Besides, diffusible ligands (ADDL) binding to particular synaptic sites and the resulting oxidative stress and synapse loss are markedly decreased by the presence of insulin. This mechanism is associated with a signal dependent down regulation of ADDL binding sites. Low peripheric insulin level may increase cerebral glucose and modulate cognitive functions. Besides, low levels of insulin contributes reverse the anamnestic effects of cholinergic blockade.

7. References

Citron, M. (2002). Alzheimer's disease: treatment in discovery and development. *Nat Neurosci.* 5:1055-7.

Peila, R.; Rodriguez, BL. & Lauren, LJ. (2002). Type-2 diabetes, diabetes, Apo E gene and the risk for dementia and related pathogenesis: the Honolulu-Asia Aging Study. *Diabetes.* 51:1256-62.

Ott, A.; Stolk, RP.; Hofman, A.; Van Harskamp, F.; Pols, HA. & Breteler MM. (1996). Diabetes mellitus and risk of dementia: the Rotterdarm Study. *Neurology* 53(9);1907-9.

Luchsinger, JA.; Tang, MX.; Shea, S. & Mayeux, R. (2004). Hyperinsulinemia and risk of Alzheimer's disease. *Neurology* 63:1187-92.

Janson, J.; Laedtke, T.; Parisi, JE.; O Brien, P.; Petersen, RC. & Butler, PC. (2004). Increased risk of type 2 diabetes in Alzheimer disease. *Diabetes* 53:474-81.

Whitmer, RA.; Sidney, S.; Selby, J.; Johnston, SC. & Yaffe, K. (2005) Midlife cardiovascular risk factors and risk of dementia in late life. *Neurology* 64:277-81

Han, W. & Li, C. (2010) Linking type 2 diabetes and Alzheimer's disease. *Proc Natl Acad Sci USA.* 107:6557-8.

Freude, S.; Schilbach, K & Schubert, M. (2009). The role of IGF-1 receptor and insulin receptor signaling for the pathogenesis of Alzheimer's disease: from model organism to human disease. *Current Alzheimer Research* 6:213-23.

Carro, E. & Torres-Aleman, I. (2004). The role of insulin and insulin-like growth factor I in the molecular and cellular mechanisms underlying the pathology of Alzheimer's disease. *Eur J of Pharmacology* 490:127-33.

Byme, JH. (2003). Learning and memory: basic mechanism. In: Squire LR, Bloom FE, Mc Connel SK, Roberts JL, Spitzer NC, Zigmond MJ, editors. Fundamental neuroscience. *San Diego (CA): Academic Press* 1276–98.

Qiu, WQ. & Folstein, MF. (2006). Insulin, insulin-degrading enzyme and amyloid-beta peptide in Alzheimer's disease: review and hypothesis. *Neurobiol Aging* 27:190-8.

Fisman, M.; Gordon, B.; Feleki, V.; Helmes, T.; Mac Donald & J, Dupre. (1988). Metabolic changes in Alzheimer's disease. *J. Am. Geriatr Soc.* 36:298-300.

Plastino, M.; Fava, A.; Pirritano, D.; Cotronei, P.; Sacco, N.; Sperlì, T.; Spanò, A.; Gallo, D.; Mungari, P.; Consoli, D &, Bosco, D. (2010). Effects of insulinic therapy on cognitive impairment in patients with Alzheimer disease and diabetes mellitus type-2. *J Neurol Sci* 288:112-6.

Craft, S.; Asthana, S.; Newcomer, JW.; Wilkinson, CW.; Matos, IT.; Baker, LD.; Cherrier, K.; Purganan, K.; Wait, C.; Petrova, A.; Plymate, S.; Raskind, M.; Grimwood, K & Veith, RC. (1999). Enhancement of Alzheimer disease with insulin and somatostatin, but not glucose. Arch Gen Psychiatry 56:1135-40.

Craft, S.; Asthana, S.; Cook, DG.; Baker, LD.; Cherrier, K.; Purgan, K.; Wait, C.; Petrova, A.; Latendresse, S.; Watson, GS.; Newcomer, JW.; Schelleenberg, GD & Kreohn, AJ. (2003). Insulin dose-response effects on memory and plasma amyloid precursor protein in Alzheimer's disease: interaction's with Apolipoprotein E genotype. *Psychoneuroendocrinology* 28:809-22.

Den Heijer, T.; Vermeer, SE.; Van Dijk, EJ.; Prins, ND.; Koudstaal, PJ.; Hofman, A & Breteler, MM. (2003). Type 2 diabetes and atrophy of medial temporal lobe structures on brain MRI, *Diabetologia* 46:1604-10.

Craft, S.; Ashana, G.; Schellenberg, G.; Baker, L.; Cherrier, M.; Boyt, AA.; Martins, RN.; Rakind, M.; Peskind, E. & Plymate, S. (2000). Insulin effects on glucose metabolism, memory and plasma amyloid precursor protein in Alzheimer's disease differ according to apolipoprotein-E-genotype. *Ann NY Acad Sci* 903:222-8.

Messier, C. (2003). Diabetes, Alzheimer's disease and apolipoprotein genotype. *Exp Gerontol.* 38:941-6.

Woods, SC.; Seeley, RJ.; Baskin, DG. & Schwartz, MW. (2003). Insulin and the blood brain barrier. *Curr Pharm Des.* 9:795-800.

Banks, WA. (2004). The source of cerebral insulin. *Eur J Pharmacol.* 490:5-12.

Schechter, R.; Whitmire, J.; Wheet, GS.; Beju, D.; Jackson, KW.; Harlow, R. & Gavin, JR. (1994). Immunohistochemical and in situ hybridization study of an insulin-like substance in fetal neuron cell cultures. Brain Res. 636:9-27.

Devaskar, SU.; Giddings, SJ.; Rajakumar, PA.; Carnaghi, LR.; Menon, RK. & Zahm, DS. (1994). Insulin gene expression and insulin synthesis in mammalian neuronal cells. *J Biol Chem.* 269:8445-54.

Havrankova, J.; Schmechel, D.; Roth, J. & Brownstein, M. (1978). Identification of insulin in rat brain. *Proc Natl Acad Sci USA.* 75:5737-41.

Unger, JW.; Livingston, JN. & Moss, AM. (1991). Insulin receptors in the central nervous system: localization, signaling mechanisms and functional aspects. *Prog Neurobiol.* 36:343-62.

Baskin, DG.; Porte, DJ.; Guest, K. & Dorsa, DM. (1983). Regional concentrations of insulin in the rat brain. *Endocrinology.* 112:898-903.

Johnston, AM.; Pirola, L. & Van Obberghen, E. (2003). Molecular mechanisms of insulin receptor substrate protein-mediated modulation of insulin signaling. *FEBS Lett.* 546:32-6.

Kahn, CR.; Bird, KI.; Jarrett, DB. & Flier, JS. (1978). Direct demonstration that receptor cross-linking or aggregation is important in insulin action. *Proc Natl Acad Sci USA.* 75:4209-13.

Sun, XJ.; Rothenberg, P.; Kahn, CR.; Backer, JM.; Araki, E.; Wilden, PA.; Cahill, DA. Goldstein, BJ & White, MF. (1978). Structure of insulin receptor substrate IRS-1 defines a unique signal transduction protein. *Nature* 352:73-7.

Giovannone, B.; Scaldaferri, ML.; Federici, M.; Porzio, O.; Lauro, D.; Fusco, A.; Sbraccia, P.; Borboni, P.; Lauro, R. & Sesti, G. (2000). Insulin receptor substrate (IRS) transduction system: distinct and overlapping signaling potential. *Diabetes Metab Res Rev* 16:434-41

Messier, C. & Teutenberg, K. (2005). The role of insulin, insulin growth factor, and insulin-degrading enzyme in brain aging and Alzheimer's disease. *Neural Plast.* 12:311-28.

Banks, WA.; Jaspan, JB.; Huang, W. & Kastin, AJ. (1997). Transport of insulin across the blood-brain barrier to insulin: saturability at euglycemic doses of insulin. *Peptides.* 1997; 18: 1423-9.

Tchilian, EZ.; Zhelezarov, IE.; Patkov, VV. & Hadjiivanova, CI. (1990). 125I-insulin binding is decreased in olfactory bulbs of aged rats. *Neuropeptides.* 17:193-6.

Adem, A.; Jossan, SS.; D'Argy, R.; Gillberg, PG.; Nordberg, A.; Winblan, B. & Sara, V. (1989). Insulin-like growth factor 1 IGF-1 receptors in the human brain: quantitative autoradiographic localization. *Brain Res.* 503:299-303.

Chung, YH.; Shin, GM.; Joo, KM & Cha, CI. (2002). Region specific alterations in insulin-like growth factor receptor type I in the cerebral cortex and hippocampus of aged rats. *Brain Res* 946:307-13.

Frolic, L.; Blum-Degen, D.; Berstein, HG.; Engelsberger, S.; Humrich, J.; Laufer, S.; Muschner, D.; Thalheimer, A.; Türk, A.; Hoyer, S.; Zöchling, R.; Boissl, KW.; Jellinger, K & Riederer, P. (1998). Brain insulin and insulin receptors in aging and sporadic Alzheimer s disease. *J Neural Transm* 105:423-38.

Banks, WA. & Kastin, AJ. (1985). Peptides and the blood-brain barrier: lipophilicity as a predictor of permeability. *Brain Res Bull.* 15:287-92.

King, GL. & Johnson, SM. (1987). Receptor-mediated transport of insulin across endothelial cells. *Science.* 227:1583-6.

Jialal, I.; King, GL.; Buchwald.; S, Kahn, CR. & Crettaz, M. (1984). Processing of insulin by bovine endothelial cells in culture. Internalization without degradation. *Diabetes.* 33:794-800.

Rotwein, P.; Burgess, SK.; Milbrandt, JD. & Krause, JE. (1988). Differential expression of insulin-like growth factor geneses in rat central nervous system. *Proc Natl Acad Sci USA.* 85:265-9.

Zhao, M.; Cribbs, DH.; Anderson, AJ.; Cummings, BJ.; Su, JH.; Wasserman, AT. & Cotman, CW. (2003). The induction of the TNF alpha death domain signaling pathway in Alzheimer's disease brain. *Neurochem Res* 28:307-18.

Baskin, DG.; Stein, LJ.; Iked, H.; Woods, SC.; Porte, DJ & Dorsa, DM. (2005). Genetically obese Zucker rats have abnormality low brain insulin content. *Life Sci* 36:627-33

Moloney, AM.; Griffin, RJ.; Timmons, S.; O'Connor, R.; Ravid, R. & O'Neill, C. (2010). Defects in IGF-1 receptor, insulin receptor and IRS-1/2 in Alzheimer's disease indicate possible resistance to IGF-1 and insulin signaling. *Neurobiol Aging* 31(2):224-43.

Messier, C & White, NM. (1987). Memory improvement by glucose, fruttose, and two glucose analogs: a possible effect peripheral glucose transport. *Behav Neural Biol* 48:104-27.

Craft, S. (2007). Insulin resistance and Alzheimer's disease. Pathogenesis: potential mechanisms and implications for treatment. *Curr Alzheimer Res.* 4(2):147-52.

Squire, LR. (1986). Mechanisms of memory. *Science.* 232:1612-9.

Svensson, J.; Diez, M.; Engel, J.; Wass, C.; Tivesten, A.; Jansson, JO.; Isaksson, O.; Archer, T.; Hökfelt, T & Ohlsson, C. (2006). Endocrine, liver-derived IGF-1 is of importance for spatial learning and memory in old mice. *J. Endocrinol* 189:617-27.

Dik, MG.; Pluijm, SM.; Jonker, C.; Deeg, DJ.; Lomrcky, MZ & Lips, P. (2003). Insulin-like growth factor-1 (IGF-1) and cognitive decline in older persons. *Neurobiol Aging* 24:573-81.

Hoyer, S. (2000). Brain glucose and energy metabolism abnormalities in sporadic Alzheimer's disease. Causes and consequences: an update. *Exp Gerontol.* 35:1363-72.

Blass, JP.; Gibson, GF. & Hoyer, S. (2002). The role of the metabolic lesion in Alzheimer's disease. *J Alzheimer Dis.* 4:225-32. .

Beeri, MS.; Schmeidler, J.; Silverman, JM.; Gandy, S.; Wysocki, M.; Hannigan, CM.; Purohit, DP.; Lesser, G.; Grossman, HT & Haroutunian, V. (2008). Insulin in combination with other diabetes medication is associated with less Alzheimer neuropathology. *Neurology* 71:750-7.

Craft, S.; Peskind, E.; Schellenberg, G.; Cherrier, M.; Baker, LD.; Newcomer, J.; Plymate, S.; Latendresse, S.; Petrova, A.; Raskind, M.; Peskind, E.; Lofgreen, C. & Grimwood, K. (1999). Cerebrospinal fluid and plasma insulin levels in Alzheimer's disease differs according to apolipoprotein E genotype and gender. *Neuroendocrinology.* 70:146-52.

Adamo, M.; Raizada, MK. & LeRoith, D. (1989). Insulin and insulin growth factors receptors in the nervous system. *Mol Neurobiol.* 3:71-100.

Squire, LR. (1992). Memory and the hippocampus: a synthesis of findings with rats, monkeys, and humans. *Psychol Rev.* 99:195-231.

Hoyer, S.; Henneberg, N.; Knapp, S.; Lannert, H. & Martin, E. (1996). Brain glucose metabolism is controlled by amplification and desensitization of the neuronal insulin receptor. *Ann NY Acad Sci.* 777:374-9.

Messier, C. & Destrade, C. (1994). Insulin attenuates scopolamine-induced memory deficits. *Psychobiology.* 22:16-21.

Skeberdis, VA.; Lan, J.; Zheng, X.; Zukin, RS. & Bennett, MV (2001). Insulin promotes rapid delivery of N-methyl-D-aspartate receptors to the cell surface by exocytosis. *Proc Natl Acad Sci USA.* 98:3561–6.

De Felice, FG.; Vieira, MN.; Bomfirm, TR.; Decker, H.; Velasco, PT.; Lambert, MP.; Viola, KL.; Zhao, WQ.; Ferreira, ST. & Klein WL. (2009). Protection of synapses against Alzheimer's linked toxins: insulin signaling prevents the pathogenic binding of A-beta oligomers. *Proc Natl Acad Sci.* USA 106:1971-6.

De la Monte, SM.; Tong, M.; Lester-Coll, N.; Plater M, Jr.; & Wands, JR. (2006). Therapeutic rescue of neurodegeneration experimental type-3 diabetes: relevance to Alzheimer's disease. *J Alzheimers Dis.* 10:89-109.

Hirai, K.; Aliev, G.; Nunomura, A.; Fujioka, H.; Russell, RL.; Atwood, CS.; Johnson, AB.; Kress, Y.; Vinters, HV.; Tabaton, M.; Shimohama, S.; Cash, AD.; Siedlak, SL.; Harris, PL.; Jones, PK.; Petersen, RB.; Perry, G & Smith, MA. (2001). Mitochondrial abnormalities in Alzheimer's disease. *J Neurosci* 21:3017-23.

Gouras, GK.; Almeida, CG. & Takahashi, RH. (2005). Intraneuronal Abeta accumulation and origin of plaques in Alzheimer's disease. *Neurobiol Aging.* 26:1235-44.

Caspersen, C.; Wang, N.; Yao, J.; Sosunov, A.; Chen, X.; Lustbader, JW.; Xu, HW.; Stern, D.; McKhann, G & Yan, SD. (2005). Mitochondrial Abeta: a potential focal point for neuronal metabolic dysfunction in Alzheimer's disease. *FASEB J.* 19:2040-1.

Smith, MA.; Perry, G.; Richey, PL.; Sayre, LM.; Anderson, VE.; Beal, MF. & Kowall, N. (1996). Oxidative damage in Alzheimer's disease. *Nature* 382: 120-1.

Smith, MA.; Richey Harris, PL.; Sayre, LM.; Beckman, JS. & Perry, G. (1997). Widespread peroxynitrite-mediated damage Alzheimer's disease. *J Neurosci.* 17:2653-7.

Mark, RJ.; Pang, Z.; Geddes, JW.; Uchida, K. & Mattson, MP. (1997). Amyloid-beta peptide impairs glucose transport in hippocampal and cortical neurons: involvement lipid peroxidation. *J Neurosci* 17:1046-54.

Nunomura, A., Perry, G.; Aliev, G.; Hirai, K.; Takeda, A.; Balraj, EK.; Jones, PK.; Ghanbari, H.; Wataya, T.; Shimohama.; S.; Chiba, S.; Atwood, CS.; Petersen, RB. & Smith, MA. (2001). Oxidative damage is the earliest event in Alzheimer's disease. *J Neuropahol Exp Neurol* 60:759-67.

Cho, DH.; Nakamura, T.; Fang, J.; Cieplak, P.; Godzik, A.; Gu, Z. & Lipton, SA. (2009). S-nitrosylation of Drp 1 mediates beta-amyloid-related mithocondrial fissation and neuronal injury. *Science.* 324:102-5.

Yan, SD.; Chen, M.; Zhu, H.; Roher, A.; Slattery, T.; Zhao, L.; Nagashima, M.; Morser, J.; Migheli, A. Nawroth P, Stern, D. & Schmidt, AM. (1996). RAGE and amyloid-beta peptide neurotoxicity in Alzheimer's disease. *Nature* 382:685-91.

Lue, LF.; Walker, DG.; Jacobson, S. & Sabbagh, M. (2009). Receptor for advanced glycation end products: its role in Alzheimer's disease and other neurological diseases. *Future Neurol.* 4:167–77.

Cho, HJ.; Son, SM.; Jin, SM.; Hong, HS.; Shin, DH.; Kim, SJ.; Huh, K. & Mook-Jung, I. (2009). RAGE regulates BACE1 and A-beta generation via NFAT1 activation in Alzheimer's disease animal model. *FASEB J* 23:2639–49.

Martin, SJ.; Grimwood, PD. & Morris, RG. (2000). Synaptic plasticity and memory: an evaluation of the hypothesis. *Annu Rev Neurosci.* 23:649-711.

Ding, Q. & Keller, JN. (2005). Splice variants of the receptor for advanced glycosylation end products (RAGE) in human brain. *Neurosci Lett.* 373:67–72.

Raucci, A.; Cugusi, S.; Antonelli, A.; Barabino, SM.; Monti, L.; Bierhaus, A.; Reiss, K.; Saftig, P. & Bianchi, ME. (2008). A soluble form of the receptor for advanced glycation endproducts (RAGE) is produced by proteolytic cleavage of the membrane-bound form by the sheddase a disintegrin and metalloprotease 10 (ADAM10). *FASEB J.* 22:3716–27.

Lue, LF.; Walker, DG.; Brachova, L.; , Beach, TG.; Rogers, J.; Schmidt, AM.; Stern, DM. & Yan, SD. (2001). Involvement of microglial receptor for advanced glycation endproducts (RAGE) in Alzheimer's disease: identification of a cellular activation mechanism. *Exp Neurol.* 171:29–45.

Deane, R.; Du Yan, S.; Submamaryan, RK.; LaRue, B.; Jovanovic, S.; Hogg, E.; Welch, D.; Manness, L.; Lin, C.; Yu, J.; Zhu, H.; Ghiso, J.; Frangione, B.; Stern, A.; Schmidt, AM.; Armstrong, DL.; Arnold, B.; Liliensiek, B.; Nawroth, P.; Hofman, F.; Kindy, M.; Stern, D. & Zlokovic, B..(2003). RAGE mediates amyloid-beta peptide transport across the blood-brain barrier and accumulation in brain. *Nat Med.* 9:907–13.

Emanuele, E.; D'angelo, A.; Tomaino, C.; Binetti, G.; Ghidoni, R.; Politi, P.; Bernardi, L.; Maletta, R.; Bruni, AC. & Geroldi, D. (2005). Circulating levels of soluble receptor for advanced glycation end products in Alzheimer disease and vascular dementia. *Arch Neurol.* 62: 1734–6.

Lee, VM.; Goedert, M. & Trojanowski, JQ. (2001). Neurodegenerative tauopathies. *Ann Rev Neurosci.* 24:1121-59.

Iqbal, K.; Alonso Adel, C.; Chen, S.; Chohan, MO.; El-Akkad, E.; Gong, CX.; Khatoon, S.; Li, B.; Liu, F.; Rahman, A.; Tanimukai, H. & Grundke-Iqbal, I. (2005).Tau pathology in Alzheimer's disease and other tauopathies. *Biochim Biophys Acta* 1793:198-210.

Delacourte, A.; Sergeant, N.; Champain, D.; Wattez, A.; Maurage, CA.; Lebert, F.; Pasquier, F. & David, JP. (2002). Nonoverlapping but synergetic tau and APP pathologies in sporadic Alzheimer's disease. *Neurology* 59:398-407.

Glenner, GG. & Wong, CW. (1984). Alzheimer disease: initial report of the purification and characterization of a novel cerebrovascular amyloid protein. *Biochem Biophys Res Commun* 120:885-90.

Flaherty, DB.; Soria, JP.; Tomasiewicz, HZ. & Wood, JG. (2000). Phosphorylation of human tau protein by microtubule associated kinases: GSK3β and cdk5 are key partecipants. *J Neurosci Res* 62:463-72.

Stoothoff, WH. & Johnson, GV. (2005). Tau phosphorylation: physiological and pathological consequences. *Biochim Biophys Acta* 1739:280-97.

Millward, TA.; Zolnierowicz, S. & Hemmings, BA. (1999). Regulation of protein kinase cascades by protein phosphatase 2A. *Trends Biochem Sci.* 24:186-91.

Doble, BW. & Woodgett, JR. (2003). GSK-3β: tricks of the trade for a multi-tasking kinase. *J Cell Sci* 116:1175-86.

Avila J. (2008). Tau kinases, phosphatases. *J Cell Mol Med.* 12:258-9.

Liu, R.; Zhou, XW.; Tanila, H.; Bjorkdahl, C., Wang, JZ.; Guan, ZZ.; Cao, Y.; Gustafsson, JA.; Winblad, B. & Pei, JJ. (2008). Phosphorylated PP2A (tyrosine 307) is associated with Alzheimer neurofibrillary pathology. *J Cell Mol Med* 12:241-57.

Hong, M. & Leev, VM. (1997). Insulin and insulin-like growth factor-1 regulate tau phosphorylation in cultured human neurons. *J. Biol. Chem* 272:19547-53.

Meske, V.; Albert, F. & Ohm, TG. (2008). Coupling of mammalian target of rapamyein with phosphoinositide 3-kinase signaling pathway regulates protein phospatase 2A and glycogen synthase kinase-3-dependent phosphorylation of tau. *J. Biol Chem* 283:100-9.

Cheng, CM.; Tseng, V.; Wang, J.; Wang, D.; Matyakhina, L. & Bondy, CA. (2005). Tau is hyperphosporylated in the insulin-like growth factor-I null brain. *Endocrinology* 146:5086-91.

Schubert, M.; Brazil, DP.; Burks, DJ.; Kushner, JA.; Ye, J.; Flint, CL.; Farhang-Fallah, J.; Dikkes, P.; Warot, XM.; Rio, C.; Corfas, G. & White, MF. (2003). Insulin receptor substrate-2 deficiency impairs brain growth and promotes tau phosporylation. *J Neurosc.* 23:7084-92.

Planel, E.; Tatebayashi, Y.; Miyasaka, T.; Liu, L.; Wang, L.; Herman, M.; Yu, WH.; Luchsinger, JA.; Wadzinski, B.; Duff, KE. & Takashima, A. (1997).Insulin dysfunction induces in vivo tau after hyperphosphorylation through distinct mechanisms. *J Neurosci* 27:13635-48.

Kolch, W. (2000). Meaningful relationships: the regulation of the RAS/RAF/MEK/ERK pathway by protein interactions. *Biochem J* 351: 289-305.

Sweatt, JD. (2001). The neuronal MAP kinase cascade: a biochemical signal integration system subserving synaptic plasticity and memory. *J Neurochem* 76:1-10

Zhuang, S. & Schnellmann, RG. (2006). A death-promoting role for extracellular signal-regulated kinase. *J Pharmacol Exp Ther* 319:991-7.

Lesort, M & Johnson, GV. (2000). Insulin-like growth factor-1 and insulin mediate transient site-selective increases in tau phosphorylation in primary cortical neurons. *Neuroscience.* 99:305–16.

Kang, J.; Lemaire, HG.; Unterbeck, A.; Salbaum, JM.; Masters, CL.; Grzeschik, KH.; Multhaup, G.; Beyreuther, K. & Müller-Hill, B. (1987). The precursor of Alzheimer-s disease amyloid A_4 protein resembles a cell-surface receptor. *Nature* 325:733-6.

Zhang, Y.; Thompson, R.; Zhang, H. & Xu, U. (2011). APP processing in Alzheimer's disease. *Mol Brain.* 4: 3.

Kimberly, WT.; LaVoie, MJ.; Ostaszewski, BL; Ye, W.; Wolfe, MS. & Selkoe DJ. (2003). Gamma-secretase is a membrane protein complex comprised of presenilin, nicastrin, Aph-1 and Pen-2. *Proc Natl Acad Sci* USA. 100: 6382-7.

Vassar, R.; Bennett, BD.; Babu-Kahn, S.; Kahn, S.; Mendiaz, EA.; Denis, P.; Teplow, DB.; Ross, S.; Amarante, P.; Loeloff, R.; Luo, Y.; Fisher, S.; Fuller, J.; Edenson, S.; Lile, J.; Jarosinski, MA.; Biere, AL.; Curran, E.; Burgess, T.; Louis, JC.; Collins, F.; Treanor, J.; Rogers, G. & Citron, M. (1999). Beta-secretase cleavage of Alzheimer's amyloid precursor protein by the transmembrane aspartic protease BACE. *Science.* 286:735-41.

Holsinger, RM.; McLean, CA.; Beyreuther, K.; Masters, CL, & Evin, G (2002). Increased expression of the amyloid precursor beta-secretase in Alzheimer's disease. *Ann Neurol.* 51:783-6.

Costantini, C.; Scrable, H. & Puglielli, L. (2006). An aging pathway controls the TrkA to p75NTR receptor switch and amyloid beta-peptide generation. *EMBO J* 25:1997-2006.

Puglielli, L. (2008). Aging of the brain, neurotrophic signaling, and Alzheimer's disease: is IGF-1R the common culprit? *Neurobiol Aging.* 29:795-811.

Puglielli, L.; Ellis, BC.; Saunders, AJ. & Kovacs, DM. (2003). Ceramide stabilizes beta-size amyloid precursor protein-cleaving enzyme I and promotes amyloid beta-peptide biogenesic. *J Biol Chem.* 278:19777-83.

Kayed, RH.; Thompson. JL.; MC Intire, TM.; Milton, SC.; Cotman, CW. & Glabe, CG. (2003). Common structure of soluble amyloid oligomers implies common mechanism of pathogenesis. *Science* 300:486-9.

Hass, C. & Sedkoe, DJ. (2007). Soluble protein oligomers in neuro-degeneration: lessons from the Alzheimer's amyloid beta-peptide. *Nat Rev Mol Cell Bio.* 8:101-2.

Kamenetz, F.; Tomita, T.; Hsieh, H.; Seabrook, G.; Borchelt, D.; Iwatsubo, T.; Sisodia, S. & Malinow, R. (2003). APP Processing and synaptic function. *Neuron.* 37:925-37.

Tanzi, RE.; Moir, RD. & Wagner, SL. (2005). Twenty years of the Alzheimer disease amyloid hypothesis: a genetic perspective. *Cell.* 120:545-55.

Selkoe, DJ. (1999). Translating cell biology in to therapeutic advances in Alzheimer's disease. *Nature.* 399:23-31.

Cheng, S.; Li, L.; He, S.; Liu, J.; Sun, Y.; He, M.; Grasing, K.; Premont, RT. & Suo, WZ. (2010). GRK5 deficiency accelerates ß-amyloid accumulation in Tg2576 mice via impaired cholinergic activity. J Biol Chem. 285:41541-8.

Carro, E.; Trejo, JL.; Spuch, C.; Heard, JM. & Torres-Aleman, I. (2006). Blockade of the insulin-like growth factor I receptor in the choroid plexus originates Alzheimer's like neuropathology in rodents; new cues into the human disease? *Neurobiol Aging* 27:1618-31.

Suh, Y.; Atzomon, G.; Cho, Mo.; Hwang, D.; Liu, B.; Leahy, DJ.; Barzilai, N. & Cohen, P. (2008). Functionally significant insulin-like growth factor I receptor mutations in centenarians. Proc Natl Acad Sci USA. 105:3438-42.

Ho, L.; Qin, W.; Pompl, PN.; Xiang, Z; Wang, J.; Zhao, Z.; Peng, Y.; Cambareri, G.; Rocher, A.; Mobbs, CV.; Hof, PR. & Pasinetti, GM. (2004). Diet-induced insulin resistance promotes amyloidosis in a transgenic mouse model of Alzheimer's disease. *FASEB J* 18:902-4.

Cao, D.; Lu, H.; Lewis, TI. & Li, L. (2007). Intake of sucrose-sweetened water induced insulin resistance and exacerbates memory deficits and amyloidosis in a transgenic mouse model of Alzheimer disease. J Biol Chem. 282:36275-82.

Freude, S.; Plum, L.; Schnitker, J.; Leeser, U.; Udelhoven, M.; Krone, W.; Bruning, JC. & Schubert, M. (2005). Peripheral hyperinsulinemia promotes tau phosphorylation in vivo. *Diabetes* 54:3343-8.

Takeda, S.; Sato, N.; Uchio-Yamada, K.; Sawada, K.; Kunieda, T.; Takeuchi, D.; Kurinami, H.; Shinohara, M.; Rakugi, H. & Morishita, R. (2010). Diabetes accelerated memory dysfunction via cerebrovascular inflammation Aβ deposition in Alzheimer mouse model with diabetes. Proc Natl Acad Sci USA 107:7036-41

Montine, TJ.; Kaye, JA.; Montine, KS.; McFarland, L.; Morrow, JD. & Quinn, JF. (2001). Cerebrospinal fluid abeta-42, tau, and f2-isoprostane concentrations in patients with Alzheimer disease, other dementias, and age-matched controls. *Arch Pathol Lab Med* 125:510-2.

Sheng, JG.; Bora, SH.; Xu, G.; Borchelt, DR.; Price, DL. & Koliatsos, VE. (2003). Lipopolysaccharide-induced-neuroinflammation increase intracellular accumulation of amyloid precursor protein and amyloid beta peptide in APPswe transgenic mice. *Neurobiol Dis* 14:133-45.

Dandona, P. (2002). Endothelium, inflammation and diabetes *Curr Diab Rep.* 2:311-5.

Krogh-Madsen, R.; Plomgaard, P.; Keller, P.; Keller, C. & Pedersen BK. (2004). Insulin stimulates interlukin-6 and tumor necrosis factor-alpha gene expression in human subcutaneous adipose tissue. *Am J Physiol Endocrinol Metab* 286:234-8.

Soop, M.; Duxubury, H.; Agwunobi, AO.; Gibson, JM.; Hopkins, SJ.; Childs, C.; Cooper, RG.; Maycock, P.; Little, RA. & Carlson, GL. (2002). Euglycemic hyperinsulinemia augments the cytokine and endocrine responses in endotoxin in humans. *Am J Physiol Endocrinol Metab* 282:1276-85.

Zhao, M.; Cribbs, DH.; Anderson, AJ.; Cummings, BJ.; Su, JH.; Wasserman, AT. & Cotman, CW. (2003). The induction of the TNF alpha death domain signaling pathway in Alzheimer's disease brain. *Neurochem Res* 28:307-18.

Dzienis-Straczkowski, M.; Szelachowska, M.; Stepien, A.; Kowalska, I. & Kinalska, I. (2003). Soluble tumor necrosis factor-alpha receptors in young obese subjects with normal and impaired glucose tolerance. *Diabetes Care* 26:875-80.

Bastard, JP.; Jardel, C.; Bruckert, E.; Vidal, H. & Hainque, B. (2000). Variations in plasma soluble tumor necrosis factor receptors after diet-induced weight loss in obesity. *Diabetes Obes Metab* 2:323-5.

Axelrod, L. (1991). Insulin, prostaglandins, and the pathogenesis of hypertension. *Diabetes.* 40:1223-7.

Facchini, FS.; Hua, NW.; Reaven, GM. & Stoohs, RA. (2000). Hyperinsulinemia: the missing link among oxidative stress and age-related disease? *Free Radic Biol Med* 29:1302-6.

Mrak, RE. & Griffin, WS. (2001). Interleukin-1, neuroinflammation, and Alzheimer's disease. *Neurobiol Aging.* 22:903-8.

White, JA.; Manelli, AM.; Holmberg, KH.; Van Eldik, LJ. & Ladu, MJ. (2005). Differential effects of oligomeric and fibrillar amyloid-beta 1-42 on astrocyte mediated inflammation. *Neurobiol Dis* 18:459-65.

Papassotiropoulos, A.; Hock, C. & Nitsch, RM. (2001). Genetics of interleukin 6: implications for Alzheimer's disease. *Neurobiol Aging.* 22:863-71.

Descamps, O.; Bilheimer, D. & Herz, J. (1993). Insulin stimulates receptor-mediated uptake of Apo E-enriched lipoproteins and activated alpha 2-macroglobulin in adypocytes. *J Biol Chem.* 268:974-81.

Fishel, MA,.; Watson, GS.; Montine, TJ.; Wang, Q.; Green, PS. & Kulstad, JJ. (2005). Hyperinsulinemia provokes synchronous increases in central inflammation and beta-amyloid in normal adults. *Arch Neurol* 62:1539-44.

Yamada, T.; Kondo, A.; Takamatsu, J.; Tateishi, J. & Goto I (1995). Apolipoprotein E mRNA in the brains of patients with Alzheimer's disease. *J Neurol Sci.* 129:56-61.

Figlewicz, DP.; Bentson, K. & Octrant I. (1993). The effect of insulin on norepinephrine uptake by PC12 cells. *Brain Res* 602:161-4.

Heneka, MT.; Galea, E.; Gavriluyk, V.; Dumitrescu-Ozimek, L.; Daeschner, J.; O'Banion, MK.; Weinberg, G.; Klockgether, T. & Feinstein, DL. (2002). Noradrenergic depletion potentiates beta-amyloid-induced cortical inflammation: implications for Alzheimer's disease. *J Neurosci* 22:2434-42.

Bondareff, W.; Mountjoy, CQ.; Roth, M.; Rossor, MN.; Iversen, LL.; Reynolds, GP. & Hauser, DL. Neuronal degeneration in locus ceruleus and cortical correlates of Alzheimer disease. *Alzheimer Dia Assoc Disord* 1987; 1:256-62.

Watson, GS.; Bernhardt, T.; Reger, MA.; Cholerton, BA.; Baker, LD. & Peskind, ER. (2006). Insulin effects on CSF norepinephrine and cognition in Alzheimer's disease. *Neurobiol Aging* 27:38-41.

Bingham, EM.; Hopkins, D.; Smith, D.; Pernet, A.; Hallett, W. & Reed, L. (2002). The role of insulin in human brain glucose metabolism: an 18fluoro-deoxyglucose positron emission tomography study. *Diabetes* 51:3384–90.

Blanchard, JG. & Duncan, PM. (1997). Effect in combinations of insulin, glucose and scopolamine on radial arm maze performance. *Pharmacol Biochem Behav* 58:209–14.

9

Structure Based 3D-QSAR Studies on Cholinesterase Inhibitors

Zaheer ul Haq and Reaz Uddin
Dr. Panjwani Center for Molecular Medicine and Drug Research, International Center for Chemical and Biological Sciences, University of Karachi
Pakistan

1. Introduction

Alzheimer's disease (AD) is a slowly progressive neurodegenerative disorder of the elderly. It is characterized by widespread loss of central cholinergic neuronal function (Butters et al., 1995). The only symptomatic treatment proven to be effective to date is the use of cholinesterase inhibitors (ChEI) to augment surviving cholinergic activity (Giacobini, 2003, Terry & Buccafusco, 2003). Two types of ChE enzyme are found in the Central Nervous System (CNS), acetylcholinesterase (AChE; EC 3.1.1.7) and butyrylcholinesterase (BuChE; EC 3.1.1.8).

AChE and BuChE share 65% amino acid sequence homology despite being encoded by different genes on human chromosomes 7(7q22) and 3(3q26), respectively (Soreq & Zaku, 1993). Acetylcholinesterase is responsible for the hydrolysis of acetylcholine at the synaptic cleft and the neuromuscular junction in response to nerve action potential (Massoulie et al., 1993) while the BuChE preferentially acts on butyrylcholine, but also hydrolyzes acetylcholine (Cokugras, 2003). In addition, both AChE and BuChE seem to be involved in roles that are independent of their catalytic activities, such as cell differentiation and development (Behra et al., 2002, Meshorer et al., 2002). BuChE and AChE are able to catalyze the hydrolysis of acetylcholine (ACh) at a rate of >10,000 molecules per second (Bazelyansky et al., 1986).

Because BuChE is relatively abundant in plasma (about 3 mg/liter), and can degrade a large number of ester-containing compounds, it plays important pharmacological and toxicological roles (Lockridge & Masson, 2000). For instance, BuChE is a potential detoxifying enzyme to be used as a prophylactic scavenger against neurotoxic organophosphates such as the nerve gas soman (Lockridge & Masson, 2000, Massoulie et al., 1993, Xie et al., 2000).

Previously, the relative contribution of BuChE to the regulation of ACh levels was largely ignored presumably due to unclear physiological function of BuChE (Chatonnet & Lockridge, 1989, Mack & Robitzki, 2000, Massoulie, Pezzementi, 1993, Xie, Stribley, 2000). However, there is growing evidence that both enzymes regulate ACh levels and may also play a part in the development and progression of AD (Greig et al., 2001).

In the normal brain, AChE represents approximately 80% of ChE activity with BuChE comprising the remainder (Giacobini, 1964). In advanced AD, however, AChE activity may be reduced to 55-67% of normal levels in specific brain regions, while BuChE activity increases (Giacobini, 1964, Greig, Utsuki, 2001, Mack & Robitzki, 2000). Cytochemical studies have revealed that in certain neuronal pathways of some species, BuChE replaces AChE (Graybiel & Ragsdale, 1982). The BuChE may also have a role in the aggregation of β-amyloid protein (Aβ) that occurs in the early stages of senile plaque formation in AD (Guillozet et al., 1997). Selective inhibition of BuChE versus AChE derives from an ability to utilize the additional space present in the gorge of BuChE.

From the resolved 3D structures of various cholinesterases, it is known that the active sites residues of these enzymes lay at the bottom of a 20 Å deep hydrophobic gorge (Bourne et al., 1995, Doorn et al., 2001, Harel et al., 1992, Nachon et al., 2005, Nachon et al., 2005, Nicolet et al., 2003, Sussman et al., 1991, Tormos et al., 2005). Due to a large cavity of this gorge BuChEs accept in comparison to AChEs, broader variety of substrates and inhibitors (Radic et al., 1993, Saxena et al., 1999, Saxena et al., 1997). For instance they metabolize butyrylcholine, the choline ester with large acyl moiety whose hydrolysis by vertebrate AChEs is negligible.

Although a similar peripheral site has been described for human BuChE but site-directed mutagenesis and photo-affinity labeling studies showed that its location and the response upon ligand binding differ significantly from those of AChE (Graybiel & Ragsdale, 1982, Perry et al., 1978).

Structure-activity analysis is the foundation for understanding the structural features of both the inhibitors and the target receptors involved in particular biological process and thus helps to design more effective inhibitors (Cho et al., 1996). It appears relatively difficult to find a reliable predictive model based on the calculated energies obtained by docking (Donini & Kollman, 2000, Tame, 1999). To overcome this problem, highly predictive QSAR i.e., CoMFA (Cramer Iii et al., 1988) and CoMSIA (Klebe et al., 1994) modeling techniques have been developed by using the technique of structure-based alignments of the substrates. These models can be used to identify important protein-ligand interactions and are found to be consistent with the crystal structure of the protein-ligand complex (Prathipati et al., 2005). The availability of X-ray crystal coordinates of inhibitors bound with the receptor have contributed to formulate effective predictive 3D-QSAR models based on (1) identification of possible conformations of related inhibitors in the active site and (2) understanding of the interactions of the inhibitors with the receptor in three-dimension (Debnath, 1999). A 3D-QSAR experiment performs two functions: the derivation of a statistically significant and highly predictive model that is used to estimate and rank new compounds for planned synthesis and the provision of an easily interpretable graphical tool which can identify a particular physicochemical property for increased affinity and selectivity (Klebe, 1998). These physicochemical properties include steric bulk, partial charge, local hydrophobicity, or hydrogen bond donor and acceptor (Bohm et al., 1999).

The level-dependent contouring of usual CoMFA-field contributions highlights those regions in space where the aligned molecules would favourably or unfavourably interact with a possible environment. The CoMSIA field contributions identify those areas within the region occupied by the ligand that "favour" or "dislike" the presence of a group with a particular physicochemical property. This association of required properties with a possible ligand shape is a more direct indicator to check whether all features important for a particular activity are present in the structures under consideration (Klebe, Abraham, 1994).

The discovery of natural cholinesterase inhibitors has been a very challenging area of drug development due to the involvement of cholinesterases in Alzheimer's disease and other related dementias. We have previously reported a number of new natural inhibitors of cholinesterases (AChE and BuChE) isolated from indigenous medicinal plants (Atta ur et al., 2000, Atta ur et al., 2004, Atta ur et al., 2004, Atta ur et al., 2002, Kalauni et al., 2001). The steady state inhibition kinetics, pharmacological profiles, SAR and molecular docking studies have been conducted on a similar series of compounds for AChE inhibition (Khalid et al., 2004, Khalid et al., 2004, Zaheer-Ul-Haq et al., 2003, Zaheer ul et al., 2003).

In the present study, two 3D-QSAR methods, CoMFA and CoMSIA, were applied and evaluated in order to accurately predict the inhibitory activity. For this reason a set of structurally similar cholinesterase inhibitors (both BuChE and AChE) were used to create a predictive model. The results from this study will be helpful for the design of new and more potent cholinesterase inhibitors.

Docking is one method in which the binding of an inhibitor to a receptor can be explored (Dominguez et al., 2003, Jain, 2003, Johnson et al., 2003, Sabnis et al., 2003, Todorov et al., 2003, Vicker et al., 2003, Wang et al., 2003, Wu et al., 2003, Zhou et al., 2003). In CoMFA or other 3D-QSAR studies, the molecule alignment and conformation determination are so important that they affect the success of a model. In the present case, a bound complex of steroidal alkaloid with cholinesterase was not available, and therefore, a computational method has to be implemented to determine possible conformations and alignment of a set of molecules so that 3D-QSAR can be carried out. Several strategies have been used in the past, to determine the conformation and alignment of molecules. Of them, docking is an attractive way to align molecules for CoMFA and/or CoMSIA. Several applications of docking alignment with CoMFA have been reported (Buolamwini & Assefa, 2002, Hu & Stebbins, 2005, Medina-Franco et al., 2004, Pan et al., 2006, Wei et al., 2005).

Recently, we used FlexX and FRED (FRED, 2007) to successfully dock a set of steroidal alkaloid inhibitors into the active site gorge of cholinesterase. A 3D-QSAR model was developed based on the docked conformation of the most active compound. In this paper we have performed CoMFA modeling utilizing the genetic algorithm (GA) in the selection of the ligand conformations. Previously this GA strategy has been utilized by Yuan and Zaheer ul Haq et al (Yuan et al., 2004, Yuan & Petukhov, 2006, Zaheer ul et al., 2008) and found that this is very efficient in terms of the reliability of the CoMFA models. GA is inspired by natural selection in evolution (Holland, 1975). GA approaches the optimum of a given function in the same way nature selects the individual fittest for the environment. The GA uses a blind search strategy, requiring no knowledge of the properties of the function to be optimized, thus enabling the algorithm to be applied to a variety of optimization problems from robot behavior to drug design (Fogel et al., 1966, Forrest, 1993, Goldberg, 1989).

2. Materials and methods

2.1 Biological data

The cholinesterase inhibitory activities, represented by IC_{50} (µM), were obtained from recently published data (Atta ur, Choudhary, 2000, Atta ur, Feroz, 2004, Atta ur et al., 2003, Atta ur et al., 1997, Atta ur, Zaheer ul, 2004, Atta ur, Zaheer ul, 2002, Kalauni, Choudhary, 2001, Khalid, Zaheer ul, 2004) (Table 1). The structures of inhibitors are presented in Table 2. The pIC_{50} (-$logIC_{50}$) values were used to derive 3D-QSAR models. From a total of forty compounds, a training set was created with thirty five compounds (with the case of BuChE) and thirty three compounds (with the case of AChE) while other 5 compounds were used as the test set (Table 1). This test set was used to validate the predictive ability of the training set.

S. No.	Comp. No.	Compound Name	IC_{50} (μM) BuChE	IC_{50} (μM) AChE	pIC_{50} BuChE	pIC_{50} AChE
1	SAR01	Isosarcodine	1.89±0.06	10.31±0.13	5.72	2.99
2	SAR02	Iso-*N*-formylchoneformine	4.07±0.11	6.36±0.22	5.39	3.20
3	SAR03	Saracodinine	12.51±0.06	40.04±0.13	4.9	2.40
4	SAR04	Sarcorine	10.33±0.02	69.99±0.056	4.99	2.15
5	SAR05	N_a-Demethylsaracodine	16.55±0.20	204.2±4.951	4.78	1.69
6	SAR06	Saracocine	3.86±0.01	20±1.30	5.41	2.70
7	SAR07	Sarcodine	18.31±0.74	49.77±1.26	4.74	2.30
8	SAR08	Salignenamide-A	4.63±0.07	50.64±0.930	5.33	2.30
9	SAR09	Vaganine-A	2.32±0.06	8.59±0.155	5.63	3.07
10	SAR10	Saligcinnamide	4.84±0.12	19.99±0.123	5.32	2.70
11	SAR11	Salignenamide-C	38.36±0.74	61.3±2.02	4.42	2.21
12	SAR12	5,6-Dehydrosarconidine	1.89±0.06	20.29±1.82	5.72	2.69
13	SAR13	Salignamine	25.7±0.63	249±10.23	4.59	1.60
14	SAR14	Salignenamide-D	23.78±0.15	185.2±7.66	4.62	1.73
15	SAR15	Salignenamide-E	3.65±0.02	6.21±0.234	5.44	3.21
16	SAR16	Salignenamide-F	4.07±0.11	6.357±0.224	5.39	3.20
17	SAR17	2β-Hydroxyepipachysamine-D	28.96±0.01	78.2±2.325	4.54	2.11
18	SAR18[a]	Salonine-B	4.50±0.07	-------	5.35	-------
19	SAR19	Salonine-A	32.70±1.20	33.4±3.21	4.49	2.48
20	SAR20	Salonine-C	32.20±0.50	7.8±0.5	4.49	3.11
21	SAR21	Salignarine-F	1.90±0.20	30.2±2.0	5.72	2.52
22	SAR22	16-Dehydrosarcorine	3.95±0.53	12.5±0.01	5.4	2.90
23	SAR23	Axillarine-C	17.99±0.22	227.92±8.677	4.74	1.64
24	SAR24	Axillarine-F	18.24±0.01	182.4±5.542	4.74	1.74
25	SAR25	Dictyophlebine	3.65±0.02	6.21±0.23	5.44	3.21
26	SAR26	Sarsalignenone	4.29±0.03	5.83±0.070	5.37	3.23
27	SAR27	Nepapakistamine	25.00±0.79	50.1±1.35	4.6	2.30
28	SAR28	Sarcoveganin-C	1.50±0.02	187.8±0.71	5.82	1.73
29	SAR29	Salignarine-C	1.25±0.01	19.7±0.05	5.9	2.71
30	SAR30	Sarsalignone	2.18±0.04	7.02±0.007	5.66	3.15
31	SAR31	*N*-Methylformamidesalonine-B	10.50±0.30	48.6±2.7	4.98	2.31
32	SAR32[a]	5,14-dehydro-N_a-demethylsaracodine	25.00±0.60	-------	4.6	-------
33	SAR33	Axilliridine-A	2.49±0.06	5.21±0.105	5.6	3.28
34	SAR34	14-Dehydro- N_a-demtehylsaracodine	10.10±0.15	183.1±2.60	5	1.74
35	SAR35[t]	Vaganine-D	10.00±0.120	46.89±1.94	5	2.33
36	SAR36[t]	2-Hydroxysalignarin E	6.91±0.06	15.99±0.13	5.16	2.80
37	SAR37[t]	Epipachysamine-D	2.82±0.02	28.93±0.54	5.55	2.54
38	SAR38[t]	2-Hydroxysalignamine	20.95±3.20	82.5±2.22	4.68	2.08
39	SAR39[t]	2,3-Dehydrosarsalignone	32.20±0.50	7.0±0.1	4.49	3.15
40	SAR40	Alkaloid C	22.13±0.14	42.2±0.26	2.65	2.37

[t] = test set

[a] = not included in AChE modelling

Table 1. Inhibitory Activities of the Compounds

2.2 Modeling tools

All molecular modeling and comparative molecular field evaluations were performed using SYBYL 7.2 (Sybyl, 2007), running on AMD Athlon (tm) workstation. The aliphatic amine groups of all compounds were considered protonated. Geometry optimizations were performed using the Tripos forcefield (Clark et al., 1989) with a distance-dependent dielectric and the Powell conjugate gradient algorithm. Gasteiger Huckel charges were used. All water molecules, sulfate and chloride anions, glycerol, fucose, *N*-acetyl-*D*-glucosamine and 2-(*N*-morpholino)-ethanesulfonic acids were removed from the original protein data bank file.

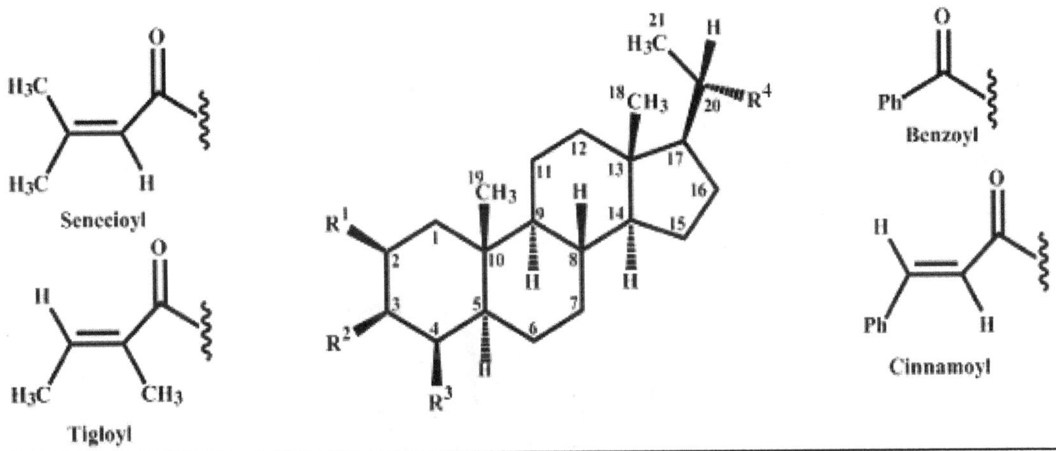

Comp. No.	R^1	R^2	R^3	R^4	Unsaturation
SAR01	H	NCH_3Ac	H	$N(CH_3)_2$	
SAR02	H	$N(CH_3)_2$	H	NHCHO	
SAR03	H	$N(CH_3)_2$	H	$N(CH_3)_2$	$\Delta^{5,6}$
SAR04	H	NHAc	H	$N(CH_3)_2$	
SAR05	H	$NHCH_3$	H	NCH_3Ac	
SAR06	H	$N(CH_3)_2$	H	NCH_3Ac	$\Delta^{5,6}$
SAR07	H	$N(CH_3)_2$	H	NCH_3Ac	
SAR08	H	$NHCOCH{=}CCH_3CH(CH_3)_2$	H	$N(CH_3)_2$	
SAR09	H	HN-Senecioyl	OAc	$N(CH_3)_2$	
SAR10	H	CH_3N-Cinnamoyl	H	$N(CH_3)_2$	
SAR11	OH	HN-Tigloyl	OAc	$N(CH_3)_2$	$\Delta^{14,15}$
SAR12	H	$NHCH_3$	H	$N(CH_3)_2$	$\Delta^{16,17}$
SAR13	H	OCH_3	H	$NHCH_3$	$\Delta^{5,6}$ & $\Delta^{16,17}$
SAR14	*a*-OH	HN-Tigloyl	H	$N(CH_3)_2$	$\Delta^{4,5}$ & $\Delta^{16,17}$
SAR15	H	$N(CH_3)COCH{=}C(CH_3)CH(CH_3)_2$	H	$N(CH_3)_2$	$\Delta^{16,17}$
SAR16	H	$N(CH_3)COCH{=}C(CH_3)CH(CH_3)_2$	H	$N(CH_3)_2$	
SAR17	OH	HN-Benzoyl	H	$N(CH_3)_2$	
SAR18	H	OCH_3	H	$N(CH_3)_2$	$\Delta^{5,6}$ & $\Delta^{16,17}$
SAR19	OH	HN-Tigloyl	OH	$N(CH_3)_2$	$\Delta^{14,15}$
SAR20	H	HN-Tigloyl	H	$N(CH_3)_2$	$\Delta^{4,5}$ & $\Delta^{14,15}$

SAR21	H	HN-Tigloyl	OH	$N(CH_3)_2$	$\Delta^{5,6}$
SAR22	H	$NHCOCH_3$	H	$N(CH_3)_2$	$\Delta^{16,17}$
SAR23	OH	HN-Benzoyl	OAc	$N(CH_3)_2$	
SAR24	OH	HN-Tigloyl	OAc	$N(CH_3)_2$	
SAR25	H	$NHCH_3$	H	$N(CH_3)_2$	
SAR27	OAc	HN-Tigloyl	OAc	$NHCH_3$	$\Delta^{16,17}$
SAR29	OH	HN-Senecioyl	H	$N(CH_3)_2$	$\Delta^{5,6}$
SAR31	H	OCH_3	H	$NCH_3(CHO)$	$\Delta^{5,6}$ & $\Delta^{16,17}$
SAR32	H	$NHCH_3$	H	NCH_3Ac	$\Delta^{5,6}$ & $\Delta^{14,15}$
SAR34	H	$NHCH_3$	H	NCH_3Ac	$\Delta^{14,15}$
SAR35	H	HN-Senecioyl	OAc	$N(CH_3)_2$	$\Delta^{16,17}$
SAR36	OH	HN-Tigloyl	H	$N(CH_3)_2$	$\Delta^{4,5}$
SAR37	H	HN-Benzoyl	H	$N(CH_3)_2$	
SAR38	OH	OCH_3	H	$N(CH_3)_2$	$\Delta^{5,6}$ & $\Delta^{16,17}$
SAR40					

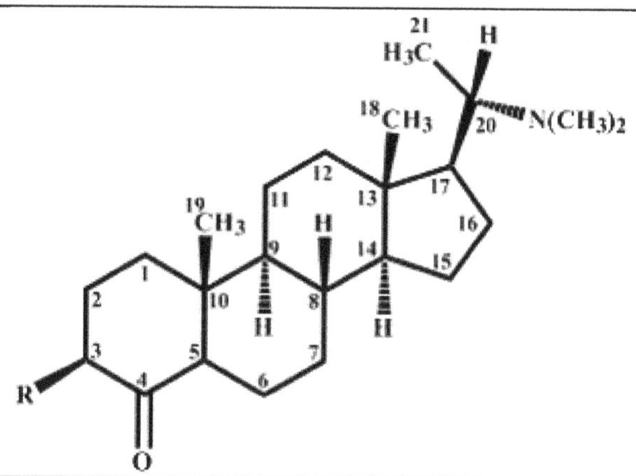

Comp. No.	R	Unsaturation
SAR26	HN-Tigloyl	$\Delta^{5,6}$ & $\Delta^{14,15}$
SAR28	HN-Tigloyl	$\Delta^{2,3}$ & $\Delta^{16,17}$
SAR30	HN-Tigloyl	$\Delta^{5,6}$
SAR33	HN-Benzoyl	$\Delta^{2,3}$
SAR39	HN-Tigloyl	$\Delta^{2,3}$ & $\Delta^{5,6}$

Table 2. Chemical Structures of the Compounds

2.3 Docking

FlexX, incremental construction algorithm (Rarey et al., 1996), was used to choose the appropriate binding conformations of the steroidal alkaloids inhibitors into the BuChE binding pocket. The crystal structure of human BuChE (pdb code: 1P0I) was used. One of the most active compound, SAR29 (see Table 2), was docked into the binding pocket and the best conformation was used as a template to align rest of the compounds. The FlexX scoring function was used to select the best conformation. Prior to dock the inhibitors with protein crystal structure, a re-docking of co-crystallized ligand with 1P0I was performed to validate the docking protocol. The top most docked solution was found in good agreement with the crystal structure of the co-crystallized ligand. The RMSD between the docking solution and the crystal structure was 1.53 Å.

Molecular docking with AChE was carried out using FRED docking program. FRED (Fast Rigid Exhaustive Docking) is a protein-ligand docking program, which takes a multiconformer library/database and receptor file as input and output molecules of the input database most likely to bind to the receptor (FRED, 2007, McGann et al., 2003).

First stage in FRED docking is a shape fitting process, which takes a set of ligand conformers as input and tests them against a "bump map" (a Boolean grid with true values where ligand atoms can potentially be placed). Orientations that clash with the protein or are distant from the active site are rejected. The crude docking solutions are further tested against a pharmacophore feature if specified and any poses that do not fit in the pharmacophore criteria are rejected. Poses surviving the shape fitting routine can then be passed through up to three scoring function filters in the screening process. Available scoring functions in FRED are ChemScore, PLP, ScreenScore, and Gaussian shape fitting (McGann, Almond, 2003).

2.4 Conformational sampling and alignment

The selected poses for SAR29 (one of the most active compound against BuChE) and SAR33 (one of the most active compound against AChE) were used as templates in structure alignment for all molecules in the respective series. For BuChE, this step was performed by using an incremental construction algorithm and a scoring function based on intermolecular interactions and overlapping density functions implemented in the Flexible Superposition (FlexS) technique (Lemmen et al., 1998). The minimum volume overlap was set at 0.6 and the number of alignments per ligand was used initially as 30 (default) but was changed for the cases where optimum alignment was not obtained. The Gasteiger Huckel charges were calculated during conformational alignment with FlexS. A top-ranked conformer for each compound was initially utilized for CoMFA modeling and then the ten best conformations were used in order to explore all possible conformational space for each compound. The ten best poses were selected based on the following:

1. FlexS ranks and
2. If the pose is correctly oriented on the template.

The Figure 1a represents the alignment of the molecules using SAR29 as a template for BuChE modeling.

In the case of AChE, the superimposition was performed using the ROCS from openeyes (OE ROCS, 2008). The ROCS is a Rapid Overlay on Crystal Structures (ROCS). ROCS method has a number of applications in virtual screening, lead hopping and in 3D-QSAR. ROCS can be utilized as an alignment method in order to produce the conformations which subsequently can be utilized in conformations sensitive 3D-QSAR i.e. CoMFA. The ROCS was used with its default settings except the maximum numbers of conformations and numbers of best hits to be saved were 30 and 1000, respectively. ROCS overlays the multiconformer compound's database in shape and chemistry with respect to the reference ligand. The overlays can be performed very quickly based on a description of the molecules as atom-centered Gaussian functions. ROCS maximizes the shared volume between a query molecule and a single conformation of a database molecule. Figure 1b represents the alignment of the molecules using SAR33 as a template for AChE modeling.

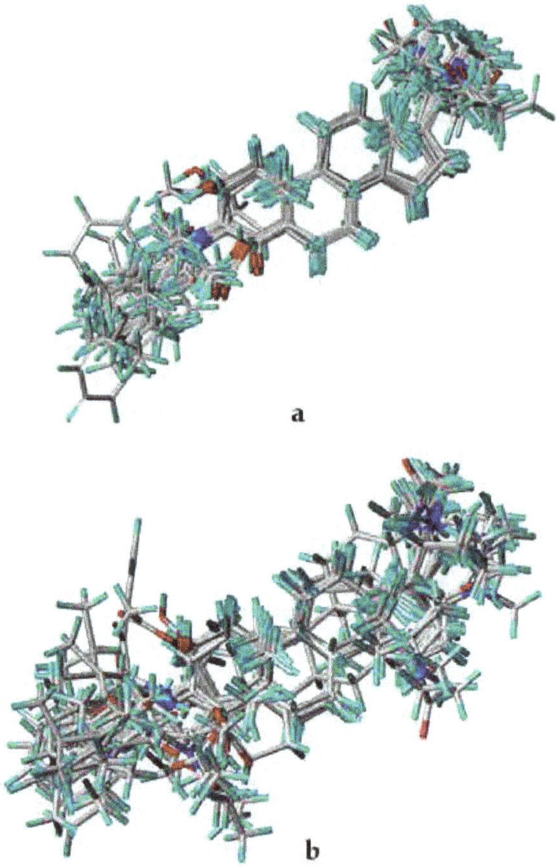

Fig. 1. Superposition of all studied inhibitors: **a**) BuChE using SAR29 as template **b**) AChE using SAR 33 as template

2.5 CoMFA modeling based on genetic algorithm

The overall strategy for CoMFA GA modeling is shown as a scheme in Figure 2. A brief description of the procedure is outlined here. To explore the multiple conformations of the ligands, a genetic algorithm analysis was applied in the selection of ligand's conformations for CoMFA. The genetic algorithm consisted of the following steps:

Initialization: This step generates an initial population P_i of CoMFA models using one randomly selected conformation among pre-filtered conformations of each ligand. The population size was set to 100.

Iterations:

Crossover: Exchange the conformations of corresponding ligands for any two models in the population P_i. The crossover ratio was set to 50:50.

Mutation: For randomly selected ligands, replace the conformations obtained in step 1 with randomly selected conformations in the database. Store the results as a temporary population P_{tmp}. The mutation rate was set to 0.05.

Selection: Generate new CoMFA models for P_{tmp}. Compare their q^2 values with those generated for population P_i and keep the best models in population P_{i+1}.

Until: The 100 generations limit is reached or the best model remains unchanged for 10 consecutive generations.

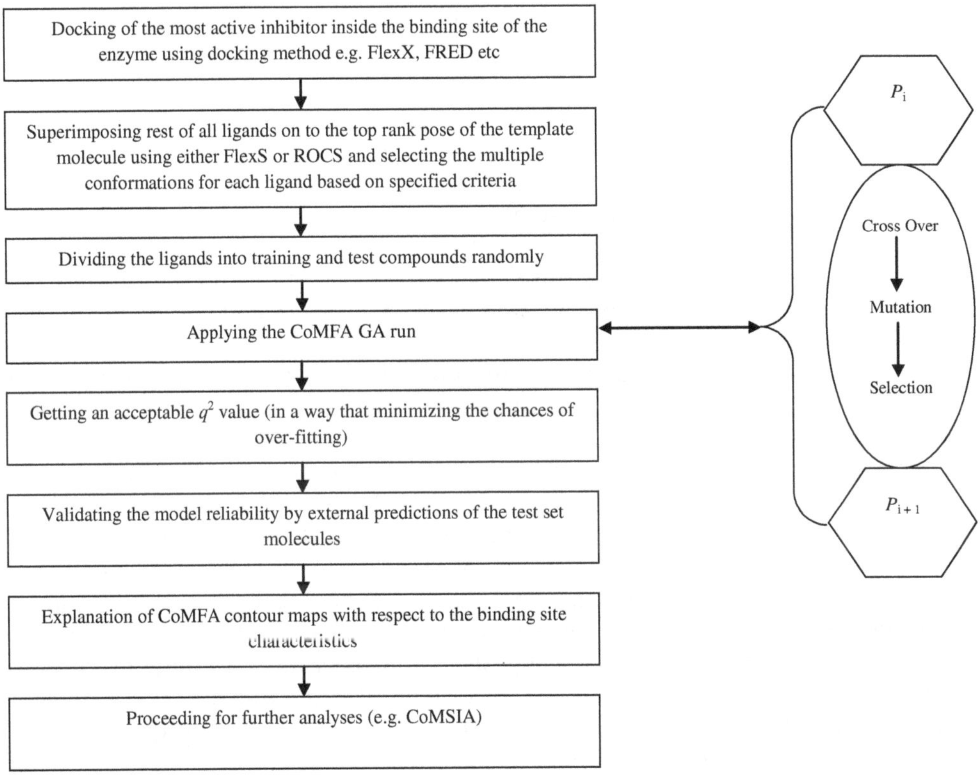

Fig. 2. Scheme for overall procedure applied during GA based 3D-QSAR modeling

2.6 CoMFA fields

Training sets of, thirty five compounds (with the case of BuChE) and thirty three compounds (with the case of AChE; see Table 1), were selected from the existing database, representing the diversity of structures and activities. After alignment, the molecules were inserted as rows of a QSAR table along with their respective IC_{50} values (as pIC_{50}). CoMFA steric and electrostatic fields were calculated as described below and entered as columns in the QSAR table. Standard steric and electrostatic CoMFA field energies of each inhibitor were calculated using an sp^3 probe atom with a +1 charge at all intersections in regularly spaced (2.0 Å) grids surrounding each molecule. Lennard Jones 6-12 potential and coulumbic potential functions, within the Tripos forcefield (Clark, Cramer, 1989) and a distance dependent (1/r) dielectric constant were used in the calculation. The grid box dimensions were determined by the "create automatically" features in the CoMFA module within the "SYBYL" program. The same grid box was used in all calculations. An energy cutoff of 30 kcal/mol for both steric and electrostatic contributions was set as threshold and the electrostatic terms were dropped within regions of steric maximum i.e., 30 kcal/mol. Five additional inhibitors (Table 1) were selected as a predictive set to test the robustness of the resulting model. They were aligned with template structures using the same alignment protocol as described earlier and finally their activities were predicted.

2.7 CoMSIA fields

Another 3D-QSAR procedure, CoMSIA can avoid some inherent deficiencies arising from the functional forms of Lennard-Jones and Coulumb potentials used in CoMFA. In CoMSIA, a distance dependent Guassian-type functional form has been introduced. This can avoid singularities at the atomic positions and the dramatic changes of potential energy due to grids in the proximity of the surface. Meanwhile, no arbitrary definition of cut-off limits is required in CoMSIA and the contour maps of the relative spatial contributions of the different fields can be substantially improved. This is essential for the interpretation in terms of separate property fields. The procedures of getting a 3D-QSAR model from a CoMSIA can be summarized into following three steps.

First, all molecules are structure-based or field-based aligned.

Then, an evenly-spaced rectangular grid is generated to enclose the molecular aggregate. A probe atom is placed at every lattice point to measure the electrostatic, steric, hydrophobic, and H-bond donor or acceptor fields.

Finally, the results from the field samplings are combined with the biological activities from the tested compounds are put into a table and partial least squares (PLS) fitting is applied to obtain the final CoMSIA model.

To choose the appropriate components and to check the statistical significance of the models, leave-one-out cross-validations were used by PLS. Then, the final 3D-QSAR model was derived from no cross-validation calculations. The CoMSIA results are finally interpreted graphically by field contribution maps using the field type "stdev*coeff".

Similar to the usual CoMFA approach, a data table has been constructed from similarity indices (Klebe, 1998) calculated via a common probe atom that is placed at the intersections of a regularly spaced lattice. A grid spacing of 2 Å has been used throughout this study. Similarity indices $A_{F,\,K}$ between the compounds of interest and a probe atom, systematically placed at the intersections of the lattice, have been calculated according to equation 1 (e.g., at grid point q for molecule j of the data set).

$$A_{FK}^{q}(j) = -\sum_{i} \omega_{probe,k} \omega_{ik} (e_{iq}^{-\alpha r})^2 \quad (1)$$

Where i = summation index over all atoms of the molecule j under investigation; ω_{ik} = actual value of the physicochemical property k of atom i; $\omega_{probe,\,k}$ = probe atom with charge +1, a = attenuation factor; and r_{iq} = mutual distance between probe atom at grid point q and atom i of the test molecule. Large values of a will result in a strong attenuation of the distance-dependent consideration of molecular similarity. Accordingly, there is little averaging of local feature matches of the molecules being compared. With small values of a, also remote parts of each molecule will be experienced by the probe and the global molecular features become more important. In the present study the a has been set at 0.3. With this selection, at a given lattice point the property value of an atom of the molecule under investigation (e.g., the partial atomic charge) is experienced in 1 Å distance by 74.1%, in 2 Å by 30.1% and in 3 Å by 6.7% of its total value. This permits a reasonable "local smearing" of the molecular similarity indices and should help to avoid extreme dependencies on small changes of the mutual alignments (Bohm, St rzebecher, 1999). In the present study five physicochemical properties k (steric, electrostatic, hydrophobic and hydrogen bond donor and acceptor) were evaluated, using a common probe atom with 1 Å radius and charge, hydrophobicity and hydrogen-bond property of +1. Steric property fields were expressed by the third power of the atomic radii. Local hydrophobicities were associated using atom-based parameters developed by Viswanadhan et al (Viswanadhan et al., 1989).

2.8 Statistical analysis/PLS

Correlations were derived using the method of Partial Least Squares (PLS) (Geladi & Kowalski, 1986) and cross validated to reduce the probability of obtaining chance correlations. As used in this report, the cross-validated q^2 refers to the squared correlation coefficient of the equation derived from the cross-validation of the training set to determine the optimum number of principal components. The conventional r^2 is the fitted correlation of the training set using the optimum number of principal components with no cross validation. The predictive r-squared was calculated by the equation 2.

$$predictive\ r-squared = \frac{SSD - PRESS}{SSD} \tag{2}$$

Where SSD is sum of squared deviations and PRESS is predictive residual sum of squares.

3. Results and discussion

3.1 Docking

The best docking poses for SAR29 and SAR33 inside the binding pockets of BuChE and AChE are shown in Figure 3a and 3b, respectively. The poses indicated that the ligands were

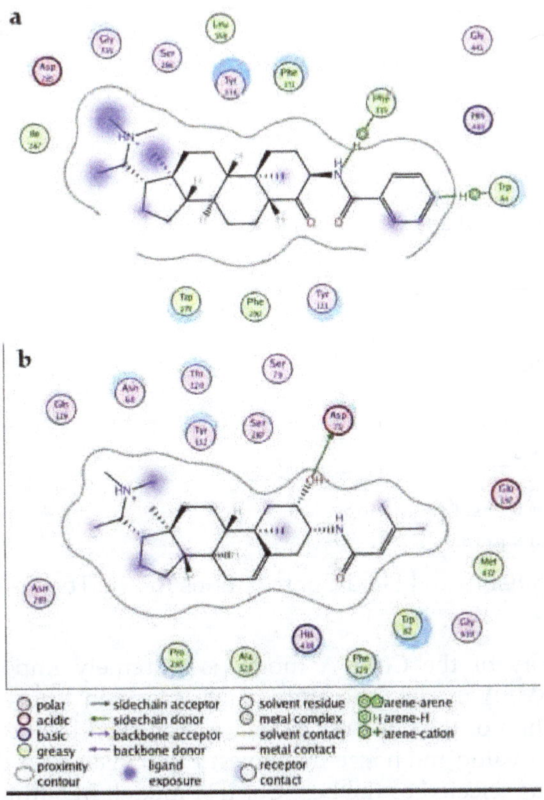

Fig. 3. Docked poses of most active compound **a**) SAR29 for BuChE and **b**) SAR33 for AChE within the surrounding binding site residues. The figures are rendered by MOE Ligand interaction

accommodated well inside the binding sites. The compound enters the cavity preferably by ring A. This might contribute highly to the stabilization of the complex since the steroid backbone of the ligand is highly hydrophobic due to its aliphatic character and therefore, not well hydrated. The main hydrophobic interactions between the hydrocarbon skeleton of the inhibitors and the cholinesterases binding sites were observed with the most common residues i.e. Thr, Tyr, Trp, Ala, and Phe.

3.2 3D-QSAR of inhibitors

3.2.1 Model selection

The CoMFA based on GA, resulted in several models and among them, the final model selection is an important issue. With the case of BuChE, four different models have been selected based on q^2 values. Among them, models 72 and 80 were obtained with the cutoff $q^2 \geq 0.65$; and the other two models 9 and 21, with the cutoff $q^2 \geq 0.90$ (Table 3).

Parameters	Model9	Model21	Model72	Model80
q^2 [a]	0.902	0.911	0.730	0.701
r^2 [b]	0.998	0.998	0.994	0.979
SEE [c]	0.022	0.020	0.040	0.072
F-value [d]	2326.92	2957.134	738.562	264.356
No. of Components [e]	6	6	6	5
Fraction [f]				
Steric	0.499	0.484	0.500	0.531
Electrostatic	0.501	0.516	0.500	0.469
Predictive *r*-Squared [g]	0.441	0.523	0.311	0.682
PRESS [h]	0.384	0.328	0.475	0.218

[a] Cross-validated correlation coefficient.
[b] Noncross-validated correlation coefficient.
[c] Standard error of estimate.
[d] *F*-test value.
[e] Optimum number of components obtained from cross-validated PLS analysis and same used in final non-cross-validated analysis.
[f] Field contributions.
[g] Correlation coefficient for test set predictions.
[h] Predicted residual sum of squares.

Table 3. Summary of Statistics and Field Contributions for the Top Four CoMFA Models with the case of BuChE

The external predictivity of the CoMFA model is extremely important in terms of the applicability of the CoMFA model. Therefore, it was decided to use the predictive-r^2 as a criterion for final selection of the one best model. As reflected by the Table 3, model 80 has the highest predictive-r^2 value and hence the lowest PRESS value for the test set predictions. Therefore, model 80 was selected as the best CoMFA model. In addition, to study the effect of charges on 3D-QSAR studies, different methods were employed to calculate the charges on ligands included in this study. Quantitative comparisons of the charges calculated by different methods are reported in Table 4. Different charges resulting from different calculation methods may influence the results of CoMFA as well as CoMSIA, but there is no significant effects of charges observed during our study for this particular steroidal class of compounds.

With the case of AChE, another way of model selection was done. In each case of GA run the predictive- r^2 was also calculated and compared it with each generation's top model. The default settings of 100 individuals and 100 generations were used but the GA resulted in early termination with 28th generation due to achieving the cutoff value of fitness function (i.e. q^2 = 0.80). The graphical representation is presented in Figure 4. The generation number six (highlighted in circle in Figure 4) was the first in identifying the acceptable q^2 as well as the predictive r^2. Hence, the model number six was utilized for further analysis with the case of AChE.

S.No.	Charges Method	CoMFA			CoMSIA		
		q^2	r^2	Components	q^2	r^2	Components
1	Gasteiger Marsilli	0.696	0.989	6	0.636	0.980	5
2	Gasteiger Huckel	0.701	0.979	5	0.627	0.982	5
3	Huckel	0.673	0.988	5	0.637	0.981	5
4	MMFF94	0.716	0.993	6	0.669	0.986	4
5	Pullman	0.697	0.989	6	0.630	0.981	5
6	Delre	0.680	0.987	5	0.634	0.980	6

Table 4. Influence of Different Charges on BuChE Predictive Model

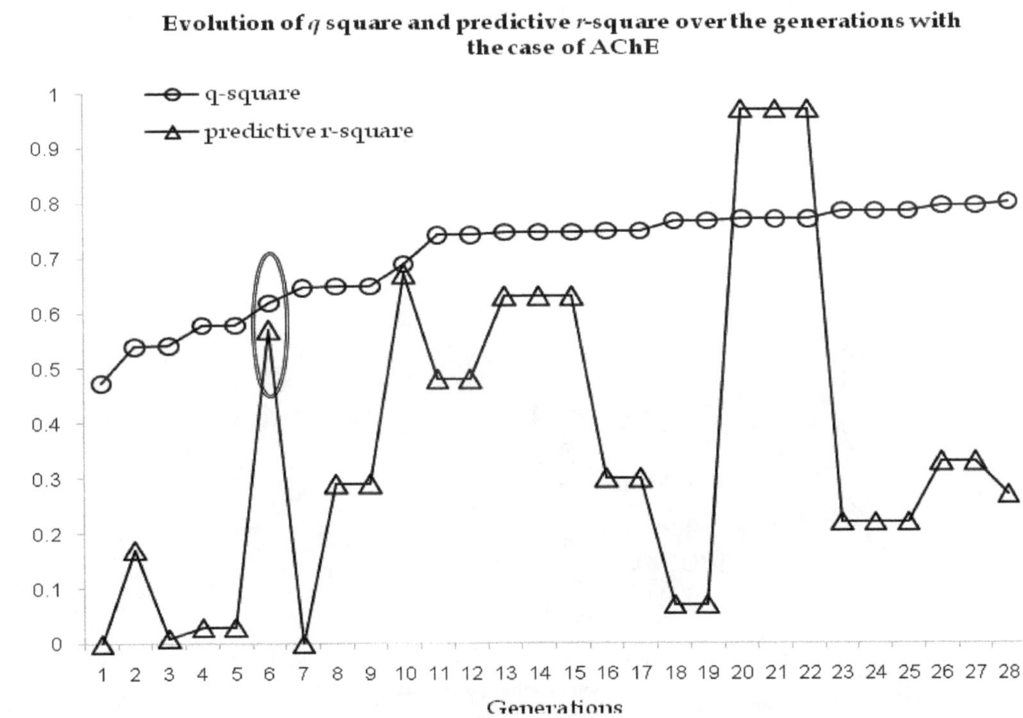

Fig. 4. Comparison between q^2 and predictive $-r^2$ over the generations with AChE modeling

3.2.2 Predictive power of the 3D-QSAR model

The final results of CoMFA and CoMSIA analysis in both cases (i.e. BuChE and AChE) with 2.0 Å grid spacing are shown in Table 5 and Table 6, respectively. PLS analysis yielded consistent results. The optimal components that produce the best cross-validation linear regression coefficient were used to produce the non-cross-validated model. The inhibitory activities (pIC_{50}) and the calculated activities using CoMFA and CoMSIA models for training set and test set are listed in Table 7. Graphic representation of observed vs calculated inhibitory activity is shown in the Figure 5. Best selected 3D-QSAR models showed good prediction for five tested compounds, which reflects that the derived models were satisfactory enough in respect to statistical significance and actual predictive ability.

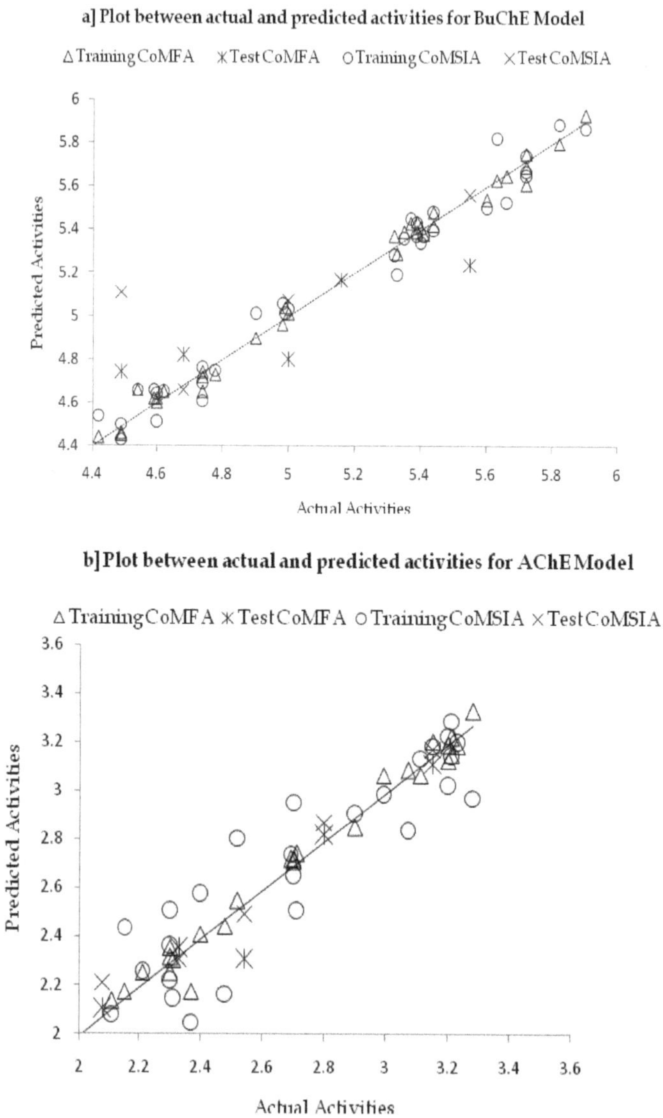

Fig. 5. Plots of the predicted versus experimental activity data of 3D-QSAR from both CoMFA and CoMSIA for training and test compounds **a**) BuChE and **b**) AChE

Parameters	CoMFA	CoMSIA				
	S, E [(h)]	S, E, H, D, A [(h)]	S, E [(h)]	S, E, H [(h)]	S, E, H, A [(h)]	S, E, H, D [(h)]
$q^{2\,a}$	0.701	0.627	0.382	0.444	0.386	0.615
SEP [b]	0.273	0.305	0.393	0.373	0.392	0.310
No. of Components [c]	5	5	5	5	5	5
r^{2d}	0.979	0.982	0.880	0.927	0.924	0.967
SEE [e]	0.072	0.085	0.174	0.135	0.138	0.090
Field Contributions	0.531, 0.469	0.064, 0.173, 0.135, 0.373, 0.255	0.330, 0.670	0.211, 0.393, 0.396	0.122, 0.237, 0.251, 0.390	0.102, 0.246, 0.197, 0.456
F-value [f]	264.356	185.867	40.877	70.649	68.035	166.192
Predictive *r*-squared [g]	0.682	0.453	0.228	0.529	0.048	0.774

[a] Cross-validated correlation coefficient.

[b] Standard error of predictions.

[c] Optimum number of components obtained from cross-validated PLS analysis and same used in final non-cross-validated analysis.

[d] Noncross-validated correlation coefficient.

[e] Standard error of estimate.

[f] *F*-test value.

[g] Correlation coefficient for test set predictions.

[h] CoMFA and CoMSIA with different field contributions such as steric (S), electrostatic (E), hydrophobic (H), donor (D), and acceptor (A) fields.

Table 5. Results of CoMFA and CoMSIA Analyses for Compounds Used in Training Set (BuChE modeling)

Parameters	CoMFA	CoMSIA				
	S, E [(h)]	S, E, H, D, A [(h)]	S, E [(h)]	S, E, H [(h)]	S, E, H, A [(h)]	S, E, H, D [(h)]
$q^{2\,a}$	0.632	0.630	0.661	0.641	0.650	0.636
SEP [b]	0.374	0.355	0.359	0.370	0.358	0.359
No. of Components [c]	6	3	6	6	5	4
r^{2d}	0.989	0.909	0.979	0.984	0.966	0.947
SEE [e]	0.066	0.176	0.090	0.078	0.111	0.136
Field Contributions	0.524, 0.476	0.066, 0.237, 0.114, 0.307, 0.276	0.201, 0.799	0.139, 0.568, 0.293	0.095, 0.349, 0.160, 0.396	0.087, 0.341, 0.172, 0.401
F-value [f]	377.882	96.415	220.40	269.126	154.86	125.930
Predictive *r*-squared [g]	0.964	0.985	0.877	0.917	0.954	0.888

[a] Cross-validated correlation coefficient.

[b] Standard error of predictions.

[c] Optimum number of components obtained from cross-validated PLS analysis and same used in final non-cross-validated analysis.

[d] Noncross-validated correlation coefficient.

[e] Standard error of estimate.

[f] *F*-test value.

[g] Correlation coefficient for test set predictions.

[(h)] CoMFA and CoMSIA with different field contributions such as steric (S), electrostatic (E), hydrophobic (H), donor (D), and acceptor (A) fields.

Table 6. Results of CoMFA and CoMSIA Analyses for Compounds Used in Training Set (AChE modeling)

S.No.	Compound	Actual pIC_{50} *BuChE*	CoMFA Predicted pIC_{50} *BuChE*	CoMSIA Predicted pIC_{50} *BuChE*	Actual pIC_{50} *AChE*	CoMFA Predicted pIC_{50} *AChE*	CoMSIA Predicted pIC_{50} *AChE*
Training set							
1	SAR01	5.72	5.61	5.65	2.99	3.07	2.98
2	SAR02	5.39	5.44	5.43	3.2	3.13	3.23
3	SAR03	4.90	4.90	5.01	2.4	2.41	2.58
4	SAR04	4.99	5.04	5.01	2.15	2.18	2.44
5	SAR05	4.78	4.73	4.75	1.69	1.69	1.75
6	SAR06	5.41	5.38	5.37	2.70	2.71	2.65
7	SAR07	4.74	4.72	4.76	2.30	2.32	2.36
8	SAR08	5.33	5.29	5.19	2.30	2.25	2.51
9	SAR09	5.63	5.63	5.82	3.07	3.09	2.84
10	SAR10	5.32	5.37	5.28	2.70	2.72	2.95
11	SAR11	4.42	4.44	4.54	2.21	2.25	2.26
12	SAR12	5.72	5.75	5.67	2.69	2.72	2.74
13	SAR13	4.59	4.62	4.66	1.60	1.76	1.72
14	SAR14	4.62	4.65	4.65	1.73	1.68	1.71
15	SAR15	5.44	5.42	5.48	3.21	3.15	3.14
16	SAR16	5.39	5.39	5.37	3.20	3.19	3.02
17	SAR17	4.54	4.66	4.66	2.11	2.13	2.08
18	SAR18[a]	5.35	5.39	5.36	-------	-------	-------
19	SAR19	4.49	4.45	4.43	2.48	2.44	2.17
20	SAR20	4.49	4.46	4.50	3.11	3.07	3.14
21	SAR21	5.72	5.69	5.74	2.52	2.55	2.81
22	SAR22	5.40	5.41	5.34	2.90	2.85	2.91
23	SAR23	4.74	4.74	4.69	1.64	1.60	1.79
24	SAR24	4.74	4.65	4.61	1.74	1.71	1.89
25	SAR25	5.44	5.48	5.40	3.21	3.22	3.29
26	SAR26	5.37	5.43	5.45	3.23	3.19	3.20
27	SAR27	4.60	4.62	4.64	2.30	2.36	2.22
28	SAR28	5.82	5.80	5.89	1.73	1.74	1.89
29	SAR29	5.90	5.93	5.87	2.71	2.74	2.51
30	SAR30	5.66	5.65	5.53	3.15	3.20	3.19
31	SAR31	4.98	4.96	5.06	2.31	2.30	2.14
32	SAR32[a]	4.60	4.60	4.51	-------	-------	-------
33	SAR33	5.60	5.54	5.50	3.28	3.33	2.97
34	SAR34	5.00	5.01	5.03	1.74	1.77	1.58
35	SAR40	2.65	2.613	2.620	2.37	2.18	2.05
Test set							
36	SAR35	5.00	4.80	5.07	2.33	2.35	2.31
37	SAR36	5.16	5.17	5.17	2.80	2.82	2.87
38	SAR37	5.55	5.24	5.56	2.54	2.31	2.49
39	SAR38	4.68	4.82	4.66	2.08	2.10	2.21
40	SAR39	4.49	4.74	5.11	3.15	3.11	3.17

[a] = not included in AChE modeling

Table 7. Comparisons of Experimental and Calculated Biological Activities of the Compounds by Using CoMFA and CoMSIA Analyses

3.2.3 Graphical interpretation of the results (CoMFA)

3.2.3.1 BuChE

CoMFA steric and electrostatic fields from the final non-cross-validated analysis were plotted as three-dimensional colored contour maps in Figure 6a. The field energies at each lattice point were calculated as the scalar results of the coefficient and the standard deviation associated with a particular column of the data table (stdev*coeff), plotted as the percentage of contribution to the CoMFA equation. These maps show regions where differences in molecular fields are associated with differences in biological activity.

The steric interactions are represented by green and yellow colors while electrostatic interactions are represented by red and blue colors (Figure 6a). In the green regions of steric contour plot, bulky substituent enhances biological activity while bulky substituent in the yellow region is likely to decrease activity. The green steric contour near the substituent at C20 of the D ring indicates that any bulky substituent is preferred at this position. This may provide more possibilities to establish hydrophobic interactions with peripheral site of the target protein. This observation is consistent with the experimental findings as compound SAR13 is less active than SAR38 because SAR13 is having less bulky substituent at C20 than SAR38.

In electrostatic contour map blue-colored contours represent regions where electropositive groups increase activity whereas red colored regions represent areas where electronegative groups enhance activity. The electrostatic contour plot on the set of compounds showed that there is a red-colored region situated close to the substituent at C3 that is to say, the negative charges at this region are in a high demand for ligand binding and a charge withdrawing group linked to this position will enhance the biological activity. This observation also correlates with the experimental determinations, for example, the compound SAR37 is more active than compound SAR17. The only difference in both of them is the presence of a hydroxyl group at C-2 in compound SAR17 which makes SAR17 less active than SAR37 since C2 position is covered by the blue contour map. On the other hand a negative group at C-4 position makes compound SAR26, SAR28, SAR30, and SAR33 the most active compounds among the listed compounds. The presence of a double bond between C-5 and C-6 makes compound SAR06 more active than compound SAR07, which has otherwise identical structure.

3.2.3.2 AChE

In Figure 7a it is possible to observe two well-defined zones (close to the substituent at position C-4 and side chain at C-3 position) in which the presence of negative density favors an increase of AChE inhibitory activity. Furthermore, the presence of a double bond in ring B, between C-5 and C-6, also increases the activity. Small zones near C-2 have an opposite effect, that is, a negative density decreases the activity: for example, the only difference between compounds SAR17 and SAR37 is the presence of a hydroxyl group at C-2, which makes compound SAR17 less active than SAR37, on the other hand a negative group at C-4 position makes compounds SAR33, SAR30 and SAR26 the most active compounds in our study. Similarly, the presence of a double bond between C-5 and C-6 makes compound SAR06 more active than compound SAR07 which has an otherwise identical structure. Figure 7a displays two big zones near position C-4 and near the side chain at C-3, where the presence of bulky substituents decreases the activity. The region between C14 and C15 is also not favorable for bulky groups, which assigns a further role to the presence of the double bond in ring D as it means the lack of a further substitution. This difference can be easily seen by comparing compounds SAR30 and SAR26.

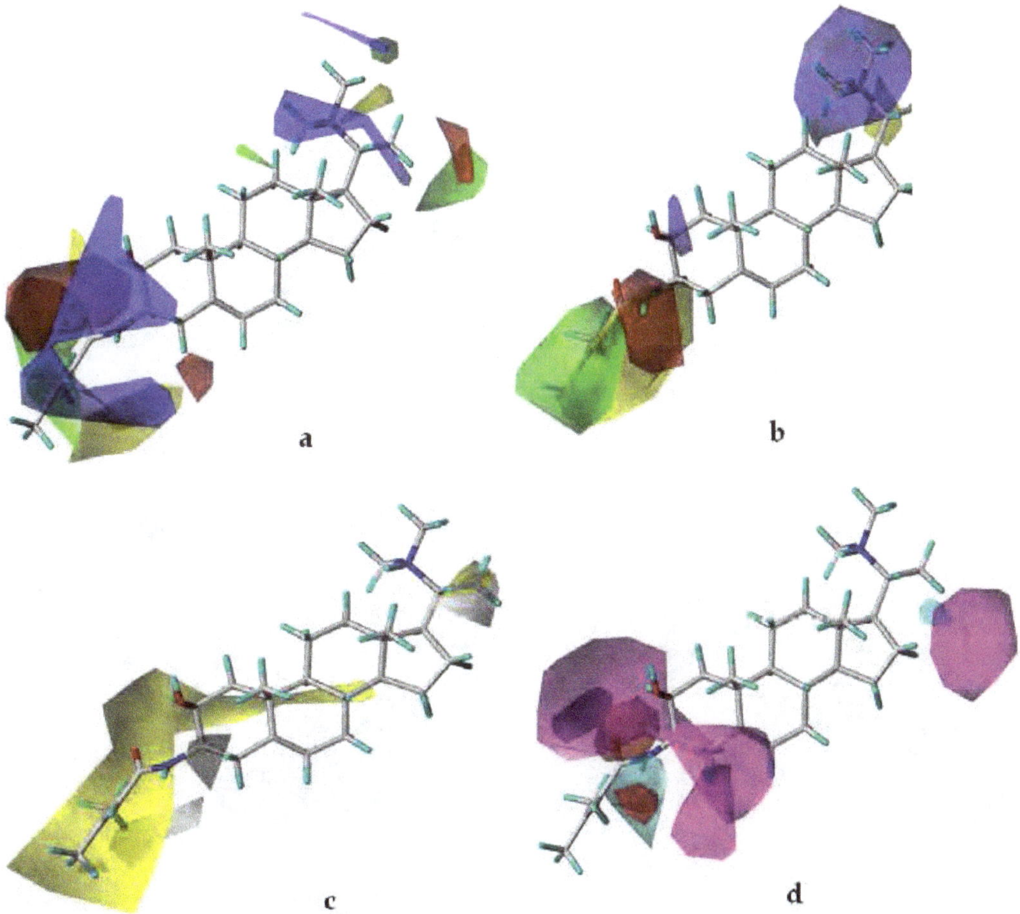

Fig. 6. **a**) The CoMFA (stdev*coeff) steric and electrostatic contour plots for BuChE modeling. The favorable steric areas in green; disfavored steric areas in yellow. The positive potential favored area in blue; positive potential disfavored areas in red. The most active compound in the series (SAR29) is shown as the reference compound. **b**) The CoMSIA (stdev*coeff) steric and electrostatic contour plots. Color scheme same as in figure 6a. The most active compound in the series (SAR29) is shown as the reference compound. **c**) The CoMSIA (stdev*coeff) hydrophobic contour plots. The favorable hydrophobic areas indicated by yellow color, whereas the disfavored hydrophobic areas are shown by white color. The most active compound (SAR29) is shown as the reference compound. **d**) The contour plots of the CoMSIA (stdev*coeff) H-bond donor and acceptor fields. The favorable H-bond donor in cyan; unfavorable H-bond donor in purple. The favorable H-bond acceptor in magenta; unfavorable H-bond acceptor in red. The most active compound (SAR29) is shown as the reference compound

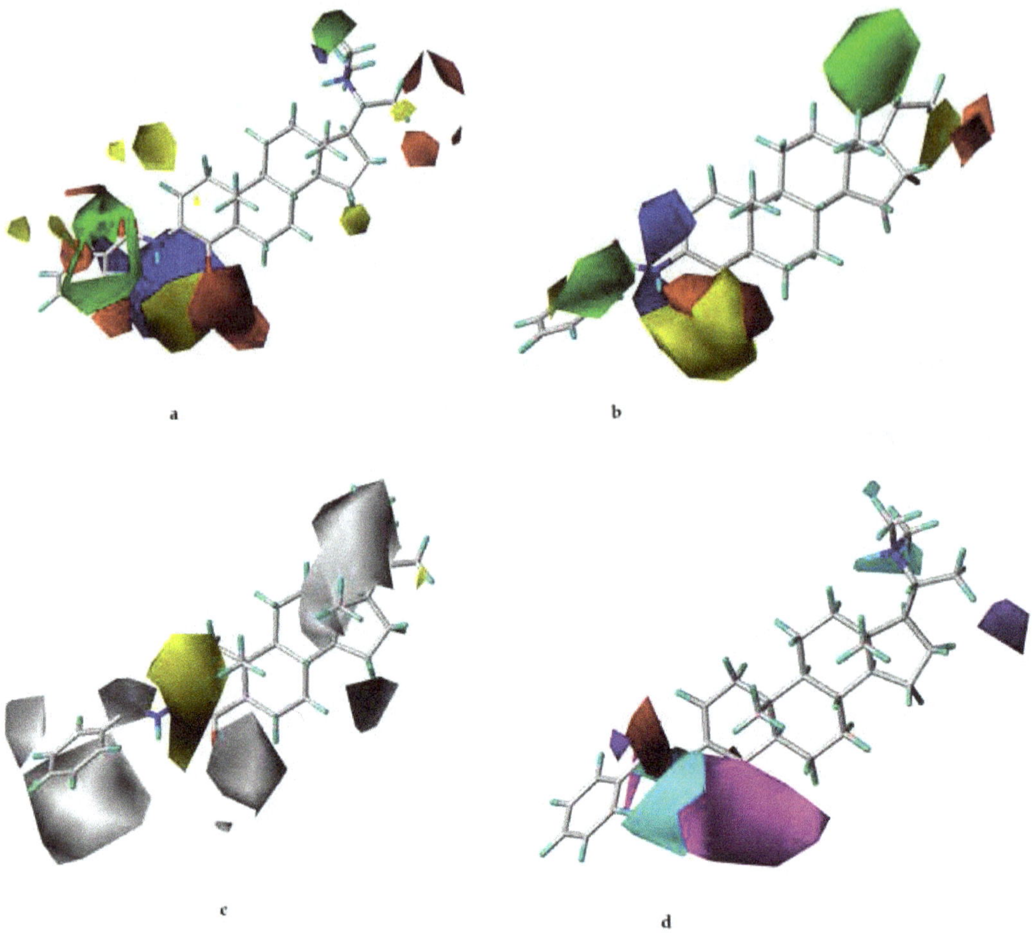

Fig. 7. **a**) The CoMFA (stdev*coeff) steric and electrostatic contour plots for AChE modeling. The favorable steric areas in green; disfavored steric areas in yellow. The positive potential favored area in blue; positive potential disfavored areas in red. The most active compound in the series (SAR33) is shown as the reference compound. **b**) The CoMSIA (stdev*coeff) steric and electrostatic contour plots. Color scheme same as in figure 7a. The most active compound in the series (SAR33) is shown as the reference compound. **c**) The CoMSIA (stdev*coeff) hydrophobic contour plots. The favorable hydrophobic areas indicated by yellow color, whereas the disfavored hydrophobic areas are shown by white color. The most active compound (SAR33) is shown as the reference compound. **d**) The contour plots of the CoMSIA (stdev*coeff) H-bond donor and acceptor fields. The favorable H-bond donor in cyan; unfavorable H-bond donor in purple. The favorable H-bond acceptor in magenta; unfavorable H-bond acceptor in red. The most active compound (SAR33) is shown as the reference compound

3.2.4 Graphical interpretation of the results (CoMSIA)

3.2.4.1 BuChE

The CoMSIA steric and electrostatic fields based on PLS analyses are represented as 3D contour plots in Figure 6b. In the electrostatic contour map, positive charge can be appeared closer to the regions of positive coefficients (blue) and negative charge can be moved closer to the regions of negative coefficients (red). A close inspection of the electrostatic contour plots (Figure 6b), reveals that for the tested molecules the electropositive groups are more preferred and appearance of the blue regions near R4 zone, indicate that more positive charge group substituted at this zone on the parent skeleton will enhance the biological activity.

In the steric contour map, it can be seen that, the areas (green contour) correspond to regions where steric occupancy with bulky groups are preferred and the areas encompassed by yellow contour should be sterically avoided. For the studied compounds on ring A, there exist two contour areas, a larger favorable area near the group substituted at the C3 on the ring A, and at the opposite site, a relatively smaller unfavorable area. Due to the steric complementarity between receptor and inhibitor, the positions which are encompassing the green region are sterically preferred to produce good steric interactions with the receptor and hence increasing the inhibitory activity. By observing the steric contour map with the compound SAR29 (one of the most active compound; Table 2), it can be readily seen that the green contour covered the whole carbonyl and double bond region at the senecioyl group while the terminal substituent on double bond in senecioyl group is covered by yellow contour. The green area is indicating that bulky substituent at double bond but adjacent to the carbonyl position will enhance the biological activity. Similarly, a smaller terminal substituent on the double bond will enhance the inhibitory activity. For example, the structure of the compound SAR12 has relatively small substituent, in the form of -NHCH3, at C3, while SAR35 has a bulky substituent in the form of senecioyl group, shows less inhibitory activity than compound SAR12. The same is observed if we compare the compound SAR25 with SAR35.

The contour map of hydrophobic properties indicates (Figure 6c) one distinct hydrophobically favorable site, a larger region near the R2 zone, which means that groups with high hydrophobicity (indicated by yellow contour in Figure 6c) will favor biological activity. It can be reasonably presumed that ring A combined with a substituent on it, is composed of a large hydrophobic core, and will produce a strong hydrophobic interaction with the receptor. This observation is also consistent with the CoMFA steric contour map (Figure 6a) in which the sterically more crowded substituent is necessary to enhance the biological activity at the same R2 zone (see Figure 8 for R zones descriptions).

The graphical interpretations of the field contributions of the H-bond properties are shown in Figure 6d as both H-bond donor and H-bond acceptor fields. In principle, they should highlight the areas beyond the ligands where putative hydrogen partners in the enzyme can form H-bonds that influence binding affinity. The hydrogen bond donor and acceptor fields showed the favorable (cyan) area near the amido group and the H-bond acceptor field showed the favorable (magenta) area around the oxygen atom in amido group (Figure 6d). This may be due to the involvement of hydrogen bonding during interaction with target.

Superimposition of the CoMFA and CoMSIA coefficient contour maps on the ligand in the active site of BuChE (Figure 9a and 9b) additionally supports the result that most of the interactions are hydrophobic in nature and the residues nearby the hydrophobic favorable area are mostly consisting of hydrophobic amino acids (i.e., Gly, Val, and Leu). As depicted in the figures 9a and 9b, the substituents at position R2 is placed in the hydrophobic pocket formed by Leu286, Gly116, Gly117, Val288, and Ala199. A green color contour map of CoMFA model (Figure 6a) and similarly of green contour of CoMSIA (Figure 6b) is appeared at this position suggesting for bulky substituents at this position. Another yellow color CoMSIA contour near the same R2 region suggesting the favorable hydrophobic interaction with the receptor hydrophobic pocket which is formed by the same amino acid residues. Most of the amino acid residues near the yellow contour regions are in hydrophobic in nature e.g., Gly, Val, and Leu. The same is true when comparing the CoMFA and CoMSIA contour maps within the active site residues of acetylcholinesterase (Figure 9c and 9d)

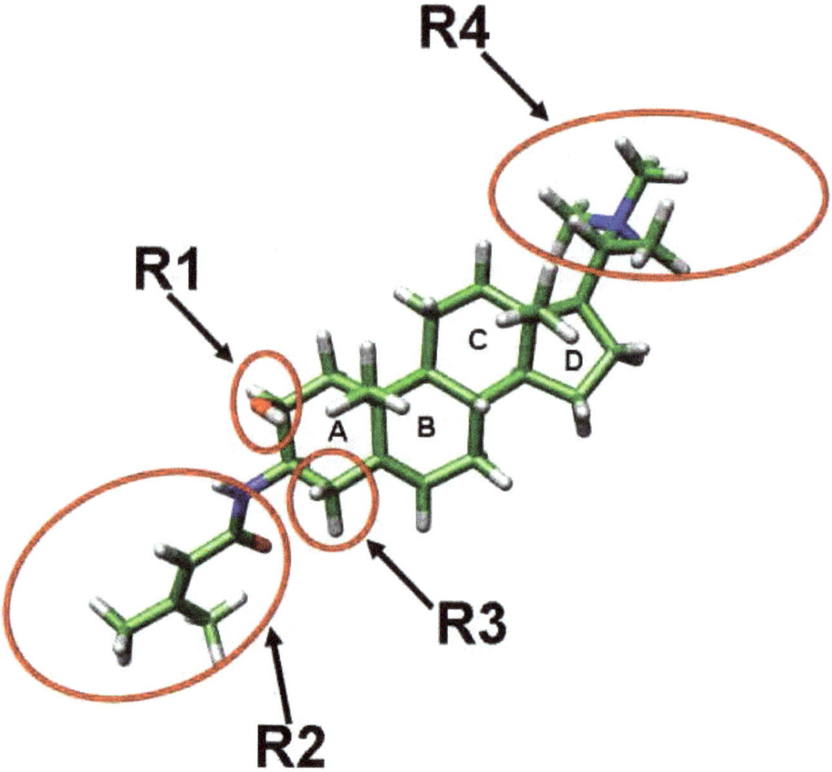

Fig. 8. An example of representative compound; showing important regions of the parent skeleton; circled here, as R1, R2, R3 and R4

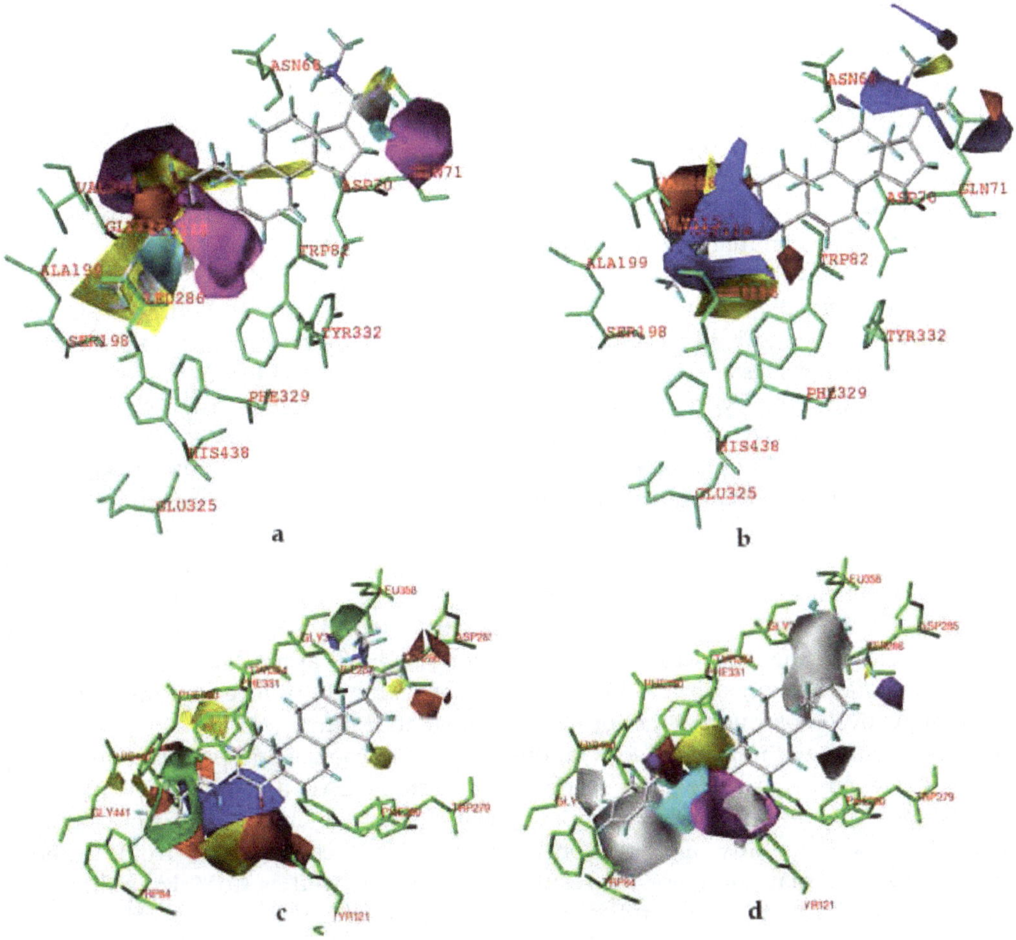

Fig. 9. **a**) CoMSIA contour plots superimposed within the active site of BuChE with compound SAR29 **b**) CoMFA contour plots superimposed within the active site of BuChE with compound SAR29 **c**) CoMFA contour plots superimposed within the active site of AChE with compound SAR33 **d**) CoMSIA contour plots superimposed within the active site of AChE with compound SAR33

3.2.4.2 AChE

The CoMSIA steric and electrostatic descriptors (Figure 7b) for the set of AChE inhibitors remain similar as the CoMFA and hence not described further. The CoMSIA hydrophobic descriptors are presented as contour maps in Figure 7c. The contour map of hydrophobic properties indicates a favourable region around the substituents as R2 (yellow contours in Figure 7c), pointing the hydrophobic groups is advantageous for the AChE inhibitory activity. The graphical interpretations of the H-bond properties are shown in Figure 7d. The contours present in the Figure 7d signify the importance of H-bond donor and acceptor characters in the region. In principle, almost all compounds have amide group present in the region and hence presence of these contours is correlated with potentially donor and acceptor amide group.

4. Conclusion

Present study correlates the cholinesterase inhibitory activities of isolated natural compounds with the steric, electrostatic and hydrophobicity parameters. Statistically significant 3D-QSAR models of the steroidal alkaloids inhibitors were designed by exploring multiple conformations of each ligand using the genetic algorithm. An alignment technique scheme was generated from the docking results and it yielded highly predictive 3D-QSAR models. The good correlation observed in all cases of 3D-QSAR supports the proposed method of alignment and selection of conformers.

Final models were validated by the prediction of inhibitory activities of the test set compounds. In terms of external predictions, CoMSIA and CoMFA both performed great. A comparison of the 3D-QSAR PLS coefficient contour maps with the structural and functional features of the binding sites also showed good correlation. It is evident from the contour plots of both analyses that the hydrophobic effect plays main contribution to the cholinesterase inhibitory activity and it's quite in agreement with the fact that the cholinesterases are having a wide active site gorge lining with hydrophobic amino acid residues. Also, bulky groups in the side chain at R2 position generally cause the increase in activity but at the same time the bulkier substituent at position R3 resulted in decreasing the activity. This R3 position is covered by a yellow steric contour and hence the bulkiness at this region is detrimental to the activity. The preference for bulky group at position R2 as described in CoMFA, seems to be correlated in CoMSIA with increased hyrdrophobicity expected at the same region. As an attempt to exploiting the cholinesterase inhibitors for 3D-QSAR approach combined with all detailed information obtained by 3D-QSAR models, we strongly believe that this study can help to design novel molecules with improved activity in near future.

The results, together with the good correlations between the actual and predicted inhibitory activities, demonstrate the power of combined docking/QSAR approach to explore the probable binding conformations of compounds at the active sites of the protein target. Additionally, present study also demonstrates that charges resulting from different calculation methods may influence the results of CoMFA as well as CoMSIA, although in our case this effect has not been significant. This is evident from the q^2 values calculated for different charge calculation methods (Table 4).

5. Acknowledgment

Financial support from Higher Education Commission, Pakistan to Uddin, R., under Split PhD program is highly acknowledged. The authors are thankful to Dr. Michael A Brunsteiner, Dr. Hongbin Yuan and Dr. Pavel A Petukhov from University of Illinois at Chicago for their help in developing the GA scripts in SPL and Perl languages. Authors are also thankful to S. T. Moin for assisting during the calculation runs. Authors are grateful to the Pakistan Science Foundation (PSF) for financial support to develop computational chemistry software facilities at the ICCBS.

Authors are also thankful to the OpenEye for providing us free academic license.

6. References

Atta ur, R.; Choudhary, M. I.; Khan, M. R.; Anjum, S.; Farooq, A. & Iqbal, M. Z. (2000). New Steroidal Alkaloids from Sarcococca saligna. *Journal of Natural Products*, Vol.63, No.10, (October 2000), pp. 1364-8, ISSN 0163-3864

Atta ur, R.; Feroz, F.; Naeem, I.; Zaheer ul, H.; Nawaz, S. A.; Khan, N.; Khan, M. R. & Choudhary, M. I. (2004). New Pregnane-type Steroidal Alkaloids from Sarcocca saligna and their Cholinesterase Inhibitory Activity. *Steroids*, Vol.69, No.11-12, (October-November 2004), pp. 735-41, ISSN 0039-128X

Atta ur, R.; Feroz, F.; Zaheer ul, H.; Nawaz, S. A.; Khan, M. R. & Choudhary, M. I. (2003). New Steroidal Alkaloids from Sarcococca saligna. *Natural Product Research*, Vol.17, No.4, (August 2003), pp. 235-41, ISSN 1478-6419

Atta ur, R.; Nasreen, A.; Akhtar, F.; Shekhani, M. S.; Clardy, J.; Parvez, M. & Choudhary, M. I. (1997). Antifungal Diterpenoid Alkaloids from Delphinium denudatum. *Journal of Natural Products*, Vol.60, No.5, (May 1997), pp. 472-474, ISSN 0163-3864

Atta ur, R.; Zaheer ul, H.; Feroz, F.; Khalid, A.; Nawaz, S. A.; Khan, M. R. & Choudhary, M. I. (2004). New Cholinesterase-Inhibiting Steroidal Alkaloids from Sarcococca saligna. *Helvetica Chimica Acta*, Vol.87, No.2, (February 2004), pp. 439, ISSN 1522-2675

Atta ur, R.; Zaheer ul, H.; Khalid, A.; Anjum, S.; Khan, M. R. & Choudhary, M. I. (2002). Pregnane-type Steroidal Alkaloids of Sarcococca saligna: A New Class of Cholinesterases Inhibitors. *Helvetica Chimica Acta*, Vol.85, No.2, (Februay 2002), pp. 678-688, ISSN 1522-2675

Bazelyansky, M.; Robey, E. & Kirsch, J. F. (1986). Fractional diffusion-limited component of reactions catalyzed by acetylcholinesterase. *Biochemistry*, Vol.25, No.1, (January 1986), pp. 125-30, ISSN 0006-2960

Behra, M.; Cousin, X.; Bertrand, C.; Vonesch, J. L.; Biellmann, D.; Chatonnet, A. & Strahle, U. (2002). Acetylcholinesterase is Required for Neuronal and Muscular Development in the Zebrafish Embryo. *Nature Neuroscience*, Vol.5, No.2, (February 2002), pp. 111-8, ISSN 1097-6256

Bohm, M.; St rzebecher, J. & Klebe, G. (1999). Three-Dimensional Quantitative Structure-Activity Relationship Analyses using Comparative Molecular Field Analysis and Comparative Molecular Similarity Indices Analysis to Elucidate Selectivity Differences of Inhibitors Binding to Trypsin, Thrombin, and Factor Xa. *Journal of Medicinal Chemistry*, Vol.42, No.3, (Febraury 1999), pp. 458-77, ISSN 0022-2623

Bourne, Y.; Taylor, P. & Marchot, P. (1995). Acetylcholinesterase Inhibition by Fasciculin: Crystal Structure of the Complex. *Cell*, Vol.83, No.3, (November 1995), pp. 503-12, ISSN 0092-8674

Buolamwini, J. K. & Assefa, H. (2002). CoMFA and CoMSIA 3D QSAR and Docking Studies on Conformationally-Restrained Cinnamoyl HIV-1 Integrase Inhibitors: Exploration of a Binding Mode at the Active Site. *Journal of Medicinal Chemistry*, Vol.45, No.4, (February 2002), pp. 841-852, ISSN 0022-2623

Butters, N.; Delis, D. C. & Lucas, J. A. (1995). Clinical Assessment of Memory Disorders in Amnesia and Dementia. *Annual Review of Psychology*, Vol.46, (February 1995), pp. 493-523, ISSN 0066-4308

Chatonnet, A. & Lockridge, O. (1989). Comparison of Butyrylcholinesterase and Acetylcholinesterase. *The Biochemical Journal*, Vol.260, No.3, (June 1989), pp. 625-34, ISSN 0264-6021

Cho, S. J.; Garsia, M. L.; Bier, J. & Tropsha, A. (1996). Structure-Based Alignment and Comparative Molecular Field Analysis of Acetylcholinesterase Inhibitors. *Journal of Medicinal Chemistry*, Vol.39, No.26, (December 1996), pp. 5064-71, ISSN 0022-2623

Clark, M.; Cramer, R. D. & Van Opdenbosch, N. (1989). Validation of the General Purpose Tripos 5. 2 Force Field. *Journal of Computational Chemistry*, Vol.10, No.8, (December 1989), pp. 982-1012, ISSN 1096-987X

Cokugras, A. N. (2003). Butyrylcholinesterase: Structure and Physiological Importance. *Turkish Journal of Biochemistry*, Vol.28, No.2, (October 2003), pp. 54-61, ISSN 0250-4685

Cramer Iii, R. D.; Patterson, D. E. & Bunce, J. D. (1988). Comparative Molecular Field Analysis (CoMFA). 1. Effect of Shape on Binding of Steroids to Carrier Proteins. *Journal of the American Chemical Society*, Vol.110, No.18, (August 1988), pp. 5959-5967, ISSN 0002-7863

Debnath, A. K. (1999). Three-Dimensional Quantitative Structure-Activity Relationship Study on Cyclic Urea Derivatives as HIV-1 Protease Inhibitors: Application of Comparative Molecular Field Analysis. *Journal of Medicinal Chemistry*, Vol.42, No.2, (January 1999), pp. 249-59, ISSN 0022-2623

Dominguez, C.; Boelens, R. & Bonvin, A. M. (2003). HADDOCK: A Protein-Protein Docking Approach Based on Biochemical or Biophysical Information. *Journal of American Chemical Society*, Vol.125, No.7, (Feb 19), pp. 1731-7, ISSN 0002-7863

Donini, O. A. & Kollman, P. A. (2000). Calculation and Prediction of Binding Free Energies for the Matrix Metalloproteinases. *Journal of Medicinal Chemistry*, Vol.43, No.22, (November 2000), pp. 4180-8, ISSN 0022-2623

Doorn, J. A.; Talley, T. T.; Thompson, C. M. & Richardson, R. J. (2001). Probing the Active Sites of Butyrylcholinesterase and Cholesterol Esterase with Isomalathion: Conserved Stereoselective Inactivation of Serine Hydrolases Structurally Related to Acetylcholinesterase. *Chemical Research in Toxicology*, Vol.14, No.7, (July 2001), pp. 807-13, ISSN 0893-228X

Fogel, L. J.; Owens, A. J. & Walsh, M. J. (1966). *Artificial Intelligence Through Simulated Evolution*, Wiley, New York

Forrest, S. (1993). Genetic Algorithms: Principles of Natural Selection Applied to Computation. *Science*, Vol.261, No.5123, (August 1993), pp. 872, ISSN 0036-8075

FRED (2007). FRED, version 2.2.3, OpenEye Scientific Software, Inc., Santa Fe, NM, USA, www.eyesopen.com, 2007. pp.

Geladi, P. & Kowalski, B. R. (1986). Partial Least Squares: A Tutorial. *Analytica Chimica Acta*, Vol.185, (July 1986), pp. 1-17, ISSN 0003-2670

Giacobini, E. (2003). Cholinesterases: New Roles in Brain Function and in Alzheimer's Disease. *Neurochemical Research*, Vol.28, No.3-4, (April 2003), pp. 515-22, ISSN 0364-3190

Giacobini, E. (1964). Metabolic Relations Between Glia and Neurons Studied in Single Cells, In: *Morphological and Biochemical Correlates of Neural Activity*, pp. 15-38, Harper & Row, ISBN 978-006-1406-40-9, New York, USA

Goldberg, D. E. (1989). *Genetic Algorithm in Search, Optimization and Machine Learning*, Addison-Wesley Professional, ISBN 978-020-1157-673, Reading, MA

Graybiel, A. M. & Ragsdale, C. W., Jr. (1982). Pseudocholinesterase Staining in the Primary Visual Pathway of the Macaque Monkey. *Nature*, Vol.299, No.5882, (September 1982), pp. 439-42, ISSN 0028-0836

Greig, N. H.; Utsuki, T.; Yu, Q.; Zhu, X.; Holloway, H. W.; Perry, T.; Lee, B.; Ingram, D. K. & Lahiri, D. K. (2001). A New Therapeutic Target in Alzheimer's Disease Treatment:

Attention to Butyrylcholinesterase. *Current Medical Research and Opinion*, Vol.17, No.3, pp. 159-65, ISSN 0300-7995

Guillozet, A. L.; Smiley, J. F.; Mash, D. C. & Mesulam, M. M. (1997). Butyrylcholinesterase in the Life Cycle of Amyloid Plaques. *Annals of Neurololgy*, Vol.42, No.6, (December 1997), pp. 909-18, ISSN 0364-5134

Harel, M.; Sussman, J. L.; Krejci, E.; Bon, S.; Chanal, P.; Massoulie, J. & Silman, I. (1992). Conversion of Acetylcholinesterase to Butyrylcholinesterase: Modeling and Mutagenesis. *Proceedings of the National Academy of Sciences of the United States of America*, Vol.89, No.22, (November 1992), pp. 10827-31, ISSN 0027-8424

Holland, J. H. (1975). *Adaptation in Natural and Artificial Systems*, University of Michigan press, ISBN 978-026-2581-11-0, Ann Arbor, MI

Hu, X. & Stebbins, C. E. (2005). Molecular Docking and 3D-QSAR Studies of Yersinia Protein Tyrosine Phosphatase YopH Inhibitors. *Bioorganic and Medicinal Chemistry*, Vol.13, No.4, (February 2005), pp. 1101-9, ISSN 0968-0896

Jain, A. N. (2003). Surflex: Fully Automatic Flexible Molecular Docking using a Molecular Similarity-Based Search Engine. *Journal of Medicinla Chemistry*, Vol.46, No.4, (February 2003), pp. 499-511, ISSN 0022-2623

Johnson, M. A.; Hoog, C. & Pinto, B. M. (2003). A Novel Modeling Protocol for Protein Receptors Guided by Bound-Ligand Conformation. *Biochemistry*, Vol.42, No.7, (February 2003), pp. 1842-53, ISSN 0006-2960

Kalauni, S. K.; Choudhary, M. I.; Shaheen, F.; Manandhar, M. D.; Atta ur, R.; Gewali, M. B. & Khalid, A. (2001). Steroidal Alkaloids from the Leaves of Sarcococca coriacea of Nepalese Origin. *Journal of Natural Products*, Vol.64, No.6, (June 2001), pp. 842-4, ISSN 0163-3864

Khalid, A.; Zaheer ul, H.; Anjum, S.; Khan, M. R.; Atta ur, R. & Choudhary, M. I. (2004). Kinetics and Structure-Activity Relationship Studies on Pregnane-Type Steroidal Alkaloids that Inhibit Cholinesterases. *Bioorganic and Medicinal Chemistry*, Vol.12, No.9, (May 1), pp. 1995-2003, ISSN 0968-0896

Khalid, A.; Zaheer ul, H.; Ghayur, M. N.; Feroz, F.; Atta ur, R.; Gilani, A. H. & Choudhary, M. I. (2004). Cholinesterase Inhibitory and Spasmolytic Potential of Steroidal Alkaloids. *Journal of Steroid Biochemistry and Molecular Biology*, Vol.92, No.5, (December 2004), pp. 477-84, ISSN 0960-0760

Klebe, G. (1998). Comparative Molecular Similarity Indices Analysis: CoMSIA, In: *3D QSAR in Drug Design: Recent Advances*, pp. 87-104, Kluwer Academic Publishers, ISBN 978-904-8149-35-3, London

Klebe, G.; Abraham, U. & Mietzner, T. (1994). Molecular Similarity Indices in a Comparative Analysis (CoMSIA) of Drug Molecules to Correlate and Predict their Biological Activity. *Journal of Medicinal Chemistry*, Vol.37, No.24, (November 1994), pp. 4130-46, ISSN 0022-2623

Lemmen, C.; Lengauer, T. & Klebe, G. (1998). FLEXS: A Method for Fast Flexible Ligand Superposition. *Journal of Medicinal Chemistry*, Vol.41, No.23, (October 1998), pp. 4502-4520, ISSN 0022-2623

Lockridge, O. & Masson, P. (2000). Pesticides and Susceptible Populations: People with Butyrylcholinesterase Genetic Variants may be at Risk. *Neurotoxicology*, Vol.21, No.1-2, (February-April 2000), pp. 113-26, ISSN 0161-813X

Mack, A. & Robitzki, A. (2000). The Key Role of Butyrylcholinesterase during Neurogenesis and Neural Disorders: An Antisense-5'Butyrylcholinesterase-DNA Study. *Progress in Neurobiology*, Vol.60, No.6, (April 2000), pp. 607-28, ISSN 0301-0082

Massoulie, J.; Pezzementi, L.; Bon, S.; Krejci, E. & Vallette, F. M. (1993). Molecular and Cellular Biology of Cholinesterases. *Progress in Neurobiology*, Vol.41, No.1, (July 1993), pp. 31-91, ISSN 0301-0082

Massoulie, J.; Sussman, J.; Bon, S. & Silman, I. (1993). Cholinergic Function and Dysfunction: Structure and Functions of Acetylcholinesterase and Butyrylcholinesterase, In: *Progress in Brain Research*, pp. 139-46, ISBN 978-044-4897-17-6,

McGann, M. R.; Almond, H. R.; Nicholls, A.; Grant, J. A. & Brown, F. K. (2003). Gaussian Docking Functions. *Biopolymers*, Vol.68, No.1, pp. 76-90, ISSN 1097-0282

Medina-Franco, J. L.; Rodríguez-Morales, S.; Juárez-Gordiano, C.; Hernández-Campos, A. & Castillo, R. (2004). Docking-Bbased CoMFA and CoMSIA Studies of Non-Nucleoside Reverse Transcriptase Inhibitors of the Pyridinone Derivative Type. *Journal of Computer-Aided Molecular Design*, Vol.18, No.5, (July 2004), pp. 345-360, ISSN 0920-654X

Meshorer, E.; Erb, C.; Gazit, R.; Pavlovsky, L.; Kaufer, D.; Friedman, A.; Glick, D.; Ben-Arie, N. & Soreq, H. (2002). Alternative Splicing and Neuritic mRNA Translocation Under Long-Term Neuronal Hypersensitivity. *Science*, Vol.295, No.5554, (January 2002), pp. 508-12, ISSN 0036-8075

Nachon, F.; Asojo, O. A.; Borgstahl, G. E.; Masson, P. & Lockridge, O. (2005). Role of Water in Aging of Human Butyrylcholinesterase Inhibited by Echothiophate: The Crystal Structure Suggests Two Alternative Mechanisms of Aging. *Biochemistry*, Vol.44, No.4, (February 2005), pp. 1154-62, ISSN 0006-2960

Nachon, F.; Nicolet, Y. & Masson, P. (2005). Butyrylcholinesterase: 3D structure, Catalytic Mechanisms. *Annales Pharmaceutiques Francaises*, Vol.63, No.3, (June 2005), pp. 194-206, ISSN 0003-4509

Nicolet, Y.; Lockridge, O.; Masson, P.; Fontecilla-Camps, J. C. & Nachon, F. (2003). Crystal Structure of Human Butyrylcholinesterase and of Its Complexes with Substrate and Products. *Journal of Biological Chemistry*, Vol.278, No.42, (October 2003), pp. 41141-7, ISSN 0021-9258

OE ROCS, v. (2008). OpenEye Scientific Software, Inc., Santa Fe, NM, USA, www.eyesopen.com, 2008. pp.

Pan, X.; Tan, N.; Zeng, G.; Han, H. & Huang, H. (2006). 3D-QSAR and Docking Studies of Aldehyde Inhibitors of Human Cathepsin K. *Bioorganic and Medicinal Chemistry*, Vol.14, No.8, (April 2006), pp. 2771-2778, ISSN 0968-0896

Perry, E. K.; Tomlinson, B. E.; Blessed, G.; Bergmann, K.; Gibson, P. H. & Perry, R. H. (1978). Correlation of Cholinergic Abnormalities with Senile Plaques and Mental Test Scores in Senile Dementia. *British Medical Journal*, Vol.2, No.6150, (November 1978), pp. 1457-1459, ISSN 1759-2151

Prathipati, P.; Pandey, G. & Saxena, A. K. (2005). CoMFA and Docking Studies on Glycogen Phosphorylase a Inhibitors as Antidiabetic Agents. *Journal of Chemical Information and Modeling*, Vol.45, No.1, (Jan-Feb 2005), pp. 136-45, ISSN 1549-9596

Radic, Z.; Pickering, N. A.; Vellom, D. C.; Camp, S. & Taylor, P. (1993). Three Distinct Domains in the Cholinesterase Molecule Confer Selectivity for Acetyl- and

Butyrylcholinesterase Inhibitors. *Biochemistry*, Vol.32, No.45, (November 1993), pp. 12074-84, ISSN 0006-2960

Rarey, M.; Kramer, B.; Lengauer, T. & Klebe, G. (1996). A Fast Flexible Docking Method Using an Incremental Construction Algorithm. *Journal of Molecular Biology*, Vol.261, No.3, (August 1996), pp. 470-489, ISSN 0022-2836

Sabnis, Y. A.; Desai, P. V.; Rosenthal, P. J. & Avery, M. A. (2003). Probing the Structure of Falcipain-3, A Cysteine Protease from Plasmodium falciparum: Comparative Protein Modeling and Docking Studies. *Protein Science*, Vol.12, No.3, (March 2003), pp. 501-9, ISSN 0961-8368

Saxena, A.; Redman, A. M.; Jiang, X.; Lockridge, O. & Doctor, B. P. (1999). Differences in Active-Site Gorge Dimensions of Cholinesterases Revealed by Binding of Inhibitors to Human Butyrylcholinesterase. *Chemico-Biological Interactions*, Vol.119-120, (May 1999), pp. 61-9, ISSN 0009-2797

Saxena, A.; Redman, A. M.; Jiang, X.; Lockridge, O. & Doctor, B. P. (1997). Differences in Active Site Gorge Dimensions of Cholinesterases Revealed by Binding of Inhibitors to Human Butyrylcholinesterase. *Biochemistry*, Vol.36, No.48, (December 1997), pp. 14642-51, ISSN 0006-2960

Soreq, H. & Zaku, H. (1993). *Human Cholinesterases and Anticholinesterases*, Academic Press, ISBN 978-012-6552-90-4, San Diego, USA

Sussman, J. L.; Harel, M.; Frolow, F.; Oefner, C.; Goldman, A.; Toker, L. & Silman, I. (1991). Atomic Structure of Acetylcholinesterase from Torpedo californica: A Prototypic Acetylcholine-Binding Protein. *Science*, Vol.253, No.5022, (August 1991), pp. 872-9, ISSN 0036-8075

Sybyl, V. (2007). 7.3, Tripos Inc, St. *Louis, MO*, pp.

Tame, J. R. (1999). Scoring Functions: A View from the Bench. *Journal of Computer-Aided Molecular Design*, Vol.13, No.2, (March 1999), pp. 99-108, ISSN 0920-654X

Terry, A. V., Jr. & Buccafusco, J. J. (2003). The Cholinergic Hypothesis of Age and Alzheimer's Disease-Related Cognitive Deficits: Recent Challenges and their Implications for Novel Drug Development. *The Journal of Pharmacology and Experimental Therapeutics*, Vol.306, No.3, (September 2003), pp. 821-27, ISSN 0022-3565

Todorov, N. P.; Mancera, R. L. & Monthoux, P. H. (2003). A New Quantum Stochastic Tunnelling Optimisation Method for Protein-Ligand Docking *Chemical Physics Letters*, Vol.369, No.3-4, (February 2003), pp. 257-263, ISSN 0009-2614

Tormos, J. R.; Wiley, K. L.; Seravalli, J.; Nachon, F.; Masson, P.; Nicolet, Y. & Quinn, D. M. (2005). The Reactant State for Substrate-Activated Turnover of Acetylthiocholine by Butyrylcholinesterase is a Tetrahedral Intermediate. *Journal of the American Chemical Society*, Vol.127, No.42, (October 2005), pp. 14538-9, ISSN 0002-7863

Vicker, N.; Ho, Y.; Robinson, J.; Woo, L. L.; Purohit, A.; Reed, M. J. & Potter, B. V. (2003). Docking Studies of Sulphamate Inhibitors of Estrone Sulphatase in Human Carbonic Anhydrase II. *Bioorganic Medicinal Chemistry Letters*, Vol.13, No.5, (March 2003), pp. 863-5, ISSN 0960-894X

Viswanadhan, V. N.; Ghose, A. K.; Revankar, G. R. & Robins, R. K. (1989). Atomic Physicochemical Parameters for Three Dimensional Structure Directed Quantitative Structure-Activity Relationships. 4. Additional Parameters for Hydrophobic and Dispersive Interactions and their Application for an Automated Superposition of

Certain Naturally Occurring Nucleoside Antibiotics. *Journal of Chemical Information and Computer Sciences*, Vol.29, No.3, (August 1989), pp. 163 - 172, ISSN 1549-9596

Wang, L.; Merz, A. J.; Collins, K. M. & Wickner, W. (2003). Hierarchy of Protein Assembly at the Vertex Ring Domain for Yeast Vacuole Docking and Fusion. *Journal of Cell Biology*, Vol.160, No.3, (February 2003), pp. 365-74, ISSN 0021-9525

Wei, H. Y.; Tsai, K. C. & Lin, T. H. (2005). Modeling Ligand- Receptor Interaction for Some MHC Class II HLA-DR4 Peptide Mimetic Inhibitors Using Several Molecular Docking and 3D QSAR Techniques. *Journal of Chemical Information and Modeling*, Vol.45, No.5, (September-October 2005), pp. 1343-1351, ISSN 1549-9596

Wu, X.; Milne, J. L.; Borgnia, M. J.; Rostapshov, A. V.; Subramaniam, S. & Brooks, B. R. (2003). A Core-Weighted Fitting Method for Docking Atomic Structures into Low-Resolution Maps: Application to Cryo-Electron Microscopy. *Journal of Structural Biology*, Vol.141, No.1, (January 2003), pp. 63-76, ISSN 1047-8477

Xie, W.; Stribley, J. A.; Chatonnet, A.; Wilder, P. J.; Rizzino, A.; McComb, R. D.; Taylor, P.; Hinrichs, S. H. & Lockridge, O. (2000). Postnatal Developmental Delay and Supersensitivity to Organophosphate in Gene-Targeted Mice Lacking Acetylcholinesterase. *Journal of Pharmacology and Experimental Therapeutics*, Vol.293, No.3, (June 2000), pp. 896-902, ISSN 0022-3565

Yuan, H.; Kozikowski, A. P. & Petukhov, P. A. (2004). CoMFA Study of Piperidine Analogues of Cocaine at the Dopamine Transporter: Exploring the Binding Mode of the 3 Alpha-Substituent of the Piperidine Ring Using Pharmacophore-Based Flexible Alignment. *Journal of Medicinal Chemistry*, Vol.47, No.25, (December 2004), pp. 6137-43, ISSN 0022-2623

Yuan, H. & Petukhov, P. A. (2006). Improved 3D-QSAR CoMFA of the Dopamine Transporter Blockers with Multiple Conformations Using the Genetic Algorithm. *Bioorganic and Medicinal Chemistry Letters*, Vol.16, No.24, (December 2006), pp. 6267-72, ISSN 0960-894X

Zaheer-Ul-Haq; Wellenzohn, B.; Liedl, K. R. & Rode, B. M. (2003). Molecular Docking Studies of Natural Cholinesterase-Inhibiting Steroidal Alkaloids from Sarcococca saligna. *Journal of Medicinal Chemistry*, Vol.46, No.23, (November 2003), pp. 5087-90, ISSN 0022-2623

Zaheer ul, H.; Uddin, R.; Yuan, H.; Petukhov, P. A.; Choudhary, M. I. & Madura, J. D. (2008). Receptor-based modeling and 3D-QSAR for a quantitative production of the butyrylcholinesterase inhibitors based on genetic algorithm. *Journal of Chemical Information and Modeling*, Vol.48, No.5, pp. 1092-1103, ISSN 1549-9596

Zaheer ul, H.; Wellenzohn, B.; Tonmunphean, S.; Khalid, A.; Choudhary, M. I. & Rode, B. M. (2003). 3D-QSAR Studies on Natural Acetylcholinesterase inhibitors of Sarcococca saligna by comparative molecular field analysis (CoMFA). *Bioorg Med Chem Lett*, Vol.13, No.24, (Dec 15), pp. 4375-80, ISSN 0960-894X

Zhou, Z.; Fisher, D.; Spidel, J.; Greenfield, J.; Patson, B.; Fazal, A.; Wigal, C.; Moe, O. A. & Madura, J. D. (2003). Kinetic and Docking Studies of the Interaction of Quinones with the Quinone Reductase Active Site. *Biochemistry*, Vol.42, No.7, (February 2003), pp. 1985-94, ISSN 0006-2960

10

Insulin Resistance, Cognitive Impairment and Neurodegeneration: Roles of Nitrosamine Exposure, Diet and Lifestyles

Suzanne de la Monte, Ming Tong and Jack R. Wands
Rhode Island Hospital and the Warren Alpert Medical School of Brown University
USA

1. Introduction

In Western societies, Alzheimer's disease (AD) is epidemic (de la Monte, Neusner et al. 2009). For decades, the prevailing theories about AD pathogenesis focused on the roles of hyper-phosphorylated and ubiquitinated cytoskeletal proteins in neuronal perikarya and dystrophic fibers, and increased expression and abnormal processing of amyloid-beta precursor protein (AβPP), leading to AβPP-Aβ peptide deposition in neurons, plaques, and vessels, as mediators of neuronal loss, neuritic pathology, synaptic disconnection, and loss of plasticity. Apart from aging, which is the most dominant risk factor, it has not been possible to define convincing roles for AβPP-Aβ or phospho-tau accumulations as principal driving forces of neurodegeneration that could account for all of the protean manifestations of AD, including neuro-inflammation, mitochondrial dysfunction, white matter fiber loss, and neurotransmitter deficiencies. This point is particularly relevant with respect to sporadic AD, which accounts for the vast majority of cases. However, it is entirely possible that the focal points of 30+ years of intense research on the accumulation, abnormal processing, and misfolding of essentially two proteins are somewhat misplaced since these process could be the end-result rather than the cause of the pathophysiological processes that trigger and propagate the neurodegeneration cascade.

Growing evidence supports the concept that AD is actually a metabolic disease in which, neurodegeneration is mediated by impairments in brain glucose utilization and energy production that begin early in the course of disease, and worsen with its progression (Frolich, Blum-Degen et al. 1998; Hoyer 2002; Hoyer 2004; Rivera, Goldin et al. 2005; Steen, Terry et al. 2005). AD-associated reductions in glucose utilization and energy metabolism are accompanied by increased oxidative stress and neuro-inflammation, which appear to be driven by insulin and insulin-like growth factor (IGF) resistance in the brain. AD can be regarded as a brain-specific form of diabetes mellitus, i.e. Type 3 diabetes. This chapter reviews the data showing that sporadic AD in humans is associated with progressive impairments in brain insulin and IGF signaling, and contrasts the roles of peripheral insulin resistance disease states versus primary brain insulin/IGF resistance using data from both human and experimental animal studies. Epidemiological and experimental evidence supporting exposures, particularly to environmental toxins such as nitrosamines, rather than only genetic factors as causal in the pathogenesis of AD are discussed. Dietary and lifestyle changes that could reduce risk for developing insulin resistance diseases, including diabetes mellitus, obesity, non-alcoholic steatohepatitis and neurodegeneration, are discussed as public health strategies that must be considered in earnest.

2. Alzheimer's disease and brain glucose metabolism

Metabolic abnormalities in AD have been linked to deficits in brain insulin and insulin-like growth factor (IGF) signaling through pathways that are critical for maintaining neuronal survival, energy production, gene expression, and plasticity (Frolich, Blum-Degen et al. 1998). Thorough consideration of the pleitropic actions of insulin and IGFs helps to clarify how impairments in these signal transduction networks could account for many, if not all of the critical features of AD-type neurodegeneration, including increased: 1) activity of kinases that aberrantly phosphorylate tau; 2) expression of AβPP and accumulation of AβPP-Aβ; 3) oxidative and endoplasmic reticulum (ER) stress; 4) the generation of reactive oxygen and reactive nitrogen species that damage proteins, RNA, DNA, and lipids; 5) mitochondrial dysfunction; and 6) activation of pro-inflammatory and pro-death cascades. Moreover, impairment or inhibition of insulin/IGF signaling disrupts cholinergic homeostasis, thereby compromising one of the most important neurotransmitter systems utilized for neuronal plasticity, memory, and cognition.

3. Brain insulin and insulin-like growth factor problems in AD

The concept that AD could represent a metabolic disease stemmed from the findings that deficits in cerebral glucose utilization are detectable in the early stages of disease (Adolfsson, Bucht et al. 1980; Fujisawa, Sasaki et al. 1991; Caselli, Chen et al. 2008; Mosconi, Pupi et al. 2008; Mosconi, Mistur et al. 2009; Langbaum, Chen et al. 2010), and as AD progresses, so do the metabolic abnormalities (Hoyer and Nitsch 1989; Hoyer, Nitsch et al. 1991). Although several studies provided initial clues that insulin resistance could be an important feature of AD (Frolich, Blum-Degen et al. 1998; Hoyer 2002; Hoyer 2004), the human postmortem brain studies were critical for definitively establishing that both insulin resistance and insulin deficiency in the brain were consistent and fundamental abnormalities in AD (Rivera, Goldin et al. 2005; Steen, Terry et al. 2005). Gene expression and receptor binding studies showed that in AD, brain insulin gene expression, insulin levels, insulin receptor levels, and insulin receptor binding were all impaired. Insulin resistance is manifested by reduced levels of insulin receptor binding and decreased responsiveness to insulin/IGF stimulation, while the trophic factor deficiency is associated with reduced levels of insulin polypeptide and gene expression in brain and cerebrospinal fluid (Blum-Degen, Frolich et al. 1995; Blass, Gibson et al. 2002; Hoyer 2004; Hoyer 2004; Rivera, Goldin et al. 2005; Steen, Terry et al. 2005). To consolidate these concepts, we proposed that AD be referred to as, "Type 3 diabetes" because it represents the conglomerate effects of Type 1 (insulin deficiency) and Type 2 (insulin resistance) diabetes, whereby the consequential metabolic abnormalities are largely restricted to the brain (Rivera, Goldin et al. 2005; Steen, Terry et al. 2005).

It has been well-established that insulin signaling mechanisms parallel, interact, or cross-talk with related insulin-like growth factor (IGF) pathways in various organ-systems, including the brain (de la Monte and Wands 2005). Despite apparent redundancy, insulin, IGF-1 and IGF-2 stimulations have differential effects on various target cells in the brain, and at different stages of development, maturation, and aging (de la Monte and Wands 2005). Ordinarily, insulin and IGF signaling networks overlap and complement one another, enabling deficits in one pathway to be compensated for by increased activation of one or both of the others, and thereby provide a kind of safety net for supporting critical neuronal and glial functions in the brain. Therefore, with regard to neurodegenerative diseases, it was of interest to determine if the impairments in insulin signaling networks in AD were selective, or whether they broadly affected IGF pathways as well.

The human postmortem studies demonstrated that, like insulin, AD is associated with significant impairments in IGF-1 and IGF-2 signaling mechanisms in the brain, and that as dementia progresses, so do the deficits in IGF signaling networks (Rivera, Goldin et al. 2005; Steen, Terry et al. 2005). AD-associated deficits in IGF signaling are marked by reduced expression of IGF trophic factors and receptors, and decreased binding to IGF receptors, reflecting IGF deficiency and resistance. Since the impairments in IGF signaling mechanisms develop and progress simultaneously with declines in insulin signaling, the scaffolding needed to support a broad range of functions, including cerebral glucose utilization, neuronal survival, myelin maintenance, metabolism, neurotransmitter function, and plasticity gets destroyed, practically en masse. Consequences include reductions in the expression of choline acetyltransferase, tau, and glyceraldehyde-3-phosphate dehydrogenase (GAPDH) genes, which mediate cholinergic/cognitive, neuronal cytoskeletal, and metabolic functions (Rivera, Goldin et al. 2005). Insulin/IGF resistance-mediated impairments in energy metabolism promote oxidative stress, accumulation of reactive oxygen species (ROS), DNA damage, and mitochondrial dysfunction, all of which drive pro-apoptosis, pro-inflammatory, and pro-AβPP-Aβ cascades.

4. Impaired insulin/IGF signaling and tau pathology in AD

Neuronal cytoskeletal lesions that correlate with severity of dementia in AD include, neurofibrillary tangles, dystrophic neurites, and neuropil threads, which contain aggregated and ubiquitinated insoluble fibrillar tau (Duyckaerts, Delatour et al. 2009; Takashima 2009). In AD, hyperphosphorylation of tau, a microtubule-associated protein, is mediated by inappropriate activation of kinases, such as glycogen synthase kinase 3β (GSK-3β). Hyper-phosphorylated tau is rendered highly susceptible to misfolding and self-aggregating into insoluble fibrils, generating dementia-associated cytoskeletal lesions (Iqbal, Liu et al. 2009). These degenerative processes lead to disruption of the neuronal cytoskeletal network and synaptic disconnection (Iqbal, Liu et al. 2009). In addition, pre-fibrillar tau aggregates to form soluble oligomers that are neurotoxic and can cause synaptic disconnection and neuronal death (Takashima 2010). Ubiquitination of hyper-phosphorylated tau (Arnaud, Robakis et al. 2006), along with dysfunction of the ubiquitin-proteasome system (Oddo 2008), result in further accumulation of insoluble fibrillar tau, oxidative stress, ROS generation, and cell loss in AD (Mandelkow, Stamer et al. 2003).

Brain insulin/IGF resistances contribute to the development and accumulation of dementia-associated neuronal cytoskeletal lesions (de la Monte, Ganju et al. 2000; de la Monte, Neely et al. 2001; de la Monte and Wands 2002; Xu, Eun Yeon et al. 2003) because tau gene expression and phosphorylation are regulated by insulin and IGF (Schubert, Brazil et al. 2003; Schubert, Gautam et al. 2004), and brain insulin and IGF resistances decrease signaling through phosphoinositol-3-kinase (PI3K), Akt (Schubert, Brazil et al. 2003; Schubert, Gautam et al. 2004), and Wnt/β-catenin (Doble and Woodgett 2003), which result in increased activation of GSK-3β (Nishimura, Yu et al. 1999; De Ferrari and Inestrosa 2000; Fraser, Yu et al. 2001; Mudher, Chapman et al. 2001; Grilli, Ferrari Toninelli et al. 2003). In addition, tau hyper-phosphorylation in AD is mediated by inhibition of protein phosphatases 1 and 2A (Hanger, Seereeram et al. 2009; Iqbal, Liu et al. 2009; Morales, Farias et al. 2010), which are regulated by insulin/IGF. Besides hyper-phosphorylation, tau pathology in AD is mediated by impaired tau gene expression due to reduced insulin and IGF signaling (de la Monte, Chen et al. 2003). Consequences include failure to generate sufficient amounts of normal soluble tau protein, vis-a-vis accumulation of hyper-phosphorylated insoluble fibillar tau, and attendant exacerbation of cytoskeletal collapse, neurite retraction, and synaptic disconnection.

5. Insulin/IGF resistance and amyloid-beta (Aβ) accumulation and neurodegeneration

Dysregulated expression and processing of amyloid precursor protein (AβPP) results in accumulation of neurotoxic AβPP-Aβ (Aβ) oligomeric fibrils and insoluble aggregated fibrils (plaques) in the brain. These lesions arise secondary to increased AβPP gene expression and abnormal AβPP proteolysis, leading to the generation of 40 or 42 amino acid length Aβ peptides that can aggregate. In sporadic AD, which accounts for 90% or more of the cases, the causes of Aβ accumulation and toxicity are not known, but over the past few years, the role of impaired insulin/IGF signaling has come into consideration. One argument is that Aβ toxicity causes insulin resistance. The opposing argument is that brain insulin resistance with attendant oxidative stress and neuro-inflammation, promotes Aβ accumulation and toxicity. The findings that insulin stimulation promotes trafficking of Aβ from the trans-Golgi network to the plasma membrane, stimulates Aβ secretion (Watson, Peskind et al. 2003), and inhibits Aβ intracellular accumulation (Gasparini, Gouras et al. 2001; Gasparini, Netzer et al. 2002) support the latter position. Moreover, experimental data indicate that impaired insulin signaling disrupts the processing of AβPP and clearance of Aβ (Messier and Teutenberg 2005), which again supports a causal role for brain insulin resistance. On the other hand, it is important to recognize that AD, and all other neurodegenerative diseases represent the effects of cascades that cause diseases to progress over time. Therefore, it is essential that we understand both initiating and propagating factors in disease because treatments can be preventive or interventional. The findings that: 1) Aβ disrupts insulin signaling by competing with insulin, or reducing the affinity of insulin binding to its own receptor (Ling, Martins et al. 2002; Xie, Helmerhorst et al. 2002); 2) AβPP oligomers inhibit neuronal transmission of insulin-stimulated signals by desensitizing insulin receptors; and 3) intracellular AβPP-Aβ interferes with PI3 kinase activation of Akt-mediated survival signaling and increases GSK-3β activation (promoting tau hyper-phosphorylation), suggest that dysregulation of AβPP expression and processing can exacerbate insulin resistance.

6. Insulin/IGF resistance, oxidative stress, and metabolic dysfunction in AD

Deficits in cerebral glucose utilization and energy metabolism occur very early in the course of AD (Iwangoff, Armbruster et al. 1980; Sims, Bowen et al. 1980; Hoyer 2004). Glucose uptake and utilization in brain are dependent upon glucose transport by glucose transporter 4 (GLUT4), which is stimulated by insulin. Therefore, impairments in brain insulin responsiveness could account for the deficits in brain glucose utilization and energy metabolism in AD. Deficiencies in energy metabolism correlate with the increased levels of oxidative stress, mitochondrial dysfunction, and pro-inflammatory cytokine activation in AD brains (Hoyer and Lannert 1999; Hoyer, Lee et al. 2000; de la Monte and Wands 2002). Oxidative stress leads to increased generation and accumulation of reactive oxygen (ROS) and reactive nitrogen species (RNS) that attack subcellular organelles, yielding DNA, RNA, lipid, and protein adducts that further compromise the structural and functional integrity of neurons. Consequences include disruption of the neuronal cytoskeleton, synaptic disconnection, neurotransmitter deficits, impaired neuronal plasticity, and reduced neuronal survival.

Mitochondrial dysfunction reduces ATP production, increases ROS, and triggers neuro-inflammatory responses through the activation of microglia and astrocytes. This cascade is propagated by neuro-inflammation inhibiting insulin/IGF signaling, and increasing stress, organelle dysfunction, pro-apoptosis signaling, AβPP expression, and aberrant AβPP cleavage with AβPP-Aβ deposition and toxic fibril formation (Lorenzo and Yankner 1996; Niikura, Hashimoto et al. 2002; Chen, Xu et al. 2003; Tsukamoto, Hashimoto et al. 2003; Blasko, Stampfer-Kountchev et al. 2004; Eikelenboom and van Gool 2004; Tuppo and Arias 2005). Persistence of oxidative stress leads to constitutive activation of kinases e.g. GSK-3β, that promote hyper-phosphorylation of tau. Therefore, oxidative stress and energy imbalances stemming from brain insulin/IGF resistance contribute to the cascade of neuronal loss, AβPP toxicity, tau cytoskeletal pathology, and neuro-inflammation (de la Monte and Wands 2005; Rivera, Goldin et al. 2005; de la Monte, Tong et al. 2006).

7. Peripheral versus central mediators of brain insulin/IGF deficiency and resistance

The molecular and biochemical abnormalities in AD brains closely mimic those present in diabetes mellitus; however, until recently, the vast majority of sporadic AD cases had no association with diabetes. In fact, prior to 1980, the epidemiological trends for AD (increasing prevalence) were opposite those of diabetes mellitus (declining as a cause of death) (de la Monte, Neusner et al. 2009). Even today, most cases of AD arise in the absence of type 2 diabetes, obesity, or metabolic syndrome, indicating that insulin/IGF resistance and deficiency can selectively involve the brain. Similarly, brain-only insulin and/or IGF resistance with cognitive impairment and AD-type neurodegeneration can be produced by intracerebroventricular (ICV) administration of small interfering (si)-RNA duplexes targeting the insulin or IGF receptors (see below), genetic depletion of insulin/IGF receptors, or ICV treatment with streptozotocin (STZ), which destroys insulin and IGF receptor bearing cells (Biju and Paulose 1998; Lannert and Hoyer 1998; Hoyer, Lannert et al. 1999; Hoyer, Lee et al. 2000; Nitta, Murai et al. 2002; Weinstock and Shoham 2004; Lester-Coll, Rivera et al. 2006; Grunblatt, Salkovic-Petrisic et al. 2007; Labak, Foniok et al. 2010; de la Monte, Tong et al. 2011). These studies support a primary role for brain insulin/IGF resistance and deficiency as the cause of AD-type neurodegeneration.

Within the past 2-3 decades, morbidity and mortality rates have trended upward for diabetes and other insulin resistance diseases, including metabolic syndrome (dyslipidemic states), non-alcoholic steatohepatitis (NASH), and obesity, despite improvements in medical treatment (de la Monte, Neusner et al. 2009). At the same time, the increasing overlap between cognitive impairment or AD and peripheral insulin resistance diseases has raised concerns about the potential contributions or even causal roles of obesity and diabetes mellitus in neurodegeneration and dementia (Qiu, De Ronchi et al. 2007; de la Monte, Neusner et al. 2009). Correspondingly, a number of human and experimental animal studies have demonstrated significant associations between peripheral insulin resistance states, obesity, or diabetes mellitus and brain insulin/IGF resistance, mild cognitive impairment (MCI), dementia, or AD (Craft 2005; Rivera, Goldin et al. 2005; Steen, Terry et al. 2005; Craft 2006; de la Monte, Tong et al. 2006; Lester-Coll, Rivera et al. 2006; Craft 2007). The debate over whether AD and cognitive impairment are caused by peripheral, brain, or both forms of insulin/IGF resistance is on-going, and essentially focused on three main questions: 1) Do T2DM and other peripheral insulin resistance states cause neurodegeneration, including AD? 2) How do T2DM and other peripheral insulin resistance disease states serve as co-factors in cognitive impairment and neurodegeneration? and 3) Is AD fundamentally a brain-specific form of diabetes mellitus? These questions are addressed below.

7.1 Potential roles of obesity and T2DM in cognitive impairment and neurodegeneration

Epidemiologic studies have shown that individuals with glucose intolerance, deficits in insulin secretion, or T2DM have a significantly increased risk for developing mild cognitive impairment (MCI) or AD-type dementia. Longitudinal studies also support roles for T2DM (Pasquier, Boulogne et al. 2006; Verdelho, Madureira et al. 2007) and obesity/dyslipidemic disorders (Martins, Hone et al. 2006) in the development of MCI, dementia, or AD (Haan and Wallace 2004; Luchsinger and Mayeux 2004; Ristow 2004; Launer 2005; Pasquier, Boulogne et al. 2006; Luchsinger, Reitz et al. 2007; Whitmer 2007). Despite these provocative observations, and an independent study demonstrating higher frequencies of peripheral insulin resistance in AD than in normal aging (Janson, Laedtke et al. 2004), postmortem human brain studies detected similar rates of AD among diabetics and controls (Nelson, Smith et al. 2008). Moreover, although experimental chronic high fat diet (HFD) feeding and diet induced obesity (DIO) with T2DM cause cognitive impairment with deficits in spatial learning and memory (Winocur and Greenwood 2005; Winocur, Greenwood et al. 2005), the resulting brain atrophy with brain insulin resistance, neuro-inflammation, oxidative stress, and deficits in cholinergic function are relatively mild and lack most of the important structural lesions that characterize AD pathology (Moroz, Tong et al. 2008; Lyn-Cook, Lawton et al. 2009). Therefore, observations in both humans and experimental models suggest that while obesity or T2DM can be associated with cognitive impairment, brain atrophy, and some aspects of AD-type neurodegeneration, these peripheral insulin resistance disease states are not sufficient to cause AD. Instead, the findings suggest that T2DM, obesity, and probably other peripheral/systemic insulin resistance states serve as co-factors that contribute to the pathogenesis or progression of neurodegeneration. The significance of this conclusion is that therapeutic strategies designed to treat T2DM, obesity, and systemic insulin resistance could help slow the progress or reduce the severity of AD, but will not likely prevent it altogether. Correspondingly, studies have already shown that treatment with hypoglycemic or insulin sensitizer agents can be protective for reducing the incidence and severity of AD (Luchsinger 2010).

7.2 Factors mediating cognitive impairment and neurodegeneration with systemic insulin resistance syndromes

Since it is clear that peripheral insulin resistance disease states can significantly and adversely alter cognitive function and contribute to the progression of AD-type neurodegeneration, efforts should be made to understand which aspects of peripheral insulin/IGF resistance are responsible for these effects. The rationale is that preventive measures could include treatments that ameliorate specific consequences of peripheral insulin resistance diseases, and the use of biomarkers that identify individuals who are at increased risk for developing MCI or AD. Moreover, treatments that restore peripheral insulin responsiveness could be used as neuroprotective agents as well. The ensuing discussion focuses on the roles of cerebral vascular disease and neurotoxic lipids.

7.2.1 Cerebral microvascular disease

How T2DM, obesity, and peripheral insulin resistance contribute to MCI, dementia, and neurodegeneration is not well understood. Factors under investigation include, chronic hyperglycemia, peripheral insulin resistance, oxidative stress, accumulation of advanced glycation end-products, increased expression and activation of insulin degrading enzyme, increased production of pro-inflammatory cytokines, and cerebral microvascular disease (Whitmer 2007). The potential contributions of cerebral microvascular disease require particular attention because chronic ischemic injury is an established mechanism of neurodegeneration, and diabetes mellitus causes significant microvascular disease. Chronic ischemic encephalopathy in AD ranges from multifocal ischemic lesions, to infarcts strategically localized in structures that are typically targeted for AD neurodegeneration, to leukoaraiosis with attrition of white matter fibers (Etiene, Kraft et al. 1998). Magnetic resonance imaging (MRI) studies have shown that lacunes and ischemic atrophy of medial temporal lobe structures (AD targets) increase with duration and progression of T2DM (Korf, White et al. 2006). Hyper-insulinemia and inheritance of the ApoE-ε4 allele also contribute to cerebrovascular disease and increase risk of AD progression. Insulin resistance and hyperinsulinemia can injure blood vessels and cause intimal thickening, scarring, and leakiness (Huang, Zou et al. ; Haudenschild, Van Sickle et al. 1981; Hotta, Taguma et al. 1996; Kubota, Kubota et al. 2003; Kincaid-Smith 2004; Matsumoto, Nakao et al. 2005). A recent study demonstrated that chronic ischemic leukoencephalopathy and leukoaraiosis in cerebral autosomal dominant arteriopathy with subacute infarcts and leukoencephalopathy (CADASIL) is associated with white matter microvascular insulin and IGF resistance (Brennan-Krohn, Salloway et al. 2010). White matter atrophy and fiber degeneration in CADASIL are associated with marked narrowing of vessel lumens, fibrotic destruction of vessel walls, and perivascular tissue attrition. In effect, the loss of vascular elasticity/compliance combined with compromised flow over time lead to chronic ischemic leukoencephalopathy. It is noteworthy that one of the earliest gross abnormalities in AD is white matter atrophy and fiber loss (de la Monte 1989). These findings suggest that, in addition to peripheral insulin resistance, systemic diseases that promote end-arterial resistance, e.g. hypertension could contribute to neurodegeneration by promoting cerebral microvascular disease. In fact, these mechanisms probably underlie the pathophysiology of vascular dementia. Future studies are needed to determine the degree to which reduced cerebral microvascular expression of insulin and IGF receptors correlates with cognitive impairment and neurodegeneration in AD and T2DM.

7.2.2 Neurotoxic lipids and neurodegeneration

Several studies have shown that cognitive impairment and neuropsychiatric dysfunction occur with liver disease caused by various agents, including alcohol abuse, obesity, chronic Hepatitis C virus infection, Reyes syndrome, or nitrosamine exposure (Schmidt, Gallo et al.

2005; Elwing, Lustman et al. 2006; Weiss and Gorman 2006; Karaivazoglou, Assimakopoulos et al. 2007; Loftis, Huckans et al. 2008; Perry, Hilsabeck et al. 2008; Kopelman, Thomson et al. 2009). These disease states are linked by the presence of hepatic steatosis or steatohepatitis with hepatic insulin resistance, endoplasmic reticulum (ER) stress, and increased generation of cytotoxic sphingolipids, including ceramides (de la Monte, Tong et al. 2006; Lester-Coll, Rivera et al. 2006; Moroz, Tong et al. 2008; Lyn-Cook, Lawton et al. 2009; Tong, Neusner et al. 2009; Tong, Longato et al. 2010). Mechanistically, inflammation, superimposed on disease states that promote lipid storage in hepatocytes, results in progressive ER stress, oxidative damage, mitochondrial dysfunction, and lipid peroxidation, which together promote hepatic insulin resistance (Capeau 2008; Kraegen and Cooney 2008). Hepatic insulin resistance stimulates lipolysis (Kao, Youson et al. 1999), and lipolysis leads to increased generation of toxic lipids e.g. ceramides, which further impair insulin signaling, mitochondrial function, and cell viability (Holland and Summers 2008; Kraegen and Cooney 2008; Langeveld and Aerts 2009).

Ceramides are lipid signaling molecules (Summers 2006) that cause insulin resistance (Liu, Obeid et al. 1997; Chalfant, Kishikawa et al. 1999; Arboleda, Huang et al. 2007) by activating pro-inflammatory cytokines (Summers 2006; Van Brocklyn 2007; Bryan, Kordula et al. 2008) and inhibiting signaling through PI3 kinase-Akt (Hajduch, Balendran et al. 2001; Bourbon, Sandirasegarane et al. 2002; Powell, Hajduch et al. 2003; Nogueira, Anhe et al. 2008). With steatohepatitis, hepatic and peripheral insulin resistance are accompanied by local and peripheral increases in ceramide levels (de la Monte, Tong et al. 2006; Lester-Coll, Rivera et al. 2006; Moroz, Tong et al. 2008; Tong, Neusner et al. 2009; Tong, Longato et al. 2010). Further studies showed that in vitro treatments with toxic ceramides cause brain insulin resistance, oxidative stress, and metabolic dysfunction (Tong and de la Monte 2009), and that in vivo administration (i.p.) of toxic ceramides causes cognitive-motor deficits, brain insulin resistance, oxidative stress, and neurodegeneration, similar to the findings in AD-type neurodegeneration. These findings led to the hypothesis that, in the settings of obesity, T2DM, and various peripheral insulin resistance states, cognitive impairment can be mediated via a liver-brain axis of neurodegeneration (de la Monte, Longato et al. 2009; de la Monte, Longato et al. 2009; de la Monte, Tong et al. 2010). We propose that livers with steatohepatitis, insulin resistance, and ER stress produce toxic lipids, in particular ceramides, that traffic through the circulation, and due to their lipid-soluble nature, cross the blood-brain barrier and exert neurotoxic and neurodegenerative effects by impairing brain and cerebral microvascular insulin signaling. This mechanism could account for the parallel and overlapping epidemics of peripheral systemic (T2DM, obesity, non-alcoholic steatohepatitis, metabolic syndrome) and brain (AD) insulin resistance diseases (de la Monte, Neusner et al. 2009).

7.3 Primary brain insulin/IGF resistance as the key pathogenic factor in AD-type neurodegeneration

The above discussion provides ample evidence that peripheral insulin resistance diseases can significantly contribute to the pathogenesis of neurodegeneration mediated through cerebral micro-vascular disease and/or liptoxicity effectuated via a liver-brain axis. However, on the whole, the neuro-behavioral, structural, biochemical, and molecular abnormalities produced by peripheral insulin resistance disease states are relatively modest compared with AD, reinforcing the concept that additional factors are needed to cause the full-blown disease. To better understand the underlying problems associated with AD and why peripheral insulin resistance diseases are themselves not sufficient to cause AD per se, the salient abnormalities in human AD brains requires scrutiny. Moreover, studies designed to produce states of brain but not peripheral insulin resistance must be examined and compared to both AD and the secondary effects of diabetes mellitus and other peripheral insulin resistance diseases.

7.3.1 Alzheimer's is a brain diabetes mellitus (type 3 diabetes)

A convincing argument could be made that AD, in its pure configuration, represents a brain form of diabetes mellitus (Rivera, Goldin et al. 2005; Steen, Terry et al. 2005) given that it is associated with progressive brain insulin/IGF resistance in the absence of T2DM, obesity, or peripheral insulin resistance (Rivera, Goldin et al. 2005; Steen, Terry et al. 2005; Craft 2006; Craft 2007). Moreover, postmortem studies demonstrated that the molecular, biochemical, and signal transduction abnormalities in AD are nearly identical to those that occur in both T1DM and T2DM (Nicolls 2004; Rivera, Goldin et al. 2005; Steen, Terry et al. 2005; Pasquier, Boulogne et al. 2006; Marchesini and Marzocchi 2007; Papandreou, Rousso et al. 2007; Pessayre 2007; Yeh and Brunt 2007). This led us to suggest the term, 'Type 3 diabetes' to better characterize the nature and pathophysiology of AD (Rivera, Goldin et al. 2005; Steen, Terry et al. 2005). These studies beg the question as to whether inhibition of brain insulin/IGF signaling is sufficient to cause neurodegeneration, particularly of the AD type? Alternatively, are factors other than brain insulin/IGF resistance required to mediate neurodegeneration? In this regard, one point that seems to get lost from the discussion is that IGF resistance and deficiency are part of the whole story, as was well documented in the human brain studies. With this in mind, data generated by siRNA inhibition of insulin, IGF-1, or IGF-2 receptor genes are presented to demonstrate the degree to which their adverse effects mimic AD. In addition, results of brain diabetes models produced by administration of streptozotocin are discussed in relation to human sporadic AD.

7.3.2 Experimental targeting of neuronal insulin/IGF receptors — in vitro model of neuronal insulin/IGF resistance

7.3.2.1 Methods

In vitro model. Primary cerebellar granule neuron cultures were generated from postnatal day 6 (P6) Long Evans rats (de la Monte and Tong 2009). Cerebellar granule neurons are a suitable model because the cells are non-transformed, they can be efficiently transfected with non-viral vectors, and they are highly dependent upon insulin and IGF signaling for function. In addition, the cerebellar cortex is a target of neurodegeneration in various diseases including, AD (Cole, Neal et al. 1993; Ishii, Sasaki et al. 1997; Larner 1997; Wegiel, Wisniewski et al. 1999). Freshly isolated cerebellar granule cells were transfected with commercially prepared small interfering RNA duplexes (si-RNA) targeting insulin receptor (siInR) [INSR NM_017071], IGF-1 receptor (siIGF-1R) [IGF1R NM_052807], IGF-2R (siIGF-IIR) [IGF2R NM_012756], or no specific gene sequences (Scrambled; si-Scr) [NM D-001210-01-20] using the Amaxa "v" nucleofector cell line reagents and the Amaxa nucleofector apparatus (Amaxa, Inc. Gaithersburg, MD). With this approach, we achieved 75-90% transfection efficiencies as determined by fluorescence microscopic imaging of cells co-transfected with recombinant plasmid expressing green fluorescent protein (GFP). Cells were seeded into 96-well plates to measure viability, mitochondrial function, and immunoreactivity, or 6-well plates to measure gene expression after 24 or 48 hours in culture. Cell density was determined by labeling the cultures with 10 μg/ml Hoechst H33342 in Tris-buffered saline (TBS), and measuring fluorescence (Ex360 nm/Em460 nm) in a Spectramax M5 microplate reader (Molecular Dynamics, Inc., Sunnyvale, CA). Mitochondrial function was measured using the 3-[4,5-dimethylthiazol-2-yl]-2,5-diphenyltetrazolium bromide (MTT) assay as previously described (de la Monte, Neely et al. 2001). Absorbances were measured at 540 nm in Spectramax M5 microplate reader. Gene expression and immunoreactivity were measured by quantitative reverse transcriptase polymerase chain reaction (qRT-PCR) amplification and cellular enzyme-linked immunosorbant assays.

Gene expression. Gene expression was measured by quantitative reverse transcriptase polymerase chain reaction (qRT-PCR) analysis, as described (Cantarini, de la Monte et al. 2006; Gundogan, Elwood et al. 2008). In brief, cells were lysed in Qiazol reagent and total RNA was isolated using the EZ1 RNA universal tissue kit and the BIO Robot EZ1 (Qiagen, Inc., Valencia, CA). RNA was reverse transcribed using random oligodeoxynucleotide primers and the AMV First Strand cDNA synthesis kit. The cDNA templates were used in qPCR amplifications with gene specific primer pairs published elsewhere (Gundogan, Elwood et al. 2008). Primers were designed using MacVector 10 software (MacVector, Inc., Cary, NC) and their target specificity was verified using NCBI-BLAST (Basic Local Alignment Search Tool). Amplified signals from triplicate reactions were detected and analyzed using the Mastercycler ep realplex instrument and software (Eppendorf AG, Hamburg, Germany). Relative mRNA abundance was calculated from the ng ratios of specific mRNA to 18S rRNA measured in the same samples. Inter-group statistical comparisons were made using calculated mRNA/18S rRNA ratios.

Immunoreactivity. Cellular enzyme-linked immunosorbant assays (ELISAs) were used to measure immunoreactivity directly in fixed cultured cells (96-well plates) (de la Monte, Ganju et al. 1999). The main modification of the original protocol was that immunoreactivity was detected with Amplex Red fluorophor (Ex 579/Em 595) instead of a colorimetric reagent. Cell density was assessed by staining the cells with Hoechst H33342 and measuring fluorescence (Ex360 nm/Em460 nm) in a Spectramax M5 microplate reader. The calculated ratios of fluorescence immunoreactivity (fluorescence light units; FLU) to H33342 were used for inter-group comparisons. Eight replicate cultures were analyzed in each experiment.

Statistics. Inter-group (N=8-12/group) comparisons were made using one-way analysis of variance (ANOVA) with the Tukey post-hoc test. Statistical analyses were performed using the GraphPad Prism 5 software (San Diego, CA) and significant P-values (<0.05) are indicated over the graphs.

Reagents. Rabbit, mouse, or goat generated monoclonal or polyclonal antibodies to tau, phospho-tau (AT8-S199, S202, T205), glial fibrillary acidic protein (GFAP), choline acetyltransferase (ChAT), Amyloid-β precursor protein (AβPP), AβPP-amyloid-β peptide (AβPP-Aβ), acetylcholinesterase (AChE), and Hu (neuronal marker) were purchased from Chemicon (Tecumsula, CA), CalBiochem (Carlsbad, CA), Molecular Probes (Eugene, OR), Invitrogen (Carlsbad, CA), or Abcam (Cambridge, MA). All other immunodetection reagents were purchased from Vector Laboratories (Burlingame, CA) or Molecular Probes (Eugene, OR). Histochoice fixative was purchased from Amresco, Inc (Solon, OH). QIAzol Lysis Reagent for RNA extraction and QuantiTect SYBR Green PCR Mix were obtained from Qiagen, Inc (Valencia, CA). The AMV 1st Strand cDNA Synthesis kit was purchased from Roche Applied Science (Indianapolis, IN). Synthetic oligonucleotides used in quantitative polymerase chain reaction (qPCR) assays were purchased from Sigma-Aldrich Co (St. Louis, MO). Fine chemicals were purchased from CalBiochem (Carlsbad, CA) or Sigma-Aldrich (St. Louis, MO).

7.3.2.2 Results

si-RNA targeting of insulin/IGF receptors broadly inhibited expression of insulin and IGF polypeptide and receptor genes. The qRT-PCR analyses demonstrated that cells transfected with si-InR, si-IGF-1R, or si-IGF-2R had significantly reduced expression of the insulin and insulin receptor mRNA transcripts relative to si-Scr transfected control cells (Figures 1A, 1B). In contrast, cells transfected with si-InR had significantly increased expression of IGF-1 and IGF-1R relative to si-Scr transfected cells (Figures 1C, 1D). si-InR transfected cells also had significantly higher levels of IGF-1R relative to both si-IGF-1R and si-IGF-2R transfected cells (Figure 1C).

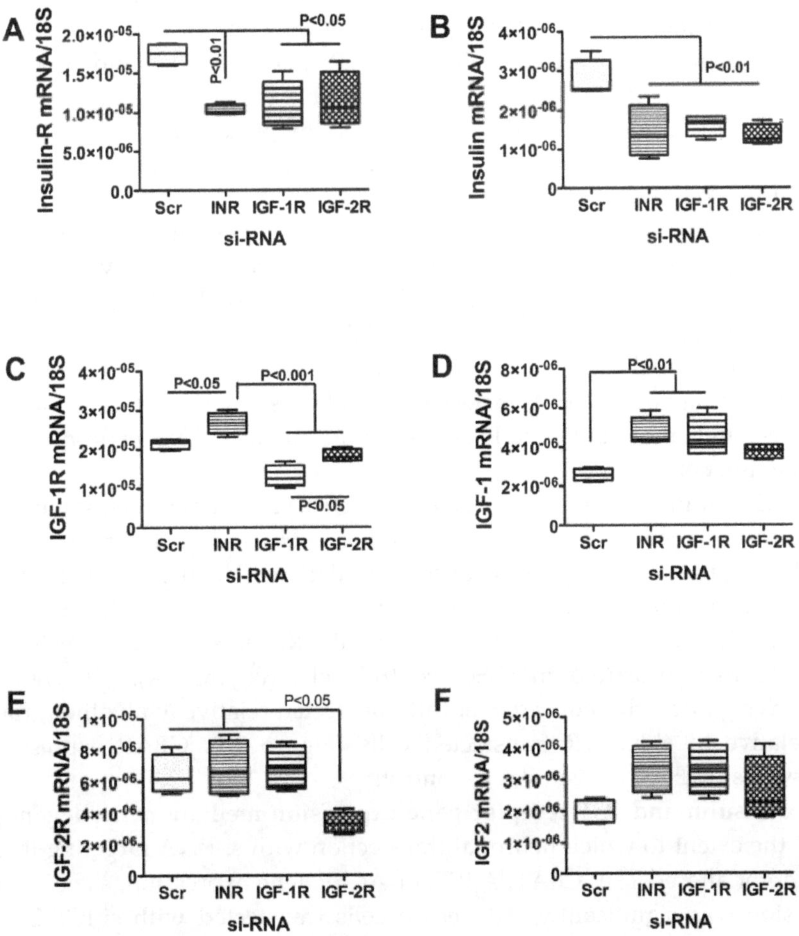

Fig. 1. Effects of si-RNA treatments on expression of insulin receptor, IGF-1, and IGF-2 receptors and polypeptide genes. mRNA levels of (A) InR, (B) insulin, (C) IGF-1R, (D) IGF-1, (E) IGF-2R, or (F) IGF-2 were measured by qRT-PCR with data normalized to 18S rRNA (N=8 per group). Inter-group comparisons were made by ANOVA and the Tukey post hoc test. P values are shown.

Cells transfected with si-IGF-1R had significantly reduced levels of IGF-1R relative to all other groups (Figure 1C) and higher levels of IGF-1 relative to si-Scr controls (Figure 1D). Cells transfected with si-IGF-2R had significantly lower mean levels of IGF-2R compared with the other groups (Figure 1E). IGF-1 (Figure 1D) and IGF-2 (Figure 1F) polypeptide expressions were generally higher in the experimental si-RNA groups relative to control, but the differences were only statistically significant with respect to IGF-1 mRNA levels in si-InR and si-IGF-1R transfected cells. Therefore, InR and insulin gene expression were inhibited in CNS neurons that were transfected with si-RNA targeting insulin, IGF-1, or IGF-2 receptors, while IGF-1R expression was selectively suppressed by transfection with si-IGF-1R, and IGF-2R expression was selectively inhibited in cells transfected with si-IGF-2R. With regard to the polypeptide genes, as noted, insulin gene expression was suppressed by si-InR, si-IGF-1R, or si-IGF-2R, whereas IGF-1 and IGF-2 mRNAs were generally increased relative to control. The latter could reflect a compensatory response to down regulation of the receptors. The aggregate results suggest that in cerebellar granule neurons, InR expression overlaps with IGF-1R and IGF-2R, and that some sub-populations express of IGF-1R and IGF-2R, while others may only express IGF-2R. Moreover, the findings suggest that the insulin polypeptide gene is expressed in insulin receptor bearing cells, whereas IGF-1 and IGF-2 are probably expressed in several different neuronal populations.

si-RNA targeting InR or IGF-2R impairs cell survival and mitochondrial function in neuronal cultures. Mitochondrial function was measured with the MTT assay, and cell density was measured by Hoechst H33342 fluorescence. MTT activity, corrected for cell density, was significantly lower in si-InR and si-IGF-2R relative to si-Scr transfected cultures (Figure 2A). In addition, the mean cell densities in cultures transfected with si-InR or si-IGF-2R were reduced relative to si-Scr transfected control cells (Figure 2B). Therefore, inhibition of signaling through the insulin or IGF-2 receptors impairs CNS neuronal viability and mitochondrial function.

Effects of si-RNA transfection on neuronal and astrocytic biomarkers. We used qRT-PCR analysis to measure gene expression corresponding to Hu and glial fibrillary acidic protein (GFAP), reflecting neuronal and astrocyte cell populations. The higher levels of Hu relative to GFAP reflect the predominantly neuronal nature of the cells isolated from cerebella (Figures 3A and 3B). Hu expression in si-InR, si-IGF-1R, and si-IGF-2R transfected cultures was similar to that measured in si-Scr control cells (Figure 3A). In contrast, GFAP expression was significantly reduced in si-InR transfected relative to all other groups, and in si-IGF-2R relative to si-IGF-1R transfected cells (Figure 3B). GFAP expression in cells transfected with si-IGF-1R was similar to control.

Inhibition of insulin and IGF receptor gene expression mediate neurodegeneration. We investigated the extent to which neuronal transfection with si-RNA targeting insulin, IGF-1 or IGF-2 receptor altered Tau, ChAT, AβPP, or AChE gene expression, as occur in AD. Tau gene expression was significantly reduced in cells transfected with si-IGF-2R relative to control (Figure 3C), corresponding with the somewhat reduced expression of Hu in the same cells (Figure 3A). In addition, AβPP mRNA was increased in si-InR transfected cells, and reduced in si-IGF-1R and si-IGF-2R transfected relative to si-Scr and si-InR transfected cells (Figure 3D). ChAT and AChE mRNA levels were significantly reduced in si-InR, si-IGF-1R, and si-IGF-2R transfected relative to si-Scr controls (Figure 3E and 3F).

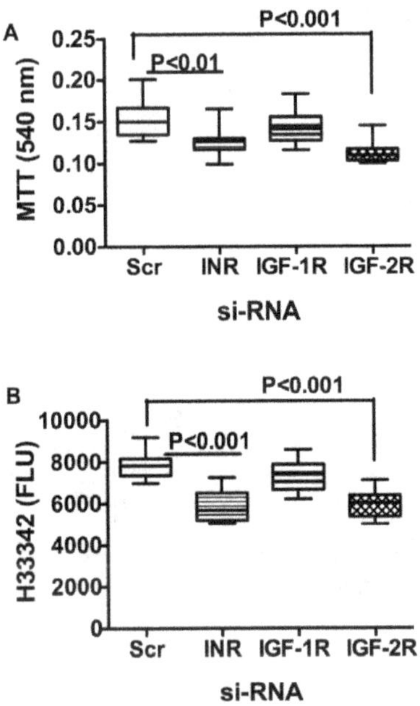

Fig. 2. Effects of siRNA treatments on mitochondrial function (MTT assay) and cell survival (H33342 fluorescence). N=8 cultures/group. Data were analyzed by ANOVA.

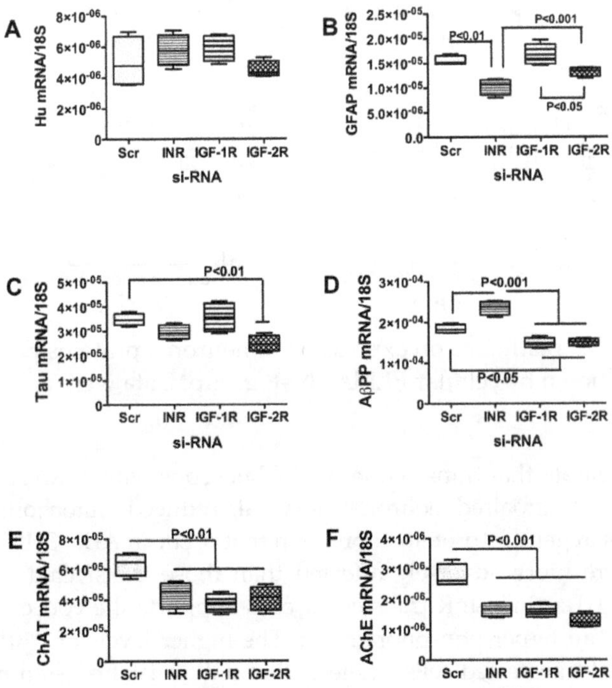

Fig. 3. Effects of siRNA treatments on expression of neuronal and glial genes shown by qRT-PCR. N=8 group. Data were analyzed by ANOVA.

Cellular ELISAs demonstrated similar mean levels of Tau and pTau among all groups, except in the si-InR relative to siScr transfected controls (Figures 4A and 4B). In addition, AβPP was significantly higher in cells transfected with si-IGF-1R or si-IGF-2R relative to si-Scr controls (Figure 4C), and AβPP-Aβ immunoreactivity was significantly increased in si-IGF-1R and si-IGF-2R relative to si-Scr and si-InR transfected cells (Figure 4D). Finally, corresponding with the qRT-PCR results, ChAT immunoreactivity was significantly lower in si-InR, si-IGF-1R, and si-IGF-2R transfected relative to controls (Figure 4E). AChE immunoreactivity was also significantly reduced in si-InR and si-IGF-1R transfected relative to control (Figure 4F).

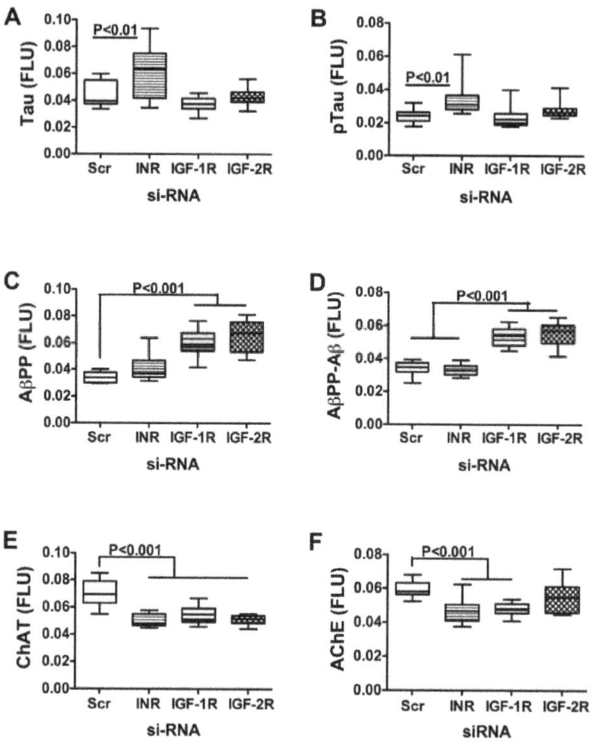

Fig. 4. Effects of siRNA treatments on expression of neuronal proteins pertinent to neurodegeneration shown by cellular ELISA. N=8 group. Data were analyzed by ANOVA.

7.3.2.3 Discussion

These studies demonstrate that transfection of CNS neurons with si-RNA targeting InR, IGF-1R, or IGF-2R leads to impaired neuronal survival, reduced mitochondrial function, and several abnormalities in gene or protein expression that occur in AD. Cells transfected with si-InR or si-IGF-2R were more adversely affected than those transfected with si-IGF-1R. The finding of increased pTau in si-InR transfected cells supports the concept that brain insulin resistance promotes Tau hyper-phosphorylation. The higher levels of AβPP and AβPP-Aβ in si-IGF-1R or si-IGF-2R transfected cells suggests that IGF resistance is an important mediator of AβPP-Aβ deposition and accumulation in brain. Cells transfected with si-InR, si-IGF-1R, or si-IGF-2R had reduced expression of AChE and/or ChAT. Altogether, these findings provide new evidence that molecular inhibition of insulin or IGF signaling in CNS neurons causes cellular, molecular, and biochemical abnormalities similar to those present in AD brains. Moreover, the findings suggest that signaling through the insulin and IGF receptors has distinct but overlapping effects; therefore, differential impairment of their functions produces different pathological and neurodegenerative effects, e.g. pTau levels increase with brain insulin resistance, AβPP expression increases and its protein is aberrantly processed with IGF-1 or IGF-2 resistance, and ChAT inhibition occurs with brain insulin and/or IGF resistance.

The overlapping inhibitory effects of the si-RNA transfections suggest that insulin and IGF-2 receptors are co-expressed in many of the same cells, and that IGF-1 and IGF-2 receptors are co-expressed in cells that have relatively low levels of insulin receptor. In addition, the reductions in insulin gene expression observed in cells that were transfected with si-InR, si-IGF-1R, or si-IGF-2R suggest that insulin polypeptide gene is expressed in insulin receptor bearing cells in the brain, and that endogenous insulin stimulation may be effectuated via autocrine or paracrine loops. Reduced cell density and mitochondrial function produced by si-InR or si-IGF-2R transfection suggest that signaling through the insulin and IGF-2 receptors is critical for CNS neuronal viability and metabolism. Moreover, the reduced Hu expression in si-InR- and si-IGF-2R- but not si-IGF-1R- transfected cells suggests that insulin and IGF-2 receptors are abundantly expressed in CNS neurons, as previously suggested (Xu, Eun Yeon et al. 2003; Soscia, Tong et al. 2006), and that signaling through either or both receptors supports neuronal survival and function. Sharply reduced levels of GFAP were detected in cells transfected with si-InR or si-IGF-2R. Since GFAP is expressed by astrocytes, the findings suggest that signaling through InR- or IGF-2R-regulated pathways is critical to glial cell survival and function. Therefore, inhibition of insulin or IGF-2 receptor signaling impairs neuronal and astrocyte survival and function, whereas inhibition of the IGF-1 receptor alone is not detrimental to CNS cell survival or energy metabolism.

We investigated the degree to which molecular abnormalities characteristically associated with AD are produced by inhibiting insulin, IGF-1, or IGF-2 receptor expression in CNS neurons. Cells transfected with si-InR, si-IGF-1R, or si-IGF-2R each had reduced levels of ChAT, corresponding with an earlier finding that ChAT is regulated by insulin and IGF (Soscia, Tong et al. 2006). ChAT generates acetylcholine, which has an important role in cognitive and motor functions (Dineley-Miller and Patrick 1992; Deutsch, Urbano et al. 2010; Peeyush, Savitha et al. 2010; Pepeu and Giovannini 2010). Since inhibition of neuronal insulin, IGF-1, or IGF-2 receptors leads to deficits in ChAT expression, impairments in cognition can be attributed to CNS insulin/IGF resistance (Rivera, Goldin et al. 2005; Lester-Coll, Rivera et al. 2006; Soscia, Tong et al. 2006; de la Monte and Wands 2008; de la Monte 2009; de la Monte, Longato et al. 2009; Lyn-Cook, Lawton et al. 2009; Tong, Longato et al. 2010). AChE expression was suppressed by the same si-RNA treatments. Although the down--regulation of AChE could represent a compensatory neuroprotective response (Noh, Koh et al. 2009) to decreased ChAT, instead it could represent a damaging effect leading to increased apoptosis (Greenberg, Toiber et al. 2010).

Transfection of CNS neurons with si-InR or si-IGF-2R inhibited Tau gene expression, while si-InR increased pTau immunoreactivity. These results corroborate previous reports that tau expression is stimulated by insulin and IGFs, while increased tau phosphorylation is mediated by impaired signaling through the insulin receptor and activation of kinases such as GSK-3β (Hong and Lee 1997). The increased levels of AβPP and AβPP-Aβ immunoreactivity in cultures transfected with si-IGF-1R and si-IGF-2R suggest that intact signaling through the IGF-1 and IGF-2 receptors may be important for regulating metabolism of AβPP and clearance of AβPP-Aβ. Since si-IGF-2R reduced expression of GFAP, astrocytes may play important roles in AβPP and AβPP-Aβ processing and clearance in the brain. On the other hand, cultures transfected with si-InR had increased AβPP gene expression, similar to the findings in AD (Rivera, Goldin et al. 2005; Steen, Terry et al. 2005). This effect could be mediated by increased oxidative stress caused by reduced energy metabolism and increased phospho-tau. Previous studies showed that oxidative stress was sufficient to increase CNS neuronal phospho-Tau and AβPP-Aβ (Chen, Xu et al. 2003). Together, the findings herein suggest that inhibition of insulin, IGF-1, and IGF-2 receptor expression and function have complimentary but overlapping roles in mediating the molecular pathogenesis of neurodegeneration, including AD. In addition, the results suggest that therapeutic measures should target all 3 receptors, since impairments of their signaling pathways would likely mediate distinct but overlapping components of the neurodegeneration cascade.

7.3.3 Experimental targeting of neuronal insulin/IGF receptors — in vivo model of brain insulin/IGF resistance

7.3.3.1 Methods

In vivo siRNA delivery. To evaluate the roles of insulin and IGF receptor resistance in relation to neurodegeneration in vivo, we generated a model in which P2 Long Evans rats were given a single intracerebroventricular (ICV) injection of si-InR [INSR NM_017071], si-IGF-1R [IGF1R NM_052807], si-IGF-2R [IGF2R NM_012756], or si-Scr (negative control) [NM D-001210-01-20]. For each rat, 0.4 nmol si-RNA plus 100 ng recombinant green fluorescent protein (GFP) expressing plasmid were combined with 10 µl of Dharmafect reagent, and injected into the right frontal region over the lateral ventricle using a Hamilton syringe with a 26-gauge needle as previously described (de la Monte, Jhaveri et al. 2007). GFP expression, which was under the control of a CMV promoter, was used to monitor success of the transfections. All rats survived the procedure, and none of them exhibited aberrant behaviors or adverse effects such as failure to thrive, poor grooming, reduced physical activity, or weight loss.

To monitor effectiveness of the transfections, rats (N=4 per group) were sacrificed at regular intervals after ICV gene delivery, and GFP expression was measured in whole brain by qRT-PCR analysis. Those studies demonstrated peak levels of GFP expression 2-3 days after ICV gene delivery, followed by a gradual decline in GFP mRNA levels. However, GFP expression persisted over the time course of the experiment as previously reported (de la Monte, Jhaveri et al. 2007). Gene expression and histological studies were performed with temporal lobe tissue. Upon sacrifice, temporal lobes were either immersion fixed in Histofix, embedded in paraffin, and used to make hematoxylin and eosin (H&E) stained histological sections (5 µm-thick), or they were snap-frozen in a dry ice/methanol bath and stored at -80°C for mRNA and protein studies. Our protocol was approved by the Institutional Animal Care and Use Committee at Lifespan-Rhode Island Hospital, and it conforms to guidelines set by the National Institutes of Health.

Morris water maze testing. We used Morris water maze tests to assess long-term effects of ICV si-InR, si-IGF-1R and si-IGF-2R on spatial learning and memory, corresponding to hippocampal function (Hamm, Dixon et al. 1992; McLay, Freeman et al. 1999; Gomez-Pinilla, So et al. 2001). Beginning on P24, rats were subjected to 3 daily trials in which latency (seconds) required to locate and land on the platform was recorded. On Day 1, the platform was visible, but on Days 2-4, the platform was submerged. On Days 3 and 4, the water entry quadrants were randomized for each trial. The data were analyzed using area-under-the-curve (AUC) calculations corresponding to performance over the 3 trials each day (de la Monte, Tong et al. 2006; Lester-Coll, Rivera et al. 2006).

Gene and protein expression. Gene and protein expression were measured by qRT-PCR analysis (see above) and direct binding ELISA. For ELISAs, temporal lobe homogenates were prepared in radioimmunoprecipitation assay (RIPA) buffer containing protease and phosphatase inhibitors (Lester-Coll, Rivera et al. 2006). Protein concentrations were determined using the BCA assay. 50 ng protein samples in Tris buffered saline, pH 7.4 (TBS) were adsorbed to flat-bottom surfaces of 96-well polystyrene plates, overnight at 4°C. Non-specific binding sites were masked by a 3-hour room temperature incubation with 300 μl/well of TBS + 0.05% Tween 20 + 3% BSA. Samples were then incubated with 0.1-0.5 μg/ml primary antibody for 1 h at 37°C. Immunoreactivity was detected with horseradish peroxidase (HRP)-conjugated secondary antibody and Amplex Red soluble fluorophore (de la Monte and Tong 2009). Fluorescence was measured (Ex 530/Em 590) in a SpectraMax M5 microplate reader. Parallel negative control assays had primary, secondary, or both antibodies omitted. Between steps, reactions were rinsed 3 times with TBS + 0.05% Tween 20 using a Nunc ELISA plate washer. Levels of immunoreactivity were normalized to protein content in the wells, which was measured using NanoOrange reagent.

Statistical analysis. Inter-group comparisons were made using repeated measures one-way ANOVA and the Dunnett post-hoc significance test for comparisons with the si-Scr control group. Statistical analyses were performed using the GraphPad Prism 5 software (San Diego, CA) and $P<0.05$ was considered significant.

7.3.3.2 Results

ICV si-RNA targeting the insulin or IGF receptors impaired spatial learning and memory. On Day 1 of testing, the mean latencies were longer for all experimental groups relative to control. However, the differences were significant only for si-InR- and si-IGF-1R-treated rats (Fig 5A). On Day 2, when the platform was submerged but entry was from a fixed position, the 95% confidence limits were broad for the 3 experimental groups, and inter-group differences were statistically significant only for the si-InR and si-IGF-1R-treated relative to controls (Figure 5B). On Day 3, the first day of randomized entry into the maze, the si-InR treated rats had significantly longer mean latencies for locating the hidden platform relative to control, whereas mean performance among si-IGF-1R and si-IGF-2R treated rats did not significantly differ from control (Figure 5C). However, performance among the si-IGF-1R treated rats was highly variable, as evidenced by the broad overlap with the si-InR and si-Scr treated groups. On Day 4, mean performances among the 4 groups were similar (Figure 5D). Therefore, the si-InR and si-IGF-1R treatments mainly impaired performance on spatial learning and memory tasks during the acquisition phases.

ICV treatment with si-InR, si-IGF-1R, or si-IGF-2R caused hippocampal hyopotrophy. Histological sections of temporal lobe, including the hippocampus, revealed normal architecture in siScr-treated controls, and pronounced hypotrophy of both the hippocampal formation and temporal cortex in rats treated with si-InR, si-IGF-1R or si-IGF-2R (Figure 6). The most striking abnormalities occurred in si-IGF-2R, followed by si-InR-treated rats, in which there were marked reductions in overall size of the temporal lobes, accompanied by conspicuously decreased neuropil volume rather than cell density (Figure 6). Since neuropil contains mainly interconnecting cell processes, the major adverse effects ICV si-InR, si-IGF-1R, and si-IGF-2R were to impair neuritic growth and synapse formation.

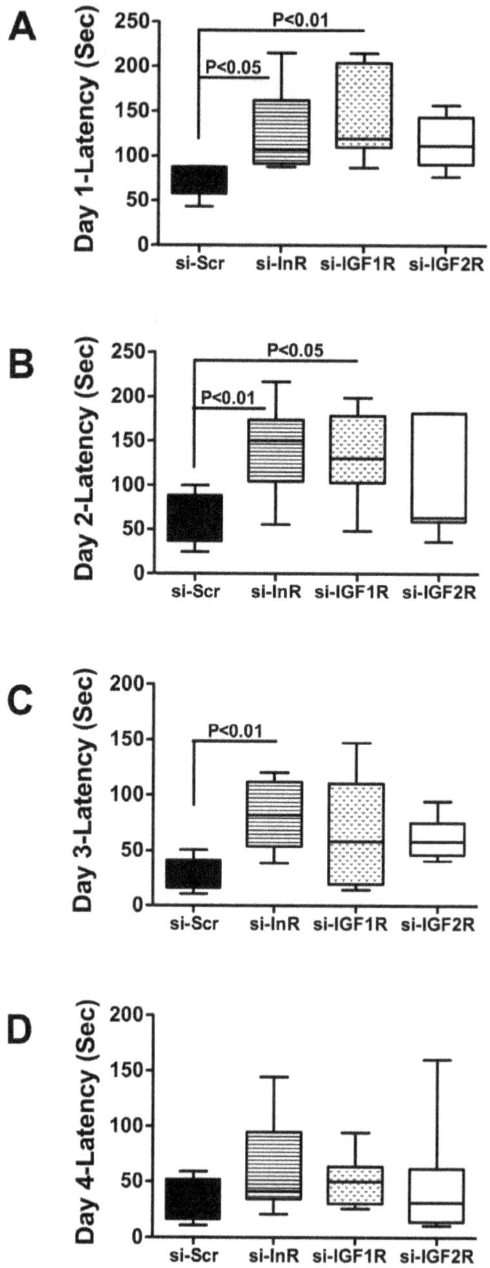

Fig. 5. Effects of ICV si-InR, si-IGF-1R, and si-IGF-2R on spatial learning and memory. P2 Long Evans rats were given ICV si-RNA targeting InR, IGF-1R, IGF-2R, or no specific gene (si-Scr). Morris Water Maze tests were performed on 4 consecutive days, beginning on P24. Data from the 3 trials/day were used to calculate area under the curve for latency. Comparisons were made by ANOVA and the Dunnett post-hoc test. Significant P values are indicated.

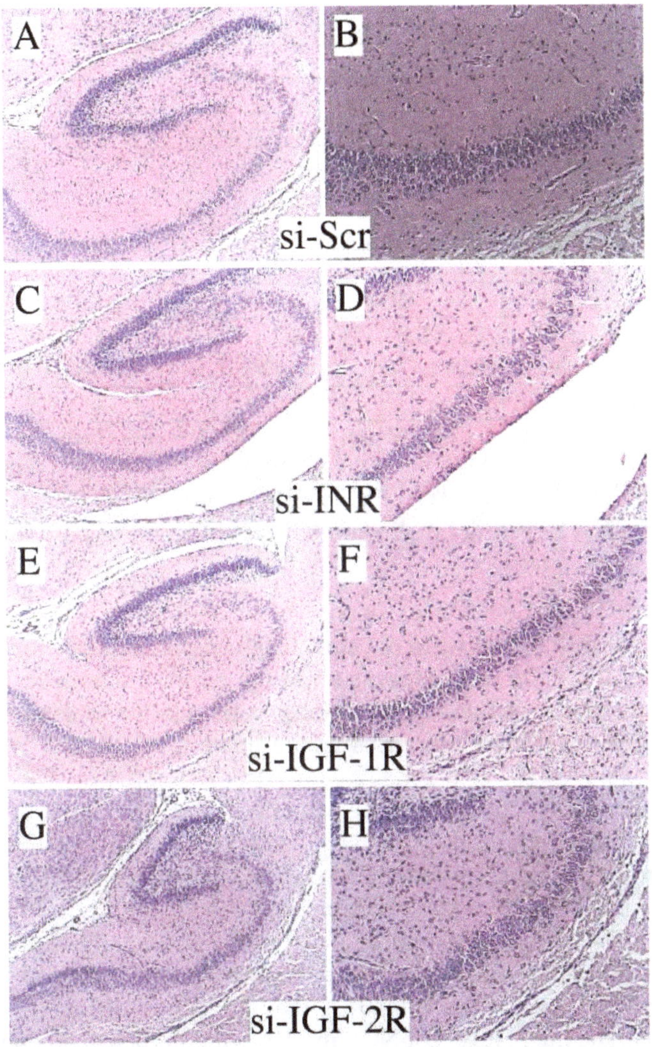

Fig. 6. ICV si-InR, si-IGF-1R, or si-IGF-2R causes hippocampal hypotrophy. Brains were harvested on P30, immersion fixed, and embedded in paraffin. Histological sections of temporal lobe, including the hippocampi, were stained with H&E. Panels A,C,E, G depict 40x original magnification images of temporal lobe and hippocampus, and Panels B,D,F,H show 100x original magnification images of the hippocampus from (A,B) si-Scr, (C,D) si-InR, (E,F) si-IGF-1R, or (G,H) si-IGF-2R transfected brains. Note extreme hypotrophy of the temporal lobe and hippocampus in si-IGF-2R and si-INR treated relative si-Scr treated controls.

Short-term effects of ICV si-InR, si-IGF-1R, and si-IGF-2R on insulin, IGF, and neurotrophin signaling (Table 1). Gene expression analysis performed on P9, i.e. 7 days after the ICV treatments, demonstrated significantly reduced temporal lobe levels of InR in the si-InR, si-IGF-1R, and si-IGF-2R treated groups (P=0.003). In addition, IGF-1R and IGF-2R expression were reduced in brains transfected with si-InR, si-IGF-1R or si-IGF-2R, although the inter-group differences were only significant for IGF-1R (P=0.008).

mRNA	si-Scr	si-InR	si-IGF-1R	si-IGF-2R	P-Value
Insulin R	15.3 ± 1.8	10.4 ± 0.6*	9.4 ± 0.8**	9.9 ± 1.1**	0.003
IGF-1R	8.3 ± 0.6	7.5 ± 0.8	7.0 ± 0.5	5.4 ± 0.4**	0.008
IGF-2R	7.9 ± 0.7	6.9 ± 0.5	6.5 ± 0.6	5.8 ± 0.6	
Insulin	0.19 ± 0.03	0.17 ± 0.04*	0.15 ± 0.02	0.16 ± 0.02	
IGF-1	2.4 ± 0.09	3.1 ± 0.17	2.6 ± 0.13	3.0 ± .29	0.008
IGF-2	49.5 ± 7.5	59.9 ± 9.4	49.1 ± 7.0	65.5 ± 5.0	
BDNF	1.6 ± 0.2	2.1 ± 0.3	1.3 ± 0.1	2.2 ± 0.3	
NGF	0.04 ± 0.004	0.06 ± 0.005	0.06 ± 0.009	0.08 ± 0.02*	0.0003
P75	14.5 ± 1.1	7.5 ± 0.8	8.2 ± 1.4	12.5 ± 2.5	0.008
NRTK	0.17 ± 0.06	0.24 ± 0.06	0.11 ± 0.04	0.16 ± 0.03	0.043
18S	2.9 ± 0.2	2.4 ± 0.7	2.8 ± 0.1	3.0 ± 0.2	

Gene expression was measured by qRT-PCR analysis. mRNA levels correspond to the mean ratio relative to 18S rRNA x10^{-6} ± S.E.M. Inter-group comparisons were made using repeated measures one-way ANOVA and the Dunnett post-hoc test for comparison with control (si-Scr). *P<0.05; **P<0.01

Table 1. Effects of siRNA targeting insulin and IGF receptors on receptor and trophic factor gene expression- P9 temporal lobe

Although insulin polypeptide gene expression was reduced in all experimental groups relative to control, the differences were not statistically significant due to the large variances and very low levels of insulin gene expression in the brain. In contrast, IGF-1 polypeptide gene expression was higher in the experimental groups relative to control (P=0.008). There were no significant inter-group differences in the mean levels of IGF-2 expression in the brain.

Neurotrophins and their receptors mediate structural and functional aspects of neuronal plasticity in the brain, their genes are regulated in part by insulin/IGF stimulation expression. Therefore, it was of interest to characterize the effects of ICV si-InR, si-IGF-1R and si-IGF-2R treatment on the expression of brain derived neurotrophic factor (BDNF), nerve growth factor (NGF), P75, and neuronal receptor tyrosine kinase (nRTK) by qRT-PCR. On P9, the mean levels of BDNF were similar among the groups, whereas for NGF (P=0.0003), P75 (P=0.008), and nRTK (P=0.043), the inter-group differences were statistically significant (Table 1). The mean levels of NGF mRNA were higher in all experimental groups relative to control, and the post hoc Dunnett test demonstrated significantly higher NGF expression in si-IGF-2R relative to si-Scr transfected brains (P<0.05). In contrast, the mean levels of P75 were lower in all experimental groups relative to control, and the post hoc Dunnett test showed that the differences were significant for the ICV si-InR and si-IGF-1R treated rats (both P<0.05). For nRTK, the mean mRNA levels were somewhat higher in the si-InR, and lower in the si-IGF-1R group relative to control, but the post hoc tests did not reach statistical significance (Table 1).

Sustained effects of ICV treatments on insulin, IGF, and neurotrophin signaling molecules in brain (Table 2). In P30 rats, 4 weeks after the ICV treatments, the mean levels of InR, IGF-1R, and IGF-2R expression were either similar, or somewhat elevated relative to si-Scr controls, but none of the inter-group differences were statistically significant. In contrast, insulin polypeptide gene expression was reduced (P=0.027), while IGF-1 expression was increased (P=0.011) in the 3 experimental groups. The mean levels of IGF-2 mRNA were also higher in experimental relative to control brains, but the differences did not reach statistical significance.

mRNA	si-Scr	si-InR	si-IGF-1R	si-IGF-2R	P-Value
Insulin R	9.9 ± 0.8	12.8 ± 1.3	11.5 ± 1.3	10.5 ± 1.1	
IGF-1R	7.1 ± 0.6	8.2 ± 0.9	8.4 ± 0.8	6.9 ± 0.7	
IGF-2R	7.0 ± 0.5	8.1 ± 0.9	7.5 ± 0.8	7.0 ± 0.7	
Insulin	0.23 ± 0.02	0.13 ± 0.02**	0.17 ± 0.03	0.16 ± 0.02	0.027
IGF-1	2.4 ± 0.09	3.4 ± 0.3**	2.8 ± 0.15	3.1 ± 0.28	0.011
IGF-2	49.5 ± 7.5	67.7 ± 12.5	52.8 ± 7.2	66.9 ± 5.0	
BDNF	1.6 ± 0.2	2.6 ± 0.3**	1.4 ± 0.14	2.5 ± 0.26*	0.0003
NGF	0.04 ± 0.003	0.07 ± 0.004	0.07 ± 0.01**	0.08 ± 0.01	<0.0001
P75	11.9 ± 1.8	9.1 ± 1.3	12.9 ± 3.5	15.5 ± 4.7	
NRTK	0.06 ± 0.01	0.28 ± 0.07**	0.12 ± 0.04	0.19 ± 0.02	0.0032

Gene expression was measured by qRT-PCR analysis. mRNA levels correspond to the mean ratio relative to 18S rRNA x10^{-6} ± S.E.M. Inter-group comparisons were made using repeated measures one-way ANOVA and the Dunnett post-hoc test for comparison with control (si-Scr). *P<0.05; **P<0.01

Table 2. Effects of siRNA targeting insulin and IGF receptors on receptor and trophic factor gene expression- P30 temporal lobe

Significant inter-group differences were observed with respect to BDNF (P=0.0003), NGF (P<0.0001), and nRTK (P=0.0032), but not P75 (Table 2). BDNF expression was significantly elevated in the si-InR (P<0.01) and si-IGF-2R (P<0.05) treated relative to control brains. The mean NGF mRNA levels were higher in all 3 experimental groups relative to control, and the post hoc Dunnett test demonstrated the differences to be significant for si-IGF-2R relative to si-Scr controls (P<0.01). Similarly, nRTK expression was higher in all three experimental groups relative to control, and the Dunnett post hoc test demonstrated the difference from control to be significant for the si-InR-treated group (P<0.01).

Sustained effects of ICV delivery of si-InR, si-IGF-1R, and si-IGF-1R on neuronal, cytoskeletal, cholinergic, and neurotrophin protein expression (Table 3): In P30 rats, Tau immunoreactivity was higher in brains transfected with si-InR or si-IGF-1R relative to control (P=0.0077).

mRNA	si-Scr	si-InR	si-IGF-1R	si-IGF-2R	P-Value
Tau	19195 ± 2951	26872 ± 1200*	23532 ± 2328	16110 ± 1946	0.008
pTau	3297 ± 467	2814 ± 164	2857 ± 128	2525 ± 119	
Actin	56026 ± 3356	63245 ± 1033*	63514 ± 997*	59794 ± 1373	0.0003
GAPDH	5244 ± 228	4856 ± 164	5214 ± 451	5172 ± 319	
ChAT	20244 ± 1863	15514 ± 606*	16660 ± 658	17375 ± 847	0.033
AChE	29347 ± 982	32767 ± 297*	34190 ±590***	31688 ± 1095	0.0013
BDNF	15932 ± 650	15563 ± 607	15353 ± 390	15936 ± 793	
NGF	38604 ± 3334	49538±1521***	45705 ± 816*	43071 ± 936	<0.0001
NT3	16714 ± 1178	11879±290***	13468 ± 499*	15528 ± 959	0.0004
NT4	7378 ± 378	9074 ± 1189	8197 ± 440	8357 ± 904	

Immunoreactivity was measured by ELISA and results were normalized to protein content in the wells. Inter-group comparisons were made by repeated measures one-way ANOVA and the Dunnett post-hoc test for comparison with control (si-Scr). *P<0.05; **P<0.01; ***P<0.001.

Table 3. Effects of siRNA targeting insulin and IGF receptors on neuronal structural and neurotrophin protein expression- P30 temporal lobe.

β-actin expression was higher in si-InR and si-IGF-1R relative to si-Scr transfected brains (P=0.0003). ICV delivery of si-InR, si-IGF-1R, or si-IGF-2R reduced temporal lobe levels of ChAT (P=0.036). In contrast, AChE immunoreactivity was elevated in si-InR, si-IGF-1R, and si-IGF-2R transfected brains (P=0.0013).

Corresponding with the qRT-PCR analyses, NGF expression was increased in the si-InR, si-IGF-1R, and si-IGF-2R treated relative to control brains (P<0.0001). The mean levels of NT3 immunoreactivity were lower in the 3 experimental groups relative to control (P=0.0004). There were no significant inter-group differences in the mean levels of pTau, GAPDH, BDNF, or NT4 in P30 rat brains.

7.3.3.3 Discussion

We used ICV injections to transfect brains with si-RNA duplex molecules targeting InR, IGF-1R, IGF-2R, or no specific genes (si-Scr). Previously, we used the same approach to generate a model of neurodegeneration, and demonstrated sustained transgene expression throughout the brain and in all cell types (de la Monte, Jhaveri et al. 2007).

Morris water maze tests demonstrated significant impairments in spatial learning in the si-InR, si-IGF-1R, and si-IGF-2R treated rats. Histopathological studies showed that the deficits in spatial learning were associated with reduced sizes of the hippocampi and temporal lobes, and hypotrophy of the neuropil, which contains interconnecting cell processes and synapses. Major abnormalities in AD include dendritic spine atrophy and synapse disruption. Since insulin and IGFs modulate neuronal plasticity and neurite outgrowth (de la Monte 2009), these findings suggest that AD-associated impairments in spatial learning and memory could be mediated by brain insulin and IGF resistance.

Gene expression studies showed that, in addition to reducing expression of the target genes, ICV si-InR, si-IGF-1R and si-IGF-2R each inhibited expression of the other two non-targeted receptors. The most likely explanation for this phenomenon is that cells in the temporal lobe express all 3 receptors at once. The inhibitory effects of the si-RNA treatments were most pronounced for si-InR. This finding, together with fact that all 3 experimental treatments resulted in hypotrophy of the temporal lobe and hippocampus, suggest that the adverse effects of the si-RNA treatments were mainly due to inhibition of insulin signaling.

Although GFP expression persisted in the brains due to continued presence of the plasmid, it is unlikely that the si-RNA molecules remained intact 1 or 2 days after transfection. The absence of any significant reduction in InR, IGF-1R, or IGF-2R expression at P30 indicates that the effects of the si-RNA treatments were transient with respect to gene expression. Therefore, the sustained effects of the si-RNA treatments on temporal lobe structure and function were mediated by short-term inhibition of gene expression during the critical postnatal period of synaptic plasticity and development. The relatively modest inhibitory effects on insulin and IGF polypeptides indicate that the structural and functional impairments caused by ICV si-InR, si-IGF-1R, or si-IGF-2R were mediated by insulin/IGF resistance rather than withdrawal of endogenously produced trophic factors.

We investigated the effects of the si-RNA treatments on neurotrophin and neurotrophin receptor expression because these molecules mediate neurite outgrowth, plasticity, neuronal survival, and other function, and insulin/IGF modulate expression and function of neurotrophins in brain (Maisonpierre, Belluscio et al. 1990; Cowansage, LeDoux et al. 2010). The studies demonstrated that the main adverse effect of the si-RNA treatments was to reduce expression of p75 neurotrophin receptor on P9. Otherwise, BDNF, NGF, p75 neurotrophin receptor, and nRTK were either increased or similarly expressed compared with si-Scr controls. ELISA studies demonstrated similar or increased expression of BDNF, NGF, and neurotrophin 4 (NT4) in P30 temporal lobes of experimental si-RNA treated rats, but significantly reduced expression of NT3 in both si-InR and si-IGF-1R treated rats. Since all neurotrophins, including NGF, BDNF, NT3 and NT4/5 function by binding to the p75 neurotrophin receptor (Frebel and Wiese 2006), early inhibition of p75 expression would have impaired neurotrophin signaling and could account for both the spatial learning deficits and hypotrophy of the temporal lobe/hippocampus in the si-RNA treated rats. NT3 regulates neuronal survival, synaptic plasticity, and neurotransmission, particularly in the hippocampus (Pae, Marks et al. 2008). Therefore, persistent reductions in NT3 expression represent local trophic factor withdrawal, which could have contributed to the cognitive impairment detected by Morris water maze testing. Although insulin/IGF regulation of neurotrophin and neurotrophin expression has not yet been characterized, the findings herein suggest that neurotrophin expression and function may be downstream of insulin/IGF signaling pathways in the brain.

In previous studies, inhibition of brain insulin and IGF signaling reduced expression of tau, ChAT, and GAPDH, increased pTau, and had variable effects on AChE expression (Soscia, Tong et al. 2006; de la Monte and Wands 2008; Tong, Longato et al. 2010). Corresponding with the normalized levels of InR and IGF-1R expression at P30, tau and GAPDH were not reduced, and pTau was not increased, but the impairments in cholinergic homeostasis were sustained in temporal lobes of si-InR and/or si-IGF-1R treated rats. ChAT is a major neurotransmitter that mediates cognitive function and plasticity throughout life (Perry, Piggott et al. 1993), and evidence suggests that besides insulin/IGF stimulation (Shi, Rabin et al. 1998), cholinergic function can be regulated by neurotrophins, including NT3 (Robertson, Baratta et al. 2006). It is noteworthy that in both si-InR and si-IGF-1R, ChAT and NT3 expression were reduced to greater extents than in si-IGF-2R treated brains.

These in vivo experiments demonstrate that sustained structural and functional developmental abnormalities can be produced by transient ICV transfection with siRNA molecules targeting insulin, IGF-1, or IGF-2 receptors. The long-term effects include deficits in spatial learning and memory, striking abnormalities in temporal lobe structure, and inhibition of mechanisms needed for cholinergic homeostasis. While these results are exciting and very much validate a role for primary brain insulin and IGF resistance as mediators of neurodegeneration and dementia, the structural changes in neurons and disorganization of the cortical laminar architecture that characterize AD-type neurodegeneration were not detected. This suggests that additional factors such as ongoing oxidative injury, are likely required to propagate the neurodegeneration cascade.

8. Experimental type 3 diabetes

The human studies provide convincing evidence that AD is associated with progressive insulin and IGF resistance and deficiency, accompanied by oxidative stress, deficits in energy metabolism, cholinergic function, neuronal survival, and synaptic plasticity in the brain. Given the fact that most cases of sporadic AD are not associated with obesity or diabetes mellitus, the said abnormalities must originate primarily in the brain. The siRNA experiments targeting the insulin or IGF receptors showed that inhibition of signaling through these receptors is sufficient to cause neurodegeneration and significantly impair a range of functions as observed in AD. On the other hand, the deficits, although sustained, were relatively static rather than progressive, suggesting that another "hit" was needed to propagate the cascade of neurodegeneration.

8.1 Toxin-induced brain diabetes mimics sporadic Alzheimer's disease

Analysis of postmortem human brains demonstrated progressive insulin and IGF resistance and deficiency with increasing severity of AD and dementia, which correlated with increased indices of oxidative stress and DNA damage, and reduced cholinergic homeostasis. Neuroinflammation and AβPP gene expression were increased early in the course of AD, but they either stabilized or declined as disease progressed. None of the subjects in those studies had diabetes mellitus, non-alcoholic steatohepatitis, or obesity. Perhaps the best model of sporadic AD is the one generated by ICV streptozotocin (STZ) treatment. STZ is a pro-diabetes drug that when injected systemically causes Type 1 diabetes mellitus (insulin deficiency) with higher doses, and Type 2 diabetes (insulin resistance) at lower doses. The i.p. or i.v. administration of STZ also causes mild hepatic steatosis and neurodegeneration (Biju and Paulose 1998; Szkudelski 2001; Bolzan and Bianchi 2002; Koulmanda, Qipo et al. 2003), but low dose ICV STZ treatment causes cognitive impairment with brain insulin resistance, brain insulin deficiency, and AD-type neurodegeneration, and not diabetes mellitus or hepatic steatosis (Biju and Paulose 1998; Hoyer, Lannert et al. 1999; Nitta, Murai et al. 2002; Weinstock and Shoham 2004; Lester-Coll, Rivera et al. 2006). STZ-induced neurodegeneration is characterized by impairments in brain insulin and IGF signaling, brain atrophy, impaired energy metabolism, mitochondrial dysfunction, oxidative stress, DNA damage, and increased AβPP, expression, AβPP-Aβ accumulation, neuroinflammation, and tau phosphorylation. Therefore, limited exposure to a single pro-diabetes drug causes neurodegeneration with all of the characteristic features of AD. Moreover, depending upon dose and route of administration, STZ treatment produces insulin resistance diseases that target the CNS, liver, pancreas, or skeletal muscle with variable degrees of overlap, or else the brain could represent the primary focus of disease.

8.2 Environmental/dietary causes of insulin/IGF resistance syndromes: Nitrosamine exposures mediate Alzheimer's, diabetes mellitus, and hepatic steatosis

Sporadic AD or Type 3 diabetes is overwhelmingly a brain-specific disease that leads to total body wasting and eventual arrival at a vegetative state. The closest experimental model of sporadic AD is that produced by ICV STZ, which does not cause systemic diabetes mellitus, i.e. Type 1 or Type 2. This very point begs the question of, what relevance could STZ possibly have in relation to the pathogenesis AD, diabetes, or hepatic steatosis in humans? After all, human are not generally exposed to STZ. The probable answer was uncovered by the realization that STZ is a nitrosamine-related compound, and that over the past several decades, Western societies have been assaulted by continuous and growing exposures to environmental and food-related nitrosamines. The epidemiological trends for AD, diabetes mellitus, obesity, and non-alcoholic steatohepatitis all show substantial increases in incidence, prevalence, morbidity, and mortality rates that correspond more with exposures than genetics as underlying causes (de la Monte, Neusner et al. 2009). For unclear reasons, although the connection between nitrosamine exposure and diabetes was entertained years ago (Berne, Gunnarsson et al. 1974; Portha, Giroix et al. 1980; Helgason, Ewen et al. 1984; Boucher, Ewen et al. 1994; Dahlquist 1994; Essien and Akpan 2006), that concept seems to have been missed, and therefore has not yet been incorporated into the conceptualization about the origins of our insulin resistance diseases epidemic.

We conducted experiments to determine if low, sub-mutagenic doses of nitrosamines that are found in processed foods, e.g. N-nitrosodiethylamine (NDEA), could cause insulin resistance diseases. The results were alarming because low-dose and very limited exposures to NDEA cause T2DM, non-alcoholic steatohepatitis, visceral obesity, cognitive impairment, and AD-type neurodegeneration with peripheral, hepatic, and brain insulin resistance (Tong, Neusner et al. 2009; Tong, Longato et al. 2010), similar to the effects of STZ. Therefore, depending on the structure of the compound, dose, and route of administration, exposures to nitrosamine-related chemicals can cause insulin resistance diseases in multiple different target organs, including brain. In addition to providing evidence that the relatively recent epidemics of sporadic AD, T2DM, and non-alcoholic steatohepatitis/metabolic syndrome could be mediated by environmental or dietary exposures (de la Monte, Neusner et al. 2009), these studies demonstrate that insulin resistance diseases with essentially the same underlying cellular abnormalities, can develop in various organs and tissues. This phenomenon could account for the overlapping increases in prevalence rates of various insulin resistance diseases within the past several decades, as well as the very frequent but incomplete overlap between AD and obesity, T2DM, and NASH (Janson, Laedtke et al. 2004), which did not exist prior to 1980, and is not accounted for by aging of the population (de la Monte, Neusner et al. 2009).

8.3 The liver-brain-axis of neurodegeneration hypothesis

Experiments with STZ and NDEA provided clear evidence that low dose exposures to nitrosamines can reproduce the molecular, biochemical, neuropathological, and neurobehavioral abnormalities observed in human sporadic cases of AD, and also cause a broad spectrum of peripheral insulin resistance diseases, including visceral obesity, diabetes, and non-alcoholic steatohepatitis (de la Monte, Tong et al. 2006; Lester-Coll, Rivera et al. 2006; de la Monte and Tong 2009; Tong, Neusner et al. 2009). Subsequent studies showed that, the adverse effects of NDEA were exacerbated by chronic high fat diet feeding (de la Monte, Tong et al. 2009; Tong, Longato et al. 2010), and that i.p. treatment with NDEA was more effective in causing neurodegeneration than ICV NDEA. Further consideration of the data revealed that the degrees of steatohepatitis, and the levels of toxic lipids, i.e. ceramides produced in liver following NDEA ± high fat diet exposures were critical variables in the equation. These findings led us to the liver-brain- axis of neurodegeneration hypothesis (de la Monte, Longato et al. 2009; de la Monte, Longato et al. 2009), which states that, chronic injury to the liver that results in steatohepatitis, hepatic insulin resistance, and ER stress, leads to dysregulated lipid metabolism and attendant elaboration of toxic lipids, including ceramides and other sphingolipids. The toxic lipids get released into the circulation due to impaired membrane integrity or cell death. Their lipid-soluble nature enables the toxic lipids to cross the blood brain barrier and exert their adverse effects on brain insulin signaling pathways that mediate neuronal and glial survival, energy metabolism, neurotransmitter function, and synaptic plasticity. This hypothesis is supported by preliminary data showing that the same profiles of sphingolipids in steatotic livers are represented in peripheral blood, and that lipids isolated from peripheral blood in insulin-resistance disease states, when applied to brain slice cultures, cause neurodegeneration with insulin resistance. Experimental in vitro and in vivo exposures to chemically defined toxic ceramides also cause neurodegeneration with brain insulin resistance (Tong and de la Monte 2009; de la Monte, Tong et al. 2010). In addition to providing a mechanism whereby environmental toxins in processed and preserved foods, and agricultural products grown with heavy doses of nitrate-containing fertilizers may be responsible for our current and growing insulin resistance diseases epidemic that is becoming pandemic with exportation of our diets and lifestyles, the liver-brain-axis hypothesis suggests how the lipotoxicity associated with visceral obesity, type 2 diabetes, and NASH could serve as co-factors in the pathogenesis of AD-type neurodegeneration.

9. Western diet and insulin/IGF resistance mediated neurodegeneration

Since aging is essential and unequivocally the most dominant risk factor for AD, critical changes associated with the loss of youthful compensatory and protective mechanisms must be responsible for the acquired permissiveness to neurodegeneration. Mechanisms of aging are still under investigation. However, strong data from organisms that span the phylogenetic tree, indicate a role for caloric restriction as preventive, and excess caloric intake as a promoter of aging. One image I find impossible to dismiss, is the one displaying two primates of approximately the same age, side by side: one monkey was chronically fed with a low calorie diet, and the other was maintained on a high calorie diet. The differences in appearance and behavior were striking. The lean monkey appeared youthful and spunky, whereas the obese monkey looked aged and sluggish (Colman, Anderson et al. 2009). In addition to obesity, high caloric intake increased the rates of diabetes, cardiovascular disease, cancer, and brain atrophy in the colony (Colman, Anderson et al. 2009; Cruzen and Colman 2009). Moreover, diets high in trans fatty acids, which are abundantly present in processed foods, caused abdominal obesity and insulin resistance (Kavanagh, Jones et al. 2007). Similar effects of nutrient poor, calorically dense diets have been demonstrated in humans (Hodge, Dowse et al. 1995; Tran, Komatsu et al. 2001; Hursting, Lavigne et al. 2003; Newby, Muller et al. 2003). In humans, caloric restriction also retards aging and reduces rates of chronic disease; therefore, this simple measure may also help to reduce risk for neurodegeneration (Qin, Chachich et al. 2006; Kim, Nguyen et al. 2007; Wang, Fivecoat et al. 2010).

Beyond avoidance of excessive caloric intake, growing evidence suggests that the source of calories is also of concern. A number of reports suggest that aging and pathophysiological states that contribute to chronic diseases are promoted by diets low in nutrient value, and high in simple sugars (fructose), starches, and trans fatty acids. Added to this is the problem associated with consumption of heavily processed foods and exposure to nitrosamines. Unfortunately, the vast majority of foods consumed in the USA are processed and contain preservatives, and over time, our exposures to nitrosamines through food processing and preservation and the heavy use of fertilizers in agriculture have increased sharply and in parallel with the insulin resistance disease epidemics (de la Monte, Neusner et al. 2009). The implications with regard to strategies for disease prevention are obvious. The implementation of measures to protect citizens of this country while not destroying lifestyle conveniences brought by modernization of culture is possible for those who are informed and proactive, but will be challenging for individuals who are unwilling to make proper choices. The larger concern is the rapid rate in which our insulin resistance disease epidemic is becoming pandemic secondary to the exportation of inexpensive Western convenience foods.

10. Sedentary lifestyles contribute to brain insulin/IGF resistance

Attempts to curb the obesity epidemic and associated health risks have focused on implementing lifestyle changes that promote healthful eating and regular exercise. Cross-cultural studies have shown that adoption of Western, go-easy lifestyles with reduced physical activity results in higher rates of obesity (Hodge, Dowse et al. 1995), and increased obesity correlates with progressive hyperlipidemia (Berns, de Vries et al. 1989). In addition, sedentary lifestyles among children lead to increased energy intake in the forms of fat, sweets, salty snacks, and carbonated beverages, and reduced intake of fruits and vegetables (Coon and Tucker 2002). In contrast, increased physical activity in the form or aerobic exercise prevents the long-term weight gain that is associated with aging (Littman, Kristal et al. 2005), and reduces risk for both cardiovascular events and cognitive impairment (Nash and Fillit 2006). More recently, clinical research demonstrated that regular physical exercise can reduce the risks for cognitive impairment and neurodegeneration (Radak, Hart et al.), or help maintain (Plassman, Williams et al. ; Deslandes, Moraes et al. 2009) or improve (Rolland, Abellan van Kan et al. ; Weih, Abu-Omar et al. 2009; Baker, Frank et al. 2010) cognitive function in the elderly. Experimentally, physical exercise was demonstrated to reduce the AβPP-Aβ burden in transgenic mouse brains (Adlard, Perreau et al. 2005), although other studies suggest that improved cognitive performance and neurotrophin function were mediated by physical activity with environmental enrichment (Wolf, Kronenberg et al. 2006). These results provide convincing evidence that regular aerobic physical exercise can help prevent neurodegeneration and preserve cognitive function. The therapeutic effects of aerobic physical exercise are likely mediated by weight loss with reduced peripheral insulin resistance, increased cerebrovascular insulin/IGF responsiveness with attendant improvements in blood flow, nutrient delivery, and metabolism, and decreased production of toxic lipids that promote neurodegeneration and brain insulin resistance.

11. Conclusions

After 30+ years of intense research, new data have emerged supporting the concept that AD is heterogeneous in nature, and mediated by brain insulin and IGF resistance with reductions in glucose utilization and energy metabolism, increased oxidative stress, and neuro-inflammation. Impairments in brain insulin and IGF signaling contribute to neuronal loss, synaptic disconnection, tau hyperphosphorylation, AβPP-Aβ accumulation, and metabolic disturbances. Peripheral insulin resistance disease states, including diabetes mellitus, obesity, and non-alcoholic steatohepatitis, contribute to brain insulin/IGF resistance and neurodegeneration, but alone, they are not sufficient to cause AD. This conclusion is supported by experiments in which brain insulin or IGF resistance were produced by ICV delivery of siRNA duplexes targeting the insulin or IGF receptors. AD fundamentally represents a brain-specific form of diabetes i.e. Type 3 diabetes that can, and often does overlap with peripheral insulin resistance diseases. Analysis of experimental streptozotocin (STZ) treatment models showed that insulin resistance and insulin deficiency states could be produced in peripheral organs, including liver, and/or the brain. The realization that STZ is a nitrosamine, led to further studies revealing that NDEA, which is one of the nitrosamines present in processed and preserved foods, or can be produced in our bodies by exposure to nitrites, also causes the full spectrum of insulin resistance diseases that are epidemic in the USA. Moreover, experimental results showed that when combined with chronic high fat dietary intake, the severity and extent of insulin resistance diseases are worsened substantially. Due to the common link of steatohepatitis with increased dysregulation of lipid metabolism and generation of toxic lipids, we proposed that AD-type neurodegeneration in the context of peripheral insulin resistance diseases is mediated via a liver-brain axis. In essence, toxic lipids generated in liver, enter the circulation, cross the blood-brain barrier, and cause brain insulin resistance by inhibiting signal transduction through the insulin receptor. This concept provides a mechanism whereby peripheral insulin resistance diseases could serve as co-factors in the pathogenesis of AD and cognitive impairment. Dietary and lifestyle measures to prevent insulin resistance diseases, including sporadic AD, were discussed, with particular emphasis on avoiding processed and preserved foods that permeate Western diets.

12. Acknowledgements

The work in our laboratory is been generously supported by grants AA-11431, AA-12908, and AA-16260 from the National Institutes of Health. The author has no competing financial interests.

13. References

Adlard, P. A., V. M. Perreau, et al. (2005). "Voluntary exercise decreases amyloid load in a transgenic model of Alzheimer's disease." J Neurosci 25(17): 4217-4221.

Adolfsson, R., G. Bucht, et al. (1980). "Hypoglycemia in Alzheimer's disease." Acta Med Scand 208(5): 387-388.

Arboleda, G., T. J. Huang, et al. (2007). "Insulin-like growth factor-1-dependent maintenance of neuronal metabolism through the phosphatidylinositol 3-kinase-Akt pathway is inhibited by C2-ceramide in CAD cells." Eur J Neurosci 25(10): 3030-3038.

Arnaud, L., N. K. Robakis, et al. (2006). "It may take inflammation, phosphorylation and ubiquitination to 'tangle' in Alzheimer's disease." Neurodegener Dis 3(6): 313-319.

Baker, L. D., L. L. Frank, et al. (2010). "Effects of aerobic exercise on mild cognitive impairment: a controlled trial." Arch Neurol 67(1): 71-79.

Berne, C., R. Gunnarsson, et al. (1974). "Letter: Diabetogenic nitrosamines?" Lancet 1(7849): 173-174.

Berns, M. A., J. H. de Vries, et al. (1989). "Increase in body fatness as a major determinant of changes in serum total cholesterol and high density lipoprotein cholesterol in young men over a 10-year period." American journal of epidemiology 130(6): 1109-1122.

Biju, M. P. and C. S. Paulose (1998). "Brain glutamate dehydrogenase changes in streptozotocin diabetic rats as a function of age." Biochem Mol Biol Int 44(1): 1-7.

Blasko, I., M. Stampfer-Kountchev, et al. (2004). "How chronic inflammation can affect the brain and support the development of Alzheimer's disease in old age: the role of microglia and astrocytes." Aging Cell 3(4): 169-176.

Blass, J. P., G. E. Gibson, et al. (2002). "The role of the metabolic lesion in Alzheimer's disease." J Alzheimers Dis 4(3): 225-232.

Blum-Degen, D., L. Frolich, et al. (1995). "Altered regulation of brain glucose metabolism as a cause of neurodegenerative disorders?" J Neural Transm Suppl 46: 139-147.

Bolzan, A. D. and M. S. Bianchi (2002). "Genotoxicity of streptozotocin." Mutat Res 512(2-3): 121-134.

Boucher, B. J., S. W. Ewen, et al. (1994). "Betel nut (Areca catechu) consumption and the induction of glucose intolerance in adult CD1 mice and in their F1 and F2 offspring." Diabetologia 37(1): 49-55.

Bourbon, N. A., L. Sandirasegarane, et al. (2002). "Ceramide-induced inhibition of Akt is mediated through protein kinase Czeta: implications for growth arrest." J Biol Chem 277(5): 3286-3292.

Brennan-Krohn, T., S. Salloway, et al. (2010). "Glial Vascular Degeneration in CADASIL." Journal of Alzheimer's disease : JAD.

Bryan, L., T. Kordula, et al. (2008). "Regulation and functions of sphingosine kinases in the brain." Biochim Biophys Acta 1781(9): 459-466.

Cantarini, M. C., S. M. de la Monte, et al. (2006). "Aspartyl-asparagyl beta hydroxylase over-expression in human hepatoma is linked to activation of insulin-like growth factor and notch signaling mechanisms." Hepatology 44(2): 446-457.

Capeau, J. (2008). "Insulin resistance and steatosis in humans." Diabetes Metab 34(6 Pt 2): 649-657.

Caselli, R. J., K. Chen, et al. (2008). "Correlating cerebral hypometabolism with future memory decline in subsequent converters to amnestic pre-mild cognitive impairment." Arch Neurol 65(9): 1231-1236.

Chalfant, C. E., K. Kishikawa, et al. (1999). "Long chain ceramides activate protein phosphatase-1 and protein phosphatase-2A. Activation is stereospecific and regulated by phosphatidic acid." J Biol Chem 274(29): 20313-20317.

Chen, G. J., J. Xu, et al. (2003). "Transient hypoxia causes Alzheimer-type molecular and biochemical abnormalities in cortical neurons: potential strategies for neuroprotection." J Alzheimers Dis 5(3): 209-228.

Cole, G., J. W. Neal, et al. (1993). "The distribution of amyloid plaques in the cerebellum and brain stem in Down's syndrome and Alzheimer's disease: a light microscopical analysis." Acta Neuropathol 85(5): 542-552.

Colman, R. J., R. M. Anderson, et al. (2009). "Caloric restriction delays disease onset and mortality in rhesus monkeys." Science 325(5937): 201-204.

Coon, K. A. and K. L. Tucker (2002). "Television and children's consumption patterns. A review of the literature." Minerva pediatrica 54(5): 423-436.

Cowansage, K. K., J. E. LeDoux, et al. (2010). "Brain-derived neurotrophic factor: a dynamic gatekeeper of neural plasticity." Curr Mol Pharmacol 3(1): 12-29.

Craft, S. (2005). "Insulin resistance and cognitive impairment: a view through the prism of epidemiology." Arch Neurol 62(7): 1043-1044.

Craft, S. (2006). "Insulin resistance syndrome and Alzheimer disease: pathophysiologic mechanisms and therapeutic implications." Alzheimer Dis Assoc Disord 20(4): 298-301.

Craft, S. (2007). "Insulin resistance and Alzheimer's disease pathogenesis: potential mechanisms and implications for treatment." Curr Alzheimer Res 4(2): 147-152.

Cruzen, C. and R. J. Colman (2009). "Effects of caloric restriction on cardiovascular aging in non-human primates and humans." Clinics in geriatric medicine 25(4): 733-743, ix-x.

Dahlquist, G. (1994). "Non-genetic risk determinants of type 1 diabetes." Diabete & metabolisme 20(3): 251-257.

De Ferrari, G. V. and N. C. Inestrosa (2000). "Wnt signaling function in Alzheimer's disease." Brain Res Brain Res Rev 33(1): 1-12.

de la Monte, S. M. (1989). "Quantitation of cerebral atrophy in preclinical and end-stage Alzheimer's disease." Ann Neurol 25(5): 450-459.

de la Monte, S. M. (2009). "Insulin resistance and Alzheimer's disease." BMB Rep 42(8): 475-481.

de la Monte, S. M., G. J. Chen, et al. (2003). "Neuronal thread protein regulation and interaction with microtubule-associated proteins in SH-Sy5y neuronal cells." Cell Mol Life Sci 60(12): 2679-2691.

de la Monte, S. M., N. Ganju, et al. (2000). "Partial rescue of ethanol-induced neuronal apoptosis by growth factor activation of phosphoinositol-3-kinase." Alcohol Clin Exp Res 24(5): 716-726.

de la Monte, S. M., N. Ganju, et al. (1999). "Microtiter Immunocytochemical ELISA Assay: A Novel and Highly Sensitive Method of Quantifying Immunoreactivity." Biotecniques 26(6): 1073-1076.

de la Monte, S. M., A. Jhaveri, et al. (2007). "Nitric oxide synthase 3-mediated neurodegeneration after intracerebral gene delivery." J Neuropathol Exp Neurol 66(4): 272-283.

de la Monte, S. M., L. Longato, et al. (2009). "The liver-brain axis of alcohol-mediated neurodegeneration: role of toxic lipids." Int J Environ Res Public Health 6(7): 2055-2075.

de la Monte, S. M., L. Longato, et al. (2009). "Insulin resistance and neurodegeneration: roles of obesity, type 2 diabetes mellitus and non-alcoholic steatohepatitis." Curr Opin Investig Drugs 10(10): 1049-1060.

de la Monte, S. M., T. R. Neely, et al. (2001). "Ethanol impairs insulin-stimulated mitochondrial function in cerebellar granule neurons." Cell Mol Life Sci 58(12-13): 1950-1960.

de la Monte, S. M., A. Neusner, et al. (2009). "Epidemilogical Trends Strongly Suggest Exposures as Etiologic Agents in the Pathogenesis of Sporadic Alzheimer's Disease, Diabetes Mellitus, and Non-Alcoholic Steatohepatitis." J Alzheimers Dis.

de la Monte, S. M. and M. Tong (2009). "Mechanisms of Nitrosamine-Mediated Neurodegeneration: Potential Relevance to Sporadic Alzheimer's Disease." J Alzheimers Dis.

de la Monte, S. M., M. Tong, et al. (2011). "si-RNA inhibition of brain insulin or insulin-like growth factor receptors causes developmental cerebellar abnormalities: relevance to fetal alcohol spectrum disorder." Molec Brain: (In Press).

de la Monte, S. M., M. Tong, et al. (2009). "Nitrosamine exposure exacerbates high fat diet-mediated type 2 diabetes mellitus, non-alcoholic steatohepatitis, and neurodegeneration with cognitive impairment." Mol Neurodegener 4: 54.

de la Monte, S. M., M. Tong, et al. (2006). "Therapeutic rescue of neurodegeneration in experimental type 3 diabetes: relevance to Alzheimer's disease." J Alzheimers Dis 10(1): 89-109.

de la Monte, S. M., M. Tong, et al. (2010). "Ceramide-mediated insulin resistance and impairment of cognitive-motor functions." J Alzheimers Dis 21(3): 967-984.

de la Monte, S. M. and J. R. Wands (2002). "Chronic gestational exposure to ethanol impairs insulin-stimulated survival and mitochondrial function in cerebellar neurons." CMLS, Cell Mol Life Sci 59: 882-893.

de la Monte, S. M. and J. R. Wands (2005). "Review of insulin and insulin-like growth factor expression, signaling, and malfunction in the central nervous system: relevance to Alzheimer's disease." J Alzheimers Dis 7(1): 45-61.

de la Monte, S. M. and J. R. Wands (2008). "Alzheimer's disease is type 3 diabetes-evidence reviewed." J Diabetes Sci Technol 2(6): 1101-1113.

Deslandes, A., H. Moraes, et al. (2009). "Exercise and mental health: many reasons to move." Neuropsychobiology 59(4): 191-198.

Deutsch, S. I., M. R. Urbano, et al. (2010). "Cholinergic abnormalities in autism: is there a rationale for selective nicotinic agonist interventions?" Clin Neuropharmacol 33(3): 114-120.

Dineley-Miller, K. and J. Patrick (1992). "Gene transcripts for the nicotinic acetylcholine receptor subunit, beta4, are distributed in multiple areas of the rat central nervous system." Brain Res Mol Brain Res 16(3-4): 339-344.

Doble, B. W. and J. R. Woodgett (2003). "GSK-3: tricks of the trade for a multi-tasking kinase." J Cell Sci 116(Pt 7): 1175-1186.

Duyckaerts, C., B. Delatour, et al. (2009). "Classification and basic pathology of Alzheimer disease." Acta Neuropathol 118(1): 5-36.

Eikelenboom, P. and W. A. van Gool (2004). "Neuroinflammatory perspectives on the two faces of Alzheimer's disease." J Neural Transm 111(3): 281-294.

Elwing, J. E., P. J. Lustman, et al. (2006). "Depression, anxiety, and nonalcoholic steatohepatitis." Psychosom Med 68(4): 563-569.

Essien, A. D. and J. O. Akpan (2006). "Diabetogenic property of charred meat on litters of pregnant albino rats." Nigerian journal of physiological sciences : official publication of the Physiological Society of Nigeria 21(1-2): 37-41.

Etiene, D., J. Kraft, et al. (1998). "Cerebrovascular Pathology Contributes to the Heterogeneity of Alzheimer's Disease." J Alzheimers Dis 1(2): 119-134.

Fraser, P. E., G. Yu, et al. (2001). "Presenilin function: connections to Alzheimer's disease and signal transduction." Biochem Soc Symp(67): 89-100.

Frebel, K. and S. Wiese (2006). "Signalling molecules essential for neuronal survival and differentiation." Biochem Soc Trans 34(Pt 6): 1287-1290.

Frolich, L., D. Blum-Degen, et al. (1998). "Brain insulin and insulin receptors in aging and sporadic Alzheimer's disease." J Neural Transm 105(4-5): 423-438.

Fujisawa, Y., K. Sasaki, et al. (1991). "Increased insulin levels after OGTT load in peripheral blood and cerebrospinal fluid of patients with dementia of Alzheimer type." Biol Psychiatry 30(12): 1219-1228.

Gasparini, L., G. K. Gouras, et al. (2001). "Stimulation of beta-amyloid precursor protein trafficking by insulin reduces intraneuronal beta-amyloid and requires mitogen-activated protein kinase signaling." J Neurosci 21(8): 2561-2570.

Gasparini, L., W. J. Netzer, et al. (2002). "Does insulin dysfunction play a role in Alzheimer's disease?" Trends Pharmacol Sci 23(6): 288-293.

Gomez-Pinilla, F., V. So, et al. (2001). "Spatial learning induces neurotrophin receptor and synapsin I in the hippocampus." Brain Res 904(1): 13-19.

Greenberg, D. S., D. Toiber, et al. (2010). "Acetylcholinesterase variants in Alzheimer's disease: from neuroprotection to programmed cell death." Neuro-degenerative diseases 7(1-3): 60-63.

Grilli, M., G. Ferrari Toninelli, et al. (2003). "Alzheimer's disease linking neurodegeneration with neurodevelopment." Funct Neurol 18(3): 145-148.

Grunblatt, E., M. Salkovic-Petrisic, et al. (2007). "Brain insulin system dysfunction in streptozotocin intracerebroventricularly treated rats generates hyperphosphorylated tau protein." J Neurochem 101(3): 757-770.

Gundogan, F., G. Elwood, et al. (2008). "Impaired placentation in fetal alcohol syndrome." Placenta 29(2): 148-157.

Haan, M. N. and R. Wallace (2004). "Can dementia be prevented? Brain aging in a population-based context." Annu Rev Public Health 25: 1-24.

Hajduch, E., A. Balendran, et al. (2001). "Ceramide impairs the insulin-dependent membrane recruitment of protein kinase B leading to a loss in downstream signalling in L6 skeletal muscle cells." Diabetologia 44(2): 173-183.

Hamm, R. J., C. E. Dixon, et al. (1992). "Cognitive deficits following traumatic brain injury produced by controlled cortical impact." J Neurotrauma 9(1): 11-20.

Hanger, D. P., A. Seereeram, et al. (2009). "Mediators of tau phosphorylation in the pathogenesis of Alzheimer's disease." Expert Rev Neurother 9(11): 1647-1666.

Haudenschild, C. C., W. Van Sickle, et al. (1981). "Response of the aorta of the obese Zucker rat to injury." Arteriosclerosis 1(3): 186-191.

Helgason, T., S. W. Ewen, et al. (1984). "N-nitrosamines in smoked meats and their relation to diabetes." IARC scientific publications(57): 911-920.

Hodge, A. M., G. K. Dowse, et al. (1995). "Modernity and obesity in coastal and Highland Papua New Guinea." International journal of obesity and related metabolic disorders : journal of the International Association for the Study of Obesity 19(3): 154-161.

Holland, W. L. and S. A. Summers (2008). "Sphingolipids, insulin resistance, and metabolic disease: new insights from in vivo manipulation of sphingolipid metabolism." Endocr Rev 29(4): 381-402.

Hong, M. and V. M. Lee (1997). "Insulin and insulin-like growth factor-1 regulate tau phosphorylation in cultured human neurons." J Biol Chem 272(31): 19547-19553.

Hotta, O., Y. Taguma, et al. (1996). "Possible relationship between hyperinsulinemia and glomerular hypertrophy in nephrosclerosis." Ren Fail 18(2): 271-278.

Hoyer, S. (2002). "The brain insulin signal transduction system and sporadic (type II) Alzheimer disease: an update." J Neural Transm 109(3): 341-360.

Hoyer, S. (2004). "Causes and consequences of disturbances of cerebral glucose metabolism in sporadic Alzheimer disease: therapeutic implications." Adv Exp Med Biol 541: 135-152.

Hoyer, S. (2004). "Glucose metabolism and insulin receptor signal transduction in Alzheimer disease." Eur J Pharmacol 490(1-3): 115-125.

Hoyer, S. and H. Lannert (1999). "Inhibition of the neuronal insulin receptor causes Alzheimer-like disturbances in oxidative/energy brain metabolism and in behavior in adult rats." Ann N Y Acad Sci 893: 301-303.

Hoyer, S., H. Lannert, et al. (1999). "Damaged neuronal energy metabolism and behavior are improved by Ginkgo biloba extract (EGb 761)." J Neural Transm 106(11-12): 1171-1188.

Hoyer, S., S. K. Lee, et al. (2000). "Inhibition of the neuronal insulin receptor. An in vivo model for sporadic Alzheimer disease?" Ann N Y Acad Sci 920: 256-258.

Hoyer, S. and R. Nitsch (1989). "Cerebral excess release of neurotransmitter amino acids subsequent to reduced cerebral glucose metabolism in early-onset dementia of Alzheimer type." J Neural Transm 75(3): 227-232.

Hoyer, S., R. Nitsch, et al. (1991). "Predominant abnormality in cerebral glucose utilization in late-onset dementia of the Alzheimer type: a cross-sectional comparison against advanced late-onset and incipient early-onset cases." J Neural Transm Park Dis Dement Sect 3(1): 1-14.

Huang, K., C. C. Zou, et al. "Carotid intima-media thickness and serum endothelial marker levels in obese children with metabolic syndrome." Arch Pediatr Adolesc Med 164(9): 846-851.

Hursting, S. D., J. A. Lavigne, et al. (2003). "Calorie restriction, aging, and cancer prevention: mechanisms of action and applicability to humans." Annual review of medicine 54: 131-152.

Iqbal, K., F. Liu, et al. (2009). "Mechanisms of tau-induced neurodegeneration." Acta Neuropathol 118(1): 53-69.

Ishii, K., M. Sasaki, et al. (1997). "Reduction of cerebellar glucose metabolism in advanced Alzheimer's disease." J Nucl Med 38(6): 925-928.

Iwangoff, P., R. Armbruster, et al. (1980). "Glycolytic enzymes from human autoptic brain cortex: normal aged and demented cases." Mech Ageing Dev 14(1-2): 203-209.

Janson, J., T. Laedtke, et al. (2004). "Increased risk of type 2 diabetes in Alzheimer disease." Diabetes 53(2): 474-481.

Kao, Y., J. H. Youson, et al. (1999). "Effects of insulin on lipid metabolism of larvae and metamorphosing landlocked sea lamprey, Petromyzon marinus." Gen Comp Endocrinol 114(3): 405-414.

Karaivazoglou, K., K. Assimakopoulos, et al. (2007). "Neuropsychological function in Greek patients with chronic hepatitis C." Liver Int 27(6): 798-805.

Kavanagh, K., K. L. Jones, et al. (2007). "Trans fat diet induces abdominal obesity and changes in insulin sensitivity in monkeys." Obesity 15(7): 1675-1684.

Kim, D., M. D. Nguyen, et al. (2007). "SIRT1 deacetylase protects against neurodegeneration in models for Alzheimer's disease and amyotrophic lateral sclerosis." EMBO J 26(13): 3169-3179.

Kincaid-Smith, P. (2004). "Hypothesis: obesity and the insulin resistance syndrome play a major role in end-stage renal failure attributed to hypertension and labelled 'hypertensive nephrosclerosis'." J Hypertens 22(6): 1051-1055.

Kopelman, M. D., A. D. Thomson, et al. (2009). "The Korsakoff syndrome: clinical aspects, psychology and treatment." Alcohol Alcohol 44(2): 148-154.

Korf, E. S., L. R. White, et al. (2006). "Brain aging in very old men with type 2 diabetes: the Honolulu-Asia Aging Study." Diabetes Care 29(10): 2268-2274.

Koulmanda, M., A. Qipo, et al. (2003). "The effect of low versus high dose of streptozotocin in cynomolgus monkeys (Macaca fascilularis)." Am J Transplant 3(3): 267-272.

Kraegen, E. W. and G. J. Cooney (2008). "Free fatty acids and skeletal muscle insulin resistance." Curr Opin Lipidol 19(3): 235-241.

Kubota, T., N. Kubota, et al. (2003). "Lack of insulin receptor substrate-2 causes progressive neointima formation in response to vessel injury." Circulation 107(24): 3073-3080.

Labak, M., T. Foniok, et al. (2010). "Metabolic changes in rat brain following intracerebroventricular injections of streptozotocin: a model of sporadic Alzheimer's disease." Acta Neurochir Suppl 106: 177-181.

Langbaum, J. B., K. Chen, et al. (2010). "Hypometabolism in Alzheimer-affected brain regions in cognitively healthy Latino individuals carrying the apolipoprotein E epsilon4 allele." Arch Neurol 67(4): 462-468.

Langeveld, M. and J. M. Aerts (2009). "Glycosphingolipids and insulin resistance." Prog Lipid Res.

Lannert, H. and S. Hoyer (1998). "Intracerebroventricular administration of streptozotocin causes long-term diminutions in learning and memory abilities and in cerebral energy metabolism in adult rats." Behav Neurosci 112(5): 1199-1208.

Larner, A. J. (1997). "The cerebellum in Alzheimer's disease." Dement Geriatr Cogn Disord 8(4): 203-209.

Launer, L. J. (2005). "Diabetes and brain aging: epidemiologic evidence." Curr Diab Rep 5(1): 59-63.

Lester-Coll, N., E. J. Rivera, et al. (2006). "Intracerebral streptozotocin model of type 3 diabetes: relevance to sporadic Alzheimer's disease." J Alzheimers Dis 9(1): 13-33.

Ling, X., R. N. Martins, et al. (2002). "Amyloid beta antagonizes insulin promoted secretion of the amyloid beta protein precursor." J Alzheimers Dis 4(5): 369-374.

Littman, A. J., A. R. Kristal, et al. (2005). "Effects of physical activity intensity, frequency, and activity type on 10-y weight change in middle-aged men and women." International journal of obesity 29(5): 524-533.

Liu, B., L. M. Obeid, et al. (1997). "Sphingomyelinases in cell regulation." Semin Cell Dev Biol 8(3): 311-322.

Loftis, J. M., M. Huckans, et al. (2008). "Depressive symptoms in patients with chronic hepatitis C are correlated with elevated plasma levels of interleukin-1beta and tumor necrosis factor-alpha." Neurosci Lett 430(3): 264-268.

Lorenzo, A. and B. A. Yankner (1996). "Amyloid fibril toxicity in Alzheimer's disease and diabetes." Ann N Y Acad Sci 777: 89-95.

Luchsinger, J. A. (2010). "Type 2 diabetes, related conditions, in relation and dementia: an opportunity for prevention?" J Alzheimers Dis 20(3): 723-736.

Luchsinger, J. A. and R. Mayeux (2004). "Cardiovascular risk factors and Alzheimer's disease." Curr Atheroscler Rep 6(4): 261-266.

Luchsinger, J. A., C. Reitz, et al. (2007). "Relation of diabetes to mild cognitive impairment." Arch Neurol 64(4): 570-575.

Lyn-Cook, L. E., Jr., M. Lawton, et al. (2009). "Hepatic ceramide may mediate brain insulin resistance and neurodegeneration in type 2 diabetes and non-alcoholic steatohepatitis." J Alzheimers Dis 16(4): 715-729.

Maisonpierre, P. C., L. Belluscio, et al. (1990). "NT-3, BDNF, and NGF in the developing rat nervous system: parallel as well as reciprocal patterns of expression." Neuron 5(4): 501-509.

Mandelkow, E. M., K. Stamer, et al. (2003). "Clogging of axons by tau, inhibition of axonal traffic and starvation of synapses." Neurobiol Aging 24(8): 1079-1085.

Marchesini, G. and R. Marzocchi (2007). "Metabolic syndrome and NASH." Clin Liver Dis 11(1): 105-117, ix.

Martins, I. J., E. Hone, et al. (2006). "Apolipoprotein E, cholesterol metabolism, diabetes, and the convergence of risk factors for Alzheimer's disease and cardiovascular disease." Mol Psychiatry 11(8): 721-736.

Matsumoto, H., T. Nakao, et al. (2005). "Insulin resistance contributes to obesity-related proteinuria." Intern Med 44(6): 548-553.

McLay, R. N., S. M. Freeman, et al. (1999). "Tests used to assess the cognitive abilities of aged rats: their relation to each other and to hippocampal morphology and neurotrophin expression." Gerontology 45(3): 143-155.

Messier, C. and K. Teutenberg (2005). "The role of insulin, insulin growth factor, and insulin-degrading enzyme in brain aging and Alzheimer's disease." Neural Plast 12(4): 311-328.

Morales, I., G. Farias, et al. (2010). "Neuroimmunomodulation in the pathogenesis of Alzheimer's disease." Neuroimmunomodulation 17(3): 202-204.

Moroz, N., M. Tong, et al. (2008). "Limited Alzheimer-type neurodegeneration in experimental obesity and Type 2 diabetes mellitus." J Alzheimers Dis 15(1): 29-44.

Mosconi, L., R. Mistur, et al. (2009). "FDG-PET changes in brain glucose metabolism from normal cognition to pathologically verified Alzheimer's disease." Eur J Nucl Med Mol Imaging 36(5): 811-822.

Mosconi, L., A. Pupi, et al. (2008). "Brain glucose hypometabolism and oxidative stress in preclinical Alzheimer's disease." Ann N Y Acad Sci 1147: 180-195.

Mudher, A., S. Chapman, et al. (2001). "Dishevelled regulates the metabolism of amyloid precursor protein via protein kinase C/mitogen-activated protein kinase and c-Jun terminal kinase." J Neurosci 21(14): 4987-4995.

Nash, D. T. and H. Fillit (2006). "Cardiovascular disease risk factors and cognitive impairment." Am J Cardiol 97(8): 1262-1265.

Nelson, P. T., C. D. Smith, et al. (2008). "Human cerebral neuropathology of Type 2 diabetes mellitus." Biochim Biophys Acta.

Newby, P. K., D. Muller, et al. (2003). "Dietary patterns and changes in body mass index and waist circumference in adults." The American journal of clinical nutrition 77(6): 1417-1425.

Nicolls, M. R. (2004). "The clinical and biological relationship between Type II diabetes mellitus and Alzheimer's disease." Curr Alzheimer Res 1(1): 47-54.

Niikura, T., Y. Hashimoto, et al. (2002). "Death and survival of neuronal cells exposed to Alzheimer's insults." J Neurosci Res 70(3): 380-391.

Nishimura, M., G. Yu, et al. (1999). "Presenilin mutations associated with Alzheimer disease cause defective intracellular trafficking of beta-catenin, a component of the presenilin protein complex." Nat Med 5(2): 164-169.

Nitta, A., R. Murai, et al. (2002). "Diabetic neuropathies in brain are induced by deficiency of BDNF." Neurotoxicol Teratol 24(5): 695-701.

Nogueira, T. C., G. F. Anhe, et al. (2008). "Involvement of phosphatidylinositol-3 kinase/AKT/PKCzeta/lambda pathway in the effect of palmitate on glucose-induced insulin secretion." Pancreas 37(3): 309-315.

Noh, M. Y., S. H. Koh, et al. (2009). "Neuroprotective effects of donepezil through inhibition of GSK-3 activity in amyloid-beta-induced neuronal cell death." Journal of neurochemistry 108(5): 1116-1125.

Oddo, S. (2008). "The ubiquitin-proteasome system in Alzheimer's disease." J Cell Mol Med 12(2): 363-373.

Pae, C. U., D. M. Marks, et al. (2008). "Does neurotropin-3 have a therapeutic implication in major depression?" Int J Neurosci 118(11): 1515-1522.

Papandreou, D., I. Rousso, et al. (2007). "Update on non-alcoholic fatty liver disease in children." Clin Nutr 26(4): 409-415.

Pasquier, F., A. Boulogne, et al. (2006). "Diabetes mellitus and dementia." Diabetes Metab 32(5 Pt 1): 403-414.

Peeyush, K. T., B. Savitha, et al. (2010). "Cholinergic, dopaminergic and insulin receptors gene expression in the cerebellum of streptozotocin-induced diabetic rats: functional regulation with Vitamin D3 supplementation." Pharmacol Biochem Behav 95(2): 216-222.

Pepeu, G. and M. G. Giovannini (2010). "Cholinesterase inhibitors and memory." Chem Biol Interact 187(1-3): 403-408.

Perry, E. K., M. A. Piggott, et al. (1993). "Transmitters in the developing and senescent human brain." Ann N Y Acad Sci 695: 69-72.

Perry, W., R. C. Hilsabeck, et al. (2008). "Cognitive dysfunction in chronic hepatitis C: a review." Dig Dis Sci 53(2): 307-321.

Pessayre, D. (2007). "Role of mitochondria in non-alcoholic fatty liver disease." J Gastroenterol Hepatol 22 Suppl 1: S20-27.

Plassman, B. L., J. W. Williams, Jr., et al. "Systematic review: factors associated with risk for and possible prevention of cognitive decline in later life." Ann Intern Med 153(3): 182-193.

Portha, B., M. H. Giroix, et al. (1980). "Diabetogenic effect of N-nitrosomethylurea and N-nitrosomethylurethane in the adult rat." Annales de la nutrition et de l'alimentation 34(5-6): 1143-1151.

Powell, D. J., E. Hajduch, et al. (2003). "Ceramide disables 3-phosphoinositide binding to the pleckstrin homology domain of protein kinase B (PKB)/Akt by a PKCzeta-dependent mechanism." Mol Cell Biol 23(21): 7794-7808.

Qin, W., M. Chachich, et al. (2006). "Calorie restriction attenuates Alzheimer's disease type brain amyloidosis in Squirrel monkeys (Saimiri sciureus)." J Alzheimers Dis 10(4): 417-422.

Qiu, C., D. De Ronchi, et al. (2007). "The epidemiology of the dementias: an update." Curr Opin Psychiatry 20(4): 380-385.

Radak, Z., N. Hart, et al. "Exercise plays a preventive role against Alzheimer's disease." J Alzheimers Dis 20(3): 777-783.

Ristow, M. (2004). "Neurodegenerative disorders associated with diabetes mellitus." J Mol Med 82(8): 510-529.

Rivera, E. J., A. Goldin, et al. (2005). "Insulin and insulin-like growth factor expression and function deteriorate with progression of Alzheimer's disease: link to brain reductions in acetylcholine." J Alzheimers Dis 8(3): 247-268.

Robertson, R. T., J. Baratta, et al. (2006). "A role for neurotrophin-3 in targeting developing cholinergic axon projections to cerebral cortex." Neuroscience 143(2): 523-539.

Rolland, Y., G. Abellan van Kan, et al. "Healthy brain aging: role of exercise and physical activity." Clin Geriatr Med 26(1): 75-87.

Schmidt, K. S., J. L. Gallo, et al. (2005). "The neuropsychological profile of alcohol-related dementia suggests cortical and subcortical pathology." Dement Geriatr Cogn Disord 20(5): 286-291.

Schubert, M., D. P. Brazil, et al. (2003). "Insulin receptor substrate-2 deficiency impairs brain growth and promotes tau phosphorylation." J Neurosci 23(18): 7084-7092.

Schubert, M., D. Gautam, et al. (2004). "Role for neuronal insulin resistance in neurodegenerative diseases." Proc Natl Acad Sci U S A 101(9): 3100-3105.

Shi, B., S. J. Rabin, et al. (1998). "Dexamethasone induces hypertrophy of developing medial septum cholinergic neurons: potential role of nerve growth factor." J Neurosci 18(22): 9326-9334.

Sims, N. R., D. M. Bowen, et al. (1980). "Glucose metabolism and acetylcholine synthesis in relation to neuronal activity in Alzheimer's disease." Lancet 1(8164): 333-336.

Soscia, S. J., M. Tong, et al. (2006). "Chronic gestational exposure to ethanol causes insulin and IGF resistance and impairs acetylcholine homeostasis in the brain." Cell Mol Life Sci 63(17): 2039-2056.

Steen, E., B. M. Terry, et al. (2005). "Impaired insulin and insulin-like growth factor expression and signaling mechanisms in Alzheimer's disease--is this type 3 diabetes?" J Alzheimers Dis 7(1): 63-80.

Summers, S. A. (2006). "Ceramides in insulin resistance and lipotoxicity." Prog Lipid Res 45(1): 42-72.

Szkudelski, T. (2001). "The mechanism of alloxan and streptozotocin action in B cells of the rat pancreas." Physiol Res 50(6): 537-546.

Takashima, A. (2009). "Amyloid-beta, tau, and dementia." J Alzheimers Dis 17(4): 729-736.

Takashima, A. (2010). "[Drug development for tauopathy and Alzheimer's disease]." Nihon Shinkei Seishin Yakurigaku Zasshi 30(4): 177-180.

Tong, M. and S. M. de la Monte (2009). "Mechanisms of ceramide-mediated neurodegeneration." J Alzheimers Dis 16(4): 705-714.

Tong, M., L. Longato, et al. (2010). "Early limited nitrosamine exposures exacerbate high fat diet-mediated type2 diabetes and neurodegeneration." BMC Endocr Disord 10(1): 4.

Tong, M., A. Neusner, et al. (2009). "Nitrosamine Exposure Causes Insulin Resistance Diseases: Relevance to Type 2 Diabetes Mellitus, Non-Alcoholic Steatohepatitis, and Alzheimer's Disease." J Alzheimers Dis.

Tran, T. M., T. Komatsu, et al. (2001). "Blood pressure, serum cholesterol concentration and their related factors in urban and rural elderly of Ho Chi Minh City." Journal of nutritional science and vitaminology 47(2): 147-155.

Tsukamoto, E., Y. Hashimoto, et al. (2003). "Characterization of the toxic mechanism triggered by Alzheimer's amyloid-beta peptides via p75 neurotrophin receptor in neuronal hybrid cells." J Neurosci Res 73(5): 627-636.

Tuppo, E. E. and H. R. Arias (2005). "The role of inflammation in Alzheimer's disease." Int J Biochem Cell Biol 37(2): 289-305.

Van Brocklyn, J. R. (2007). "Sphingolipid signaling pathways as potential therapeutic targets in gliomas." Mini Rev Med Chem 7(10): 984-990.

Verdelho, A., S. Madureira, et al. (2007). "Differential impact of cerebral white matter changes, diabetes, hypertension and stroke on cognitive performance among non-disabled elderly. The LADIS study." J Neurol Neurosurg Psychiatry 78(12): 1325-1330.

Wang, J., H. Fivecoat, et al. (2010). "The role of Sirt1: at the crossroad between promotion of longevity and protection against Alzheimer's disease neuropathology." Biochim Biophys Acta 1804(8): 1690-1694.

Watson, G. S., E. R. Peskind, et al. (2003). "Insulin increases CSF Abeta42 levels in normal older adults." Neurology 60(12): 1899-1903.

Wegiel, J., H. M. Wisniewski, et al. (1999). "Cerebellar atrophy in Alzheimer's disease-clinicopathological correlations." Brain Res 818(1): 41-50.

Weih, M., K. Abu-Omar, et al. (2009). "[Physical activity and prevention of Alzheimer's dementia: current evidence and feasibility of an interventional trial]." Fortschr Neurol Psychiatr 77(3): 146-151.

Weinstock, M. and S. Shoham (2004). "Rat models of dementia based on reductions in regional glucose metabolism, cerebral blood flow and cytochrome oxidase activity." J Neural Transm 111(3): 347-366.

Weiss, J. J. and J. M. Gorman (2006). "Psychiatric behavioral aspects of comanagement of hepatitis C virus and HIV." Curr HIV/AIDS Rep 3(4): 176-181.

Whitmer, R. A. (2007). "Type 2 diabetes and risk of cognitive impairment and dementia." Curr Neurol Neurosci Rep 7(5): 373-380.

Winocur, G. and C. E. Greenwood (2005). "Studies of the effects of high fat diets on cognitive function in a rat model." Neurobiol Aging 26 Suppl 1: 46-49.

Winocur, G., C. E. Greenwood, et al. (2005). "Memory impairment in obese Zucker rats: an investigation of cognitive function in an animal model of insulin resistance and obesity." Behav Neurosci 119(5): 1389-1395.

Wolf, S. A., G. Kronenberg, et al. (2006). "Cognitive and physical activity differently modulate disease progression in the amyloid precursor protein (APP)-23 model of Alzheimer's disease." Biol Psychiatry 60(12): 1314-1323.

Xie, L., E. Helmerhorst, et al. (2002). "Alzheimer's beta-amyloid peptides compete for insulin binding to the insulin receptor." J Neurosci 22(10): RC221.

Xu, J., J. Eun Yeon, et al. (2003). "Ethanol impairs insulin-stimulated neuronal survival in the developing brain: Role of PTEN phosphatase." J Biol Chem 278(29): 26929-26937.

Yeh, M. M. and E. M. Brunt (2007). "Pathology of nonalcoholic fatty liver disease." Am J Clin Pathol 128(5): 837-847.

Permissions

All chapters in this book were first published in ADPCCSPTT, by InTech Open; hereby published with permission under the Creative Commons Attribution License or equivalent. Every chapter published in this book has been scrutinized by our experts. Their significance has been extensively debated. The topics covered herein carry significant findings which will fuel the growth of the discipline. They may even be implemented as practical applications or may be referred to as a beginning point for another development.

The contributors of this book come from diverse backgrounds, making this book a truly international effort. This book will bring forth new frontiers with its revolutionizing research information and detailed analysis of the nascent developments around the world.

We would like to thank all the contributing authors for lending their expertise to make the book truly unique. They have played a crucial role in the development of this book. Without their invaluable contributions this book wouldn't have been possible. They have made vital efforts to compile up to date information on the varied aspects of this subject to make this book a valuable addition to the collection of many professionals and students.

This book was conceptualized with the vision of imparting up-to-date information and advanced data in this field. To ensure the same, a matchless editorial board was set up. Every individual on the board went through rigorous rounds of assessment to prove their worth. After which they invested a large part of their time researching and compiling the most relevant data for our readers.

The editorial board has been involved in producing this book since its inception. They have spent rigorous hours researching and exploring the diverse topics which have resulted in the successful publishing of this book. They have passed on their knowledge of decades through this book. To expedite this challenging task, the publisher supported the team at every step. A small team of assistant editors was also appointed to further simplify the editing procedure and attain best results for the readers.

Apart from the editorial board, the designing team has also invested a significant amount of their time in understanding the subject and creating the most relevant covers. They scrutinized every image to scout for the most suitable representation of the subject and create an appropriate cover for the book.

The publishing team has been an ardent support to the editorial, designing and production team. Their endless efforts to recruit the best for this project, has resulted in the accomplishment of this book. They are a veteran in the field of academics and their pool of knowledge is as vast as their experience in printing. Their expertise and guidance has proved useful at every step. Their uncompromising quality standards have made this book an exceptional effort. Their encouragement from time to time has been an inspiration for everyone.

The publisher and the editorial board hope that this book will prove to be a valuable piece of knowledge for researchers, students, practitioners and scholars across the globe.

List of Contributors

Rakez Kayed
University of Texas Medical Branch, USA

Rita Moretti, Francesca Esposito, Paola Torre, Rodolfo M. Antonello and Giuseppe Bellini
Medicina Clinica, Ambulatorio Complicanze Internistiche Cerebrali, Dipartimento, Universitario Clinico di Scienze Mediche Tecnologiche e Traslazionali, Università degli, Studi di Trieste, Italy

Emel Koseoglu
Erciyes University, Medicine Faculty, Neurology Department, Kayseri, Turkey

Lima and P.D.L.
Molecular Biology Laboratory, Center of Biological and Health Sciences, State University of Pará, Brazil

Vasconcellos and M.C.
Biological Activities Laboratory, Federal University of Amazonas, Brazil

Montenegro, R.C., Burbano and R.R.
Human Cytogenetics Laboratory, Institute Biological Institute of Biological Science, Federal University of Pará, Brazil

Stefanie A.G. Black and R. Jane Rylett
Molecular Brain Research Group, Robarts Research Institute, Schulich School of Medicine & Dentistry, University of Western Ontario, London, ON, Canada

Christian Hölscher
Ulster University, Neuroscience department, School of Biomed Sci, Northern Ireland, United Kingdom

Rosanna Squitti
Departement of Neuroscience, AFaR – Fatebenefratelli Hospital, Isola Tiberina, Rome, Italy
Clinica Neurologica, Università Campus Biomedico, Rome, Italy

Carlo Salustri
Institute of Cognition Sciences and Technologies (CNR), Fatebenefratelli Hospital, Isola Tiberina, Rome, Italy

Domenico Bosco, Massimiliano Plastino and Antonio Spanò
Department of Neuroscience, "S. Giovanni di Dio" Hospital, Crotone, Italy

Caterina Ermio
Department of Neuroscience, "S. Giovanni Paolo II" Hospital, Lamezia Terme, Italy

Antonietta Fava
Clinical Nutrition Unit, Medical School, University of Catanzaro, Italy

Zaheer ul Haq and Reaz Uddin
Dr. Panjwani Center for Molecular Medicine and Drug Research, International Center for Chemical and Biological Sciences, University of Karachi, Pakistan

Suzanne de la Monte, Ming Tong and Jack R. Wands
Rhode Island Hospital and the Warren Alpert Medical School of Brown University, USA

Index

www.ingramcontent.com/pod-product-compliance
Lightning Source LLC
LaVergne TN
LVHW080640210926
848485LV00003B/301